Taoism and Self Knowledge

# Sinica Leidensia

*Edited by*

Barend J. ter Haar
Maghiel van Crevel

*In co-operation with*

P.K. Bol, D.R. Knechtges, E.S. Rawski,
W.L. Idema, H.T. Zurndorfer

VOLUME 142

The titles published in this series are listed at *brill.com/sinl*

# Taoism and Self Knowledge

*The Chart for the Cultivation of Perfection*
(Xiuzhen Tu)

*By*

Catherine Despeux

*Translated by*

Jonathan Pettit

BRILL

LEIDEN | BOSTON

This work originally appeared as *Taoïsme et connaissance de soi* in 2012. Guy Trédaniel Editeur © Paris, 2012.

Cover illustration: Manifestation of the "Supreme Emperor of the Dark Heaven" (Xuantian Shangdi 玄天上帝), i.e., Zhenwu 真武, above the Mount Wudang in 1413. *Da Ming Xuantian shangdi ruiying tulu* 大明玄天上帝瑞應圖錄 (DZ 959), 16a–b. BNF 9546/952.

Library of Congress Cataloging-in-Publication Data

Names: Despeux, Catherine, author. | Pettit, J. E. E., translator.
Title: Taoism and self knowledge : the chart for the cultivation of perfection (Xiuzhen tu) / by Catherine Despeux ; translated by Jonathan Pettit.
Other titles: Taoisme et connaissance de soi. English
Description: Leiden ; Boston, MA : Brill, [2019] | Series: Sinica leidensia, ISSN 0169–9563 ; volume 142 | In English translated from the original French. | "This work originally appeared as Taoisme et connaissance de soi in 2012. Guy Tredaniel Editeur (c) Paris, 2012"— Title verso. | Includes bibliographical references and index.
Identifiers: LCCN 2018047060 (print) | LCCN 2018049610 (ebook) | ISBN 9789004383456 (E-book) | ISBN 9789004322158 (hardback : alk. paper)
Subjects: LCSH: Taoism and science. | Xiuzhen tu. | Human body—Religious aspects—Taoism. | Alchemy—Religious aspects—Taoism. | Human anatomy—Atlases.
Classification: LCC BL1942.85.S35 (ebook) | LCC BL1942.85.S35 D4713 2018 (print) | DDC 299.5/1444—dc23
LC record available at https://lccn.loc.gov/2018047060

Typeface for the Latin, Greek, and Cyrillic scripts: "Brill". See and download: brill.com/brill-typeface.

ISSN 0169-9563
ISBN 978-90-04-32215-8 (hardback)
ISBN 978-90-04-38345-6 (e-book)



This book is printed on acid-free paper and produced in a sustainable manner.

# Contents

# Illustrations

Some illustrations included in texts from the Taoist Canon are taken from a valuable woodblock printing of 1598, ink on paper, unfortunately incomplete, which is stired in the Department of Oriental Manuscripts at the French National Library (BNF). We indicated the odds of them. We thank Nathalie Monnet, chief curator of this department, for facilitating us the possibility of reproducing these illustrations. Other reproductions come from the publishing [*Chongyin Zhengtong*] *Daozang* 重印正统道藏, a rotogravure of the *Zhengtong Daozang* edition of the Taoist canon compiled in 1445, Shanghai: Shangwu yinshuguan, 1923–1926; 1120 booklets. This edition is conserved at the Library of the Institute of Advanced Chinese Studies / Collège de France, under the odd IHEC D XV 4–1 (1–285). We thank Madame Delphine Spicq, lecturer and curator of the IHEC, for having facilitated these reproductions. Other drawings were photographed from materials of the author.

BNF: Bibliothèque Nationale de France
IHEC: Institut des hautes études chinoises

# Introduction

Mental and visual representations of the body are the result of personal and collective experiences, and notions of what constitutes the body vary from one culture to another. The ways in which we isolate the objects of knowledge or perception depend on the conceptions we have of them. In the West, for example, the body is delimited by the skin and forms an entity in itself, but this is not necessarily so for a Taoist adept. Sometimes, it is difficult to understand how other cultures have apprehended representations of the body and have translated them into illustrations. These representations are very different from their Western counterparts. It is thus imperative to examine our own conceptions and to keep a certain distance from them.

In China, visual representations of the body are rare. Whenever such images appear (e.g., in painting, in sculpture, in Taoist scriptures), the depictions evoke the lightness of the human being. The lines are under emphasized, and they often undulate as they are drawn to depict body movements. These representations are closer to medieval, or even earlier, Western drawings than the sculptures of Michelangelo or Rodin, exalting muscle and power. Even though the knowledge of the body has greatly evolved over the past few centuries in China, it has nevertheless remained relatively constant when compared to Western knowledge during this same time. Descriptions and representations are relatively rare, and surprising in their simplicity.

Despite the relatively small number of images, Taoist writers often emphasize the significance of the human body. The thirteenth chapter of the *Book of the Way and its Virtue*, for instance, reads, "If I suffered so many evils, is it not because I have a body?" In ancient China, *xing* 形, a term designating the body structure, does not appear in classical texts such as the *Analects* or *Mencius*. *Xing*, however, is commonplace in early Taoist texts. It appears nearly two hundred times in Zhuangzi's self-titled Taoist treatise from the fourth century BCE. What is immediately striking, both in medical and Taoist representations, is the ovoid shape of the body, mostly drawn without the limbs. This kind of closed and delimited space evokes the Chinese Creation myths and the Chinese conception of the world as Chaos, a mixed, undivided whole, sometimes described as having the shape of an egg.

There are several different terms in Chinese to describe the body such as the body/person (*shen* 身), the physical body (*ti* 體) or its structural appearance (*xing* 形). Very early in ancient China, thinkers developed the analogy between the body and the universe, which became so common that we now speak of microcosm and macrocosm. There are many more analogies and approaches

 | DOI:10.1163/9789004383456_002

to the body, which is also the place where the individual and social identity take shape. But in China, there are few graphic representations of the body prior to the Song period (960–1279). Recently drawings representing gymnastic movements (*daoyin* 導引) were recovered during the 1973 Mawangdui (Hunan) excavations, and there are some manuscripts and diagrams of the body in the Dunhuang manuscripts.[1] There are sixteen texts related to moxibustion and representing simply the outline of the body, and several diagrams of the whole body or of the face, in documents relating to divination.

No extant Taoist text composed before the Song dynasty contains a graphic representation of the body. The catalogues of the imperial library in the official histories of these periods mention some titles of "diagrams" (*tu* 圖), which are all related to the five viscera or the acupuncture points.[2] The other components of the body or the body as a whole do not seem to have been the object of specific representations. The human body was also not a common feature in painting more generally. With the exception of portraits, which first appeared in the Tang, the reproduction of the human is not a common subject.

In Taoism, the earliest known visual representations of the body were created in the middle of the tenth century. They inaugurated a series of drawings, all related to the Internal Alchemical techniques developed during the late ninth and the tenth centuries. Like grimoires, these charts combine inscriptions and drawings often very schematic. These representations proceed from an organicist and ritualized worldview, including an order, an invisible inner structure and processes. Therefore, the body, discretely represented, is integrated into an ensemble of transformations and organization: it becomes the field of life.

Inner Alchemy, literally "inner cinnabar" (*neidan* 内丹), is a synthesis of ancient gymnastic, dietetics, breathing and meditation practices. The practices featured cosmological concepts adapted from operative alchemy, the "outer cinnabar" (*waidan* 外丹). The manipulations of Inner Alchemy take place in the laboratory of the alchemist, i.e., within the human body. Before the appearance of the Inner Alchemical system, however, the vocabulary of operative alchemy was already used in Taoism as a metaphorical resource for describing the techniques and the experiences of meditation.[3]

1 He and Lo 1996, 81–124.

2 Catalogues list several "Mingtang tu" 明堂圖 [Map of hall of light] dating from the Six Dynasties and giving the location of acupuncture points or "Wuzang tu" 五藏圖 [Charts of the five viscera]. See especially the bibliographic chapters in *Jiu Tangshu*, 47.23 and *Xin Tangshu*, 59.41 and 59.46.

3 Goossaert 1998: 498n7.

During the transition from operative alchemy to Internal Alchemy—the two are not mutually exclusive but may be performed concomitantly—several changes occured. There was first a phenomenon of internalization and transposition of the laboratory within the body. Here, the adept envisioned the cauldron and the furnace, the basic utensils of the alchemist, as metaphors for the main places to which the adept transferred his attention. These places varied depending on the stage of progress. It was either the kidneys (a term used in traditional Chinese writings to designate both kidneys and genitals) and the heart, or the lower part of the abdomen and the head. Eventually, the concrete manipulations of operative alchemy were replaced by the mental manipulations in Internal Alchemy. In the latter, an adept uses the power of imagination and visualization to induce changes in his person and his relation to the world.

One of the most common features of Inner Alchemical texts is the adaptation of cosmological concepts and models to describe the human body and the individual. In Chinese alchemy, the inner transformation is modelled on the evolution of nature. As was the case in operative alchemy, the analogy between microcosm and macrocosm is prior to Internal Alchemy; this correspondence can be found as early as the Han dynasty. Microcosm and macrocosm work in the same way: the body becomes a microcosm in which we find heaven and earth, sun and moon, stars, mountains and valleys, rivers and oceans, wind, clouds, rain, dew, and snow.

Abolishing the distinction between inside and outside, the Taoist transposes in the body both the natural world, as well as the sacred world of heavens, hells, gods and demons. The visualization practices of the body deities and the efforts to keep them in oneself are common procedures in most of the Taoist currents, notably in the Upper Clarity tradition (*Shangqing* 上清). Keeping the deities in his body permits a long life and the attainment of immortality. But the deities are also placed inside the body by the officiant during the rituals he performs to remedy the disorders not for himself but for the community or for a particular person, whether the problems or diseases or epidemics, or natural disasters, to mention only the main situations envisaged.

This book analyses the many versions of a body map called the *Chart for the Cultivation of Perfection*. These maps have emerged in different parts of China, and include a wide variety of texts, inscriptions, and figurative elements. For most maps, we do not know the author or under what circumstances they were made. This representation of the body is the culmination of a long tradition of schematic drawings that guided the meditator and the practitioner of rituals. The earliest manuscripts incorporating this kind of body maps were made in the tenth century. We also have partial maps from later centuries preserved in the Taoist Canon. But the popularity of these kinds of maps spread beyond canonical anthologies. Handwritten versions were cicrulated among members of temple groups large and small. This same broad appeal exists today. as is evidenced by Brigitte Baptandier's recent study.[4] Patrice Fava discovered a manuscript that demonstrates how people carry maps of the body and a map of the skeleton of the Lord Lao (Laojun gulu 老君骷髏).[5] A better understanding of the various versions of body maps in this book will clarify different ways that groups transmit this information.

The research into the history of representations of the body and alchemical processes prior to this *Chart for the Cultivation of Perfection* enables us to retrace its origins. The inventory of the various copies we possess, less than a dozen, illuminated the Taoist context in which it was used. The recent discovery of a version from a private collection has enriched this knowledge. The few, albeit minimal, variations between these different examples nevertheless show a flexible use of this map. In addition to the pictographic elements, the inscriptions and texts of the chart also were compared with those found in the known literature of the Taoist Canon and its complements.

In order to make more comprehensible the inscriptions and texts of this chart that we will translate throughout this study, I have grouped them according to three topics. The first topic is the body and its main sites for alchemical transmutations. This refers to the cosmological body becoming a spatio-temporal area in which the various alchemical operations will take place during meditation. Second, I address the body as a sacred world of paradises and hells, with its different palaces and divinities. Third, I present the inscriptions, texts and pictograms evoking the main processes of Internal Alchemy and the processes related to the thunder rites. I will explain the preliminary indications of this chart in the light of fundamental writings of Internal Alchemy and the thunder rites, in addition to the translation of the texts on the map.

4 See Baptandier 2016.

5 This manuscript is titled *Lingbao Taiji lianfa* 靈寶太極煉法, a register of He Huaide 何懷德. The manuscript dates from the thirty-sixth year of the Kangxi era (1698) and was written by a disciple Zhang Fazheng 張法正.

CHAPTER 1

# Chinese Inner Alchemy and Body Maps

In the 1980s, after many decades of neglect, Chinese scholars and practitioners rediscovered versions of the Taoist *Chart for the Cultivation of Perfection* (*Xiuzhen tu* 修真圖). This chart is a representation of the body, of the alchemical processes and of the rites that allow the realization of the Way. These processes were thought to enable the adept to achieve a transcendent state, and the performance of the accompanying exorcist rituals would benefit others. It is the result of a long evolution of diagrams and drawings relating to the body and its representations in Taoism. It appears in the context of Inner Alchemy and thunder rites that were in expansion in the tenth and eleventh centuries. At that time, body maps accompanied by captions and small texts, explaining the methods used to achieve the Way, appeared and it became a habit to transcribe, by the means of charts with iconography and accompanying texts, the processes of individual and collective practices in Taoist Inner Alchemy.

Representations of the body had featured elements of these charts as early as the 10th century when Taoists developed diagrams illustrating the alchemical importance of some areas of the body or certain phases of the alchemical process, which were inserted into Taoist scriptures. Several texts composed by famous experts of Inner Alchemy of this era are interspersed with illustrations and diagrams, prefiguring overall body maps, notably the *Chart for the Cultivation of Perfection*.[1]

1 An important writing of this type is the *Xiuzhen taiji hunyuan tu* 修真太極混元圖 [Diagrams on the mystery of ultimate and primordial chaos for cultivating perfection] (DZ 149) by Xiao Daocun 蕭道存 (fl. 13th cen.). The text is interspersed with explanatory diagrams. The *Dadan zhizhi* 大丹直指 [Clear directions on the great elixir] (DZ 244, 1.15a) has a representation of the twenty four degrees of the spinal column by Qiu Chuji 邱處機 (Changchun 長春) (1148–1227), one of the seven Complete Perfection masters. The *Yuqing jinsi qinghua biwen jinbao neilian danjue* 玉清金笥青華秘文金寶內鍊丹訣 [Alchemical formula of the inner refinement of the gold treasure in Qinghua's secret writings of the golden box of the Jade Purity Heavens] (DZ 240), a text attributed to Zhang Boduan 張伯端 (987–1082) but likely written later during the Song, includes a representation of the Median Cinnabar Field (2.9b), surrounded by eight trigrams in the human body (2.13a) and a representation of the light emanating from the moon toad in the human body. The *Xiuzhen shishu* [Ten books on the cultivation of perfection] has a representation of the body as bellows, with the tiger and the dragon, the serpent and the turtle, sun and moon. See Schipper and Verellen 2004 for index of *zhengtong* Daoist Canon. It will hereafter be abbreviated with DZ. (DZ 263, 9.7a). The *Qiaoqiao dongzhang* 敲蹻洞章 [Cavernous Stanzas of Master Qiaoqiao] includes a

© KONINKLIJKE BRILL NV, LEIDEN, 2019 | DOI:10.1163/9789004383456_003

There are four main types of extant body maps dating from the 10th through 12th centuries. The earliest maps, a set of six diagrams, are attributed to Yanluozi 煙蘿子 [Master of smokescreen] and date from the tenth century. These six illustrations are based on crude anatomical representations of the body, and detail the main places at which a person focuses his or her meditation, as well as the psychic forces and deities of the body. The second group of charts, composed in the late 13th century, was a synthesis of these six diagrams that featured a three-quarter view of the body. A third group (early 13th century), associated to the tradition of the cultivation of perfection (*xiuzhen* 修真), no longer refers to the anatomical body, but rather represents the body as a mountain with streams running down it; this symbolizes the breath circulating in the circuit of two meridians of the body. The names of the main alchemical sites are contained in cartouches. Finally, the fourth group appears during the Qing Dynasty (1644–1911). It combines the image of the body as a mountain and the three-quarter view of the physiological body. Anatomical references such as inner organs or the spine are either absent or very stylized. It is to this latter group that the *Chart for the Cultivation of Perfection* that we will present in detail in the next chapter belongs. In this chapter, I will discuss the other body charts of the first four groups, from the oldest of the tenth century to the most recent (1886), the *Chart of the Inner Landscape* (*Neijing tu* 內景圖) preserved in the White Cloud Temple (Baiyun guan 白雲觀) of Beijing.

## 1 From Anatomy to the Taoist Construction of the Body: Diagrams of Yanluozi (Tenth Century)

The oldest representations of the body that remain in the Taoist context are six drawings of the Yanluozi (fig. 1.1–1.6),[2] an otherwise unknown Taoist who lived near Mount Wangwu 王屋山 (Henan), and reached transcendence during the *tianfu* era (936–941) by eating ginseng root.[3] Very little in extant literature is

representation of the body with a Taiji in the three cinnabar fields and the twelve phases of the moon around the body, etc.

2 These representations were briefly presented in Needham 1983: 107–111.

3 According to the *Wangwushan zhi* 王屋山志 [Monograph on Mount Wangwu], "The Perfect Yan of Mount Wangwu obtained 'formulas for consuming purple clouds to nourish the Way.' Then, in a well dug near his home, he found a strange ginseng root." According to *juan* 8 of the *Shunzhi Huaiqing fuzhi* 順治懷慶府志 [Monograph of the Huaiqing prefecture in the Shunzhi era (1644–1661)], "Yanluozi, whose name was Yan, was a native of Mount Wangwu. In the *tianfu* era of Jin, while ploughing next to the Yang Terrace Palace (Yangtai gong 陽臺宮), he found and consumed a strange ginseng root. He immediately ascended to heaven in broad daylight." According to *juan* 11 of the *Qianlong Jiyuan xianzhi* 乾隆济源縣志 [Monograph on

attributed to enigmatic Yanluozi. Two short texts are featured alongside the six drawings in the *Ten Books on the Cultivation of Perfection*, a Taoist compilation completed around 1250.[4] There are also some fragments in the *Pivot of the Way*, a compilation of alchemical texts from the middle twelfth century.[5] The six drawings illustrate respectively the head (two), the right and left sides of the trunk (two), and the trunk with its organs from front and back (two). The two diagrams of the right and left sides of the trunk are not immediately recognizable, but a closer look reveals a fairly accurate drawing of the viscera and the arc of the spine; this enables the viewer to identify the nature of the object represented. The captions of the drawings and the accompanying texts nevertheless provide useful, if not indispensable, tools for the understanding of these diagrams. The title of these drawings features the expression *neijing* 内境 [Inner landscape] suggesting that those who possessed such charts to understand the alchemical processes thought to occur when the reader visualized their organs. This use of the text is underscored by the diagrams of the Yanluozi text, which are intended for "inner contemplation" (*neiguan* 内觀).

The first drawing represents the head as a heavenly paradise; accompanying captions identify palaces where well-known gods of the Taoist pantheon such as the Jade Emperor (Yudi 玉帝) and the Heavenly Sovereign (Tianhuang 天皇) lived. Two legends bear respectively the names of the deity of the liver, the Non-pareil Lordling (Wuying gongzi 無英公子), and of the lungs, the Perfected Man of the White Prime (Baiyuan zhenren 白元真人). Ponds and various secretions of the head, which play a significant role in Taoist practices, and specifically in Inner Alchemy, are also mentioned (fig. 1.1).

The second drawing shows the head and the main spirits that constitute the person and that can regularly escape from the body. The main one is the

Jiyuan district in the Qianlong era], "Yanluozi was a native of Wangwu. During the Tianfu era, while ploughing the fields near the Taoist Temple of the Yang Terrace, he found formulas for consuming purple clouds to nourish the Way." See Ch'en 1975: 284, appendix 2.

4 *Xiuzhen shishu* 修真十書 (DZ 263), 18.1a–6a. It consists of ten writings associated with Bai Yuchan (1194–1229?) and his circle. The texts, mostly from the southern tradition of Inner Alchemy, date from two generations before Zhang Boduan 張伯端 (987?–1082) considered as the ancestor of this lineage, to two generations after Bai Yuchan 白玉蟾 (1194–1229). These practices involve inner cultivation and meditation, but also rituals. See Skar 2004: 1118–1119.

5 See *Shangqing jinbi pian* 上清金碧篇, ed. Zeng Zao 曾慥 (c. 12th century), in *Daoshu* 道樞 [Pivot of the Way] (DZ 1017), 29.1a. Here, Yanluozi says, "Metal is the principal of the five agents, the root of the five vital forces, the origin of the five breaths." Later on (35.10a), he states "The breath is what Yanluozi refines." Several lost books are assigned in catalogues to Yanluozi, including a *Xuanzhu jing* 玄珠經 [Book on the obscure pearl]. See Van der Loon 1984: 180 (text catalogued in *Bishusheng mu* 秘書省目, 2.24b); Ch'en 1975: 284.

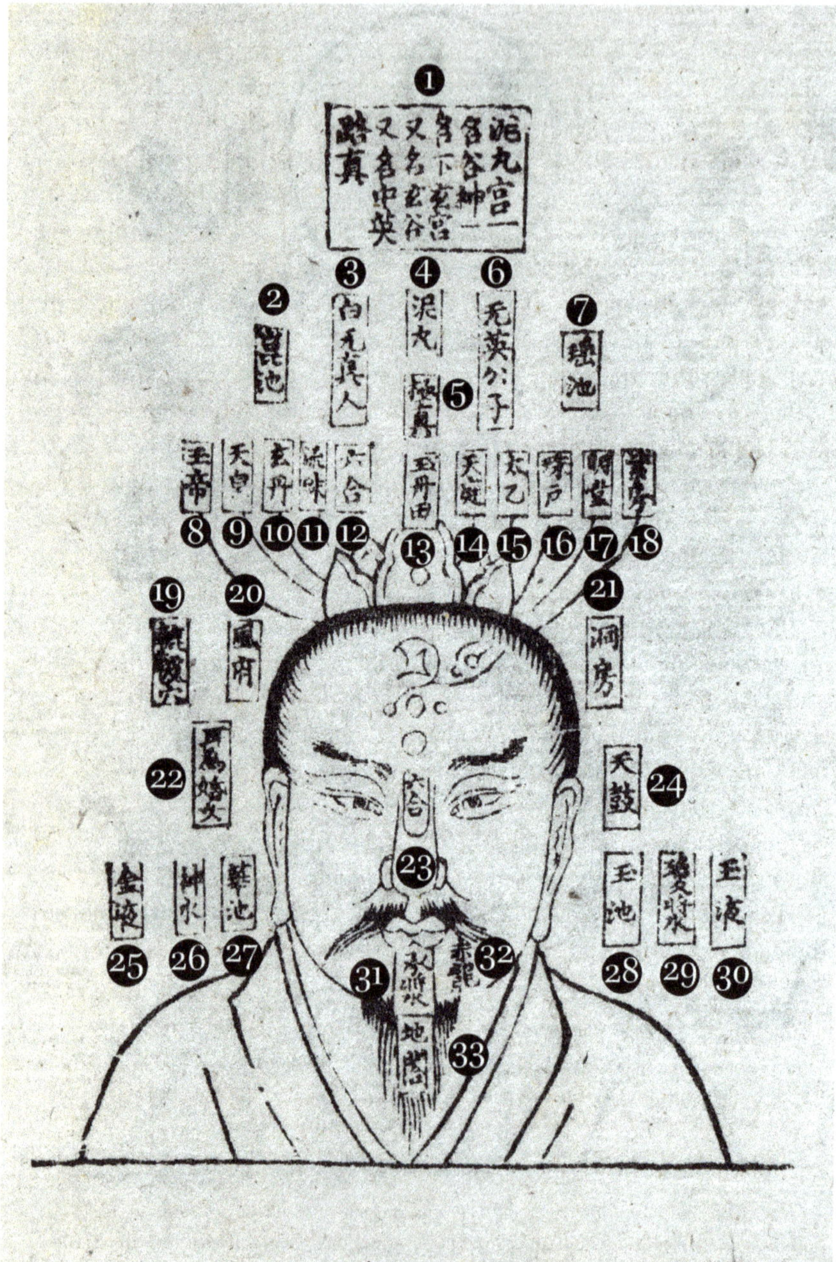


FIGURE 1.1 "Representation of the head according to Yanluozi" (*Yanluozi shoubu tu* 煙蘿子首部圖). *Xiuzhen shishu* 修真十書 (DZ 263), 18.2a

1. Muddy Pellet Palace; also called the Valley Spirit (*gushen* 谷神), the Inferior Obscure Palace (*xia xuangong* 下玄宫), the Obscure Valley (*xuangu* 玄谷), or the Perfected of Zhongying Way (Zhongying lu zhen 中英路真)
2. Mount Kun[lun] Pond (Kunchi 崑池)
3. Perfected of the White Prime (Baiyuan zhenren 白元真人)
4. Muddy Pellet (Niwan 泥丸)
5. Extreme Perfected (Jizhen 極真)
6. Non-pareil Lordling (Wuying gongzi 無英公子)
7. Yao-gem Pond (*yaochi* 瑤池)
8. Jade Emperor (Yudi 玉帝)
9. Heavenly Sovereign (Tianhuang 天皇)
10. Obscure Cinnabar (*xuandan* 玄丹)
11. Flowing Flavor (*liuwei* 流味) or the Streaming Pearls (*liuzhu* 流珠)
12. Six Unions (*liuhe* 六合)
13. Extreme Cinnabar Field (*zhi dantian* 至丹田)
14. Heavenly Court (*tianting* 天庭)
15. Great Oneness (*taiyi* 太乙)
16. Chiseled Jade Gate (*zhuohu* 琢戶)
17. Hall of Light (*mingtang* 明堂)
18. Purple Room (*zifang* 紫房)
19. Cavity of the Winches (*lulu xue* 轆轆穴)
20. Wind Palace (*fengfu* 風府)
21. Cavern Room (*dongfang* 洞房)
22. Ear is the Married Girl (*er wei hunnü* 耳為婚女)
23. Six Unions (*liuhe* 六合)
24. Heavenly Drum (*tiangu* 天鼓)
25. Golden Liquor (*jinye* 金液)
26. Divine Water (*shenshui* 神水)
27. Flowery Pond (*huachi* 華池)
28. Jade Pond (*yuchi* 玉池)
29. Rose-gem Nectar (*qiongjiang* 瓊漿)
30. Jade Liquor (*yuye* 玉液)
31. Receiving the Nectar (*chengjiang* 承漿)
32. Red Dragon (*chilong* 赤龍)
33. Terrestrial Gallery (*digo* 地閣)

Real Spirit or the Muddy Pellet Perfected (Niwan) that resides at the centre of the head, but can get out by the top; he is represented in a bright circle above the head. The other deities are the three corpses (*sanshi* 三尸), drawn to the left of the head on the upper right of the drawing, which are sort of morbidity principles sitting respectively in abdomen, heart and head. They are compared with vermin gnawing the vital principle and ascending regularly to heaven to report the good or bad behaviour of their host. To the right of the head (on the left of the drawing) are drawn the seven *po* souls associated with the lungs, whose nature is ambiguous because they can sometimes be harmful. Finally, one can see around the head the Four Numinous Spirits of the four directions (Azure Dragon, White Tiger, Vermilion Sparrow, Dark Warrior) playing in Taoism a protective role (fig. 1.2).

The third and fourth drawings of the left and right sides of the body, on which the organs are highly stylized, carry inscriptions depicting the three Cinnabar Fields (*dantian* 丹田), the main sites of alchemical transmutation, namely the respectively located in the abdomen, the region of the heart and the head.

All of these drawings contain symbols for the transformation process. For example, the Dragon and Tiger, placed face to face, symbolize the exchange between lung and liver breath in the Median Cinnabar Field. The presence of the twenty-four degrees of the spinal column evokes the constant correlation between the rhythm of alchemical processes and the mechanisms of the universe. Along the backbone, three chariots, sheep, deer and buffalo, symbolize three types of energy deployed in the three steps of the path to reverse the tide and achieve longevity (fig. 1.3 and 1.4). While rigorously taking into account the features of the anatomical body, these diagrams are more a representation of the person with his psychic powers and of the relationship between his psychological or spiritual transformations and the specific locations of the body or the organs which, in Chinese medicine and Taoism, are the seat of emotions and specific psychic forces.

Looking at the fifth and sixth drawings showing the trunk front and back with its principal organs, the anatomical references there are fundamental. We can distinguish the five viscera (liver, heart, spleen, lungs, kidneys), the gallbladder, the esophagus, the stomach, the large intestine, the small intestine, the bladder, a conduit connecting the kidneys and heart, and doors for the evacuation of urine and feces. Note that the liver is drawn on the left part of the body, a choice that accorded with conventional correlative theories in China, which linked the liver with wood, the spring season, and the east. These associations made it necessary to depict the liver on the left in an effort to observe the spatio-temporal correspondence with the five agents (fig. 1.5 and 1.6).

Although the name of Yanluozi is only found in the title of the first two diagrams concerning the head, it is very likely that the four other drawings of the trunk are also by him. He is identified as their author in a later text, written in 1113, after a series of dissections, by a certain Jia Weijie 賈偉節 of Luoyang. When writing about the later physician Yang Jie 楊介 (see below), Jia claims that Yang merely "modified the diagrams of Yanluozi" by adding the twelve meridians.[6] This would suggest that the set of drawings were understood as the creation of Yanluozi. Unfortunately, the scant evidence about Yanluozi makes it is difficult to know about the circumstances under which his conceptions of the body emerged. In the *Ten Books on the Cultivation of Perfection*, his charts are followed by a text entitled "Treaty on the Inner Aspect [of the Body] from the Attendant Zhu." This man named Zhu, otherwise unknown, is probably a man of the Song dynasty who lived before 1250. He would have seen the plates made after dissection, since he mentions that recently dissections of bandits were made on the market and those who have seen their body note that liver diseases were cared for by considering the left, yet positioned the liver was on the right. He added that, thanks to the recent dissections, this error and others of the traditional medical knowledge could be corrected such as those considering the existence of three holes in the throat, one for liquid, one for air and a third for food, while there are in fact only two.[7] He compares these descriptions with the Yanluozi's chart.

The Taoist diagrams were certainly not the only kinds of body maps in the Song Dynasty. In 1041 CE, for instance, there was a series of dissections at which painters were commissioned to draw the body. This event caused quite a stir and was reported by several scholars of the time.[8] These paintings were later called the "Drawings of the Five Viscera by Ou Xifan" (*Ou Xifan wuzang tu* 歐希范五臟圖). A second series of dissections was conducted in

6 Preface to the "Drawings of the circulation in the human body and the visualization of its true aspect" (*Cunzhen huanzhong tu* 存真環中圖) by Yang Jie, dated the third year of *zhenghe* era (1113) and signed by Jia Weijie. See Miyashita 1967: 148–149.

7 *Zhu tidian neijing lun* 朱提點内境論. In *Xiuzhen shishu* (DZ 263), 18.3b–5b.

8 Story reported in *Mengqi bitan* 夢溪筆談 [Brush talks from the dream brook] (*juan* 26, 480) by Shen Gua 沈括 (fl. 1094); Hu 2011: 827–829. See also Ye Mengde's 葉夢得 (1077–1148) *Yanxia fangyan* 巖下放言 [Unstrained words from the foot of a precipice) (SKQS), 3.11; Zhao Yushi's 趙與時 (1175–1231) *Bintui lu* 賓退錄 [Records after the guest has left] (SKQS), 4.2. In this last text, Lingjian 靈簡 is the official name. For an overview all these sources, see Okanishi 1969: 297.

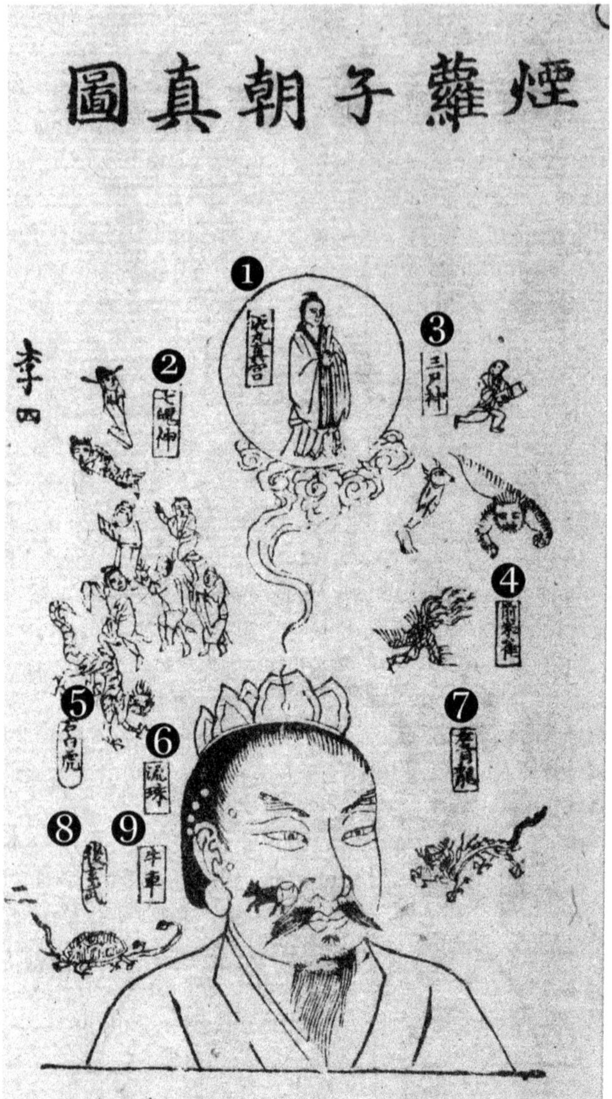


FIGURE 1.2 "Representation of the Audience to Perfection according to Yanluozi" (*Yanluozi chaozhen tu* 煙蘿子朝真圖). *Xiuzhen shishu* (DZ 263), 18.2b

1. Perfected Palace of the Muddy Pellet (*Niwan zhengong* 泥丸真宮)
2. Seven *Po* Souls (*qipo shen* 七魄神)
3. Spirits of the Three Corpses (*sanshi shen* 三尸神)
4. In front, Vermilion Sparrow (*qian zhuque* 前朱雀)
5. On the right, White Tiger (*you baihu* 右白虎)
6. Streaming Pearls (*liuzhu* 流珠)
7. On the left, Azure Dragon (*zuo qinglong* 左青龍)
8. Behind, Dark Warrior (*hou Xuanwu* 後玄武)
9. Buffalo Chariot (*niuche* 牛車)

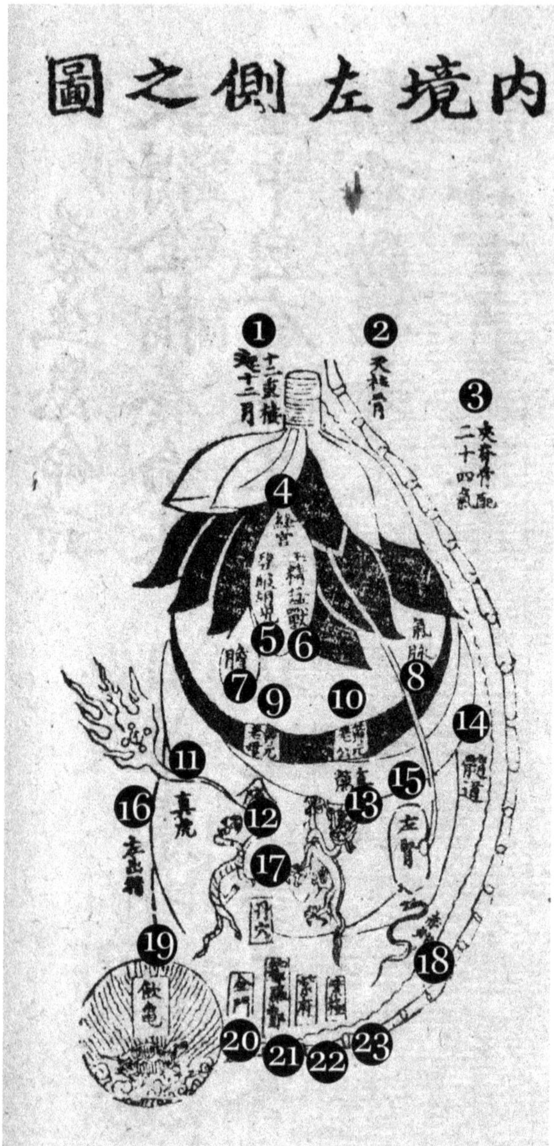


FIGURE 1.3 "Drawing of the left side of the inner aspect of the body [by Yanluozi]" (*Neijing zuoce zhi tu* 内境左側之圖). *Xiuzhen shishu* (DZ 263), 18.2b

1. Twelve-storey pagoda [associated with] the Twelve Months (*shier chonglou yu shier yue* 十二重樓與十二月)
2. Bone of Heaven's Pillar (*tianzhu gu* 天柱骨)
3. Vertebra that are correlated with the Twenty-Four Breaths (*jiajigu pei ershisi qi* 夾脊骨配二十四氣)
4. Scarlet Palace (*jianggong* 絳宮)
5. Foreign Monk with Cyan Eyes (*biyan hu'er* 碧眼胡兒)
6. Fierce Animal of the Jade Essence (*yujing mengshou* 玉精猛獸)
7. Gallbladder (*dan* 膽)
8. Breath Channels (*qimai* 氣脈)
9. Venerable Mother of the Yellow Origin (*Huangyuan laomu* 黃元老母)
10. Venerable Father of the Yellow Origin (*Huangyuan laogong* 黃元老公)
11. Perfected Tiger (*zhenhu* 真虎)
12. Umbilicus (*qi* 臍)
13. Perfected Dragon (*zhenlong* 真龍)
14. Spinal Cord (*suidao* 髓道)
15. Left Kidney (zuo shen 左腎)
16. Emanating Essence on the Left (*zuo jing chu* 左出精)
17. Cinnabar Cavity (*danxue* 丹穴)
18. Red Snake (*chishe* 赤蛇)
19. Drinking Turtle (*yingui* 飲龜)
20. Metal Gate (*jinmen* 金門)
21. Luofeng the Northern Metropolis (*Beidu Luofeng* 北都羅酆)
22. Purple Palace (*Zifu* 紫府)
23. Metal Pass (*Ziji* 紫極)

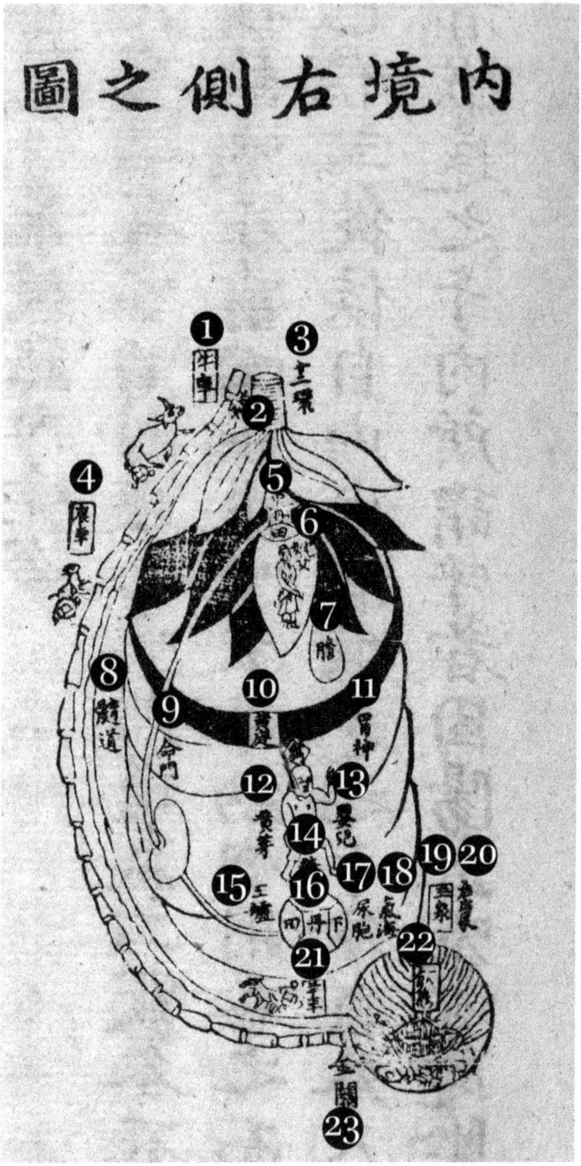


FIGURE 1.4 "Drawing of the right side of the inner aspect of the body [by Yanluozi]" (*Neijing youce zhi tu* 内境右側之圖). *Xiuzhen shishu* (DZ 263), 18.3a

1. Buffalo Chariot (*niuche* 牛車)
2. Obscure Pearl (*xuanzhu* 玄珠)
3. Twelve Rings (*shier huan* 十二環)
4. Deer Chariot (*luche* 鹿車)
5. Median Cinnabar Field (*zhong dantian* 中丹田)
6. Maiden (*Chanu* 姹女)
7. Gallbladder (*dan* 膽)
8. Spinal Cord (*suidao* 髓道)
9. Gate of the Vital Force (*mingmen* 命門)
10. Yellow Court (*huangting* 黄庭)
11. Stomach Deity (*wei shen* 胃神)
12. Yellow Sprout (*huangya* 黄芽)
13. Infant (*ying'er* 嬰兒)
14. Vital Essence (*jing* 精)
15. Jade Furnace (*yulu* 玉爐)
16. Lower Cinnabar Field (*xia dantian* 下丹田)
17. Bladder (*niaobao* 尿胞)
18. Breath ocean (*qihai* 氣海)
19. Jade Spring (*yuquan* 玉泉)
20. Urine coming out of the Right (*you chu niao* 右出尿)
21. Sheep Chariot (*yangche* 羊車)
22. Drinking Turtle (*yingui* 飲龜)
23. Metal Pass (*jinguan* 金關)

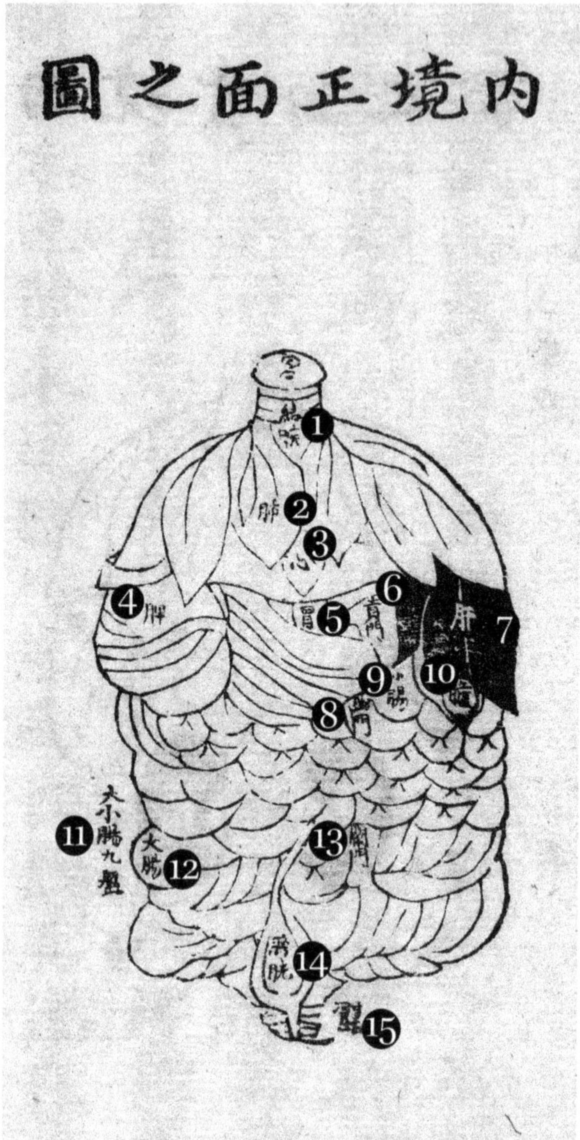


FIGURE 1.5 "Drawing of the Inner Aspect of the Body Viewed from the Front [by Yanluozi]" (*Neijing zhengmian zhi tu* 內境正面之圖). *Xiuzhen shishu* (DZ 263), 18.3a

1. Adam's Apple (*jiehou* 結喉)
2. Lungs (*fei* 肺)
3. Heart (*xin* 心)
4. Spleen (*pi* 脾)
5. Stomach (*wei* 胃)
6. Cardia (*penmen* 賁門)
7. Liver (*gan* 肝)
8. Pylorus (*youmen* 幽門)
9. Small Intestine (*xiaochang* 小腸)
10. Gallbladder (*dan* 膽)
11. Nine convolutions of the intestines (*da xiaochang jiupan* 大小腸九盘)
12. Large Intestine (*dachang* 大腸)
13. Ileocecal Valve (*lanmen* 闌門)
14. Bladder (*pangguang* 膀胱)
15. Place for Urination (*niao zici chu* 尿自此 出)

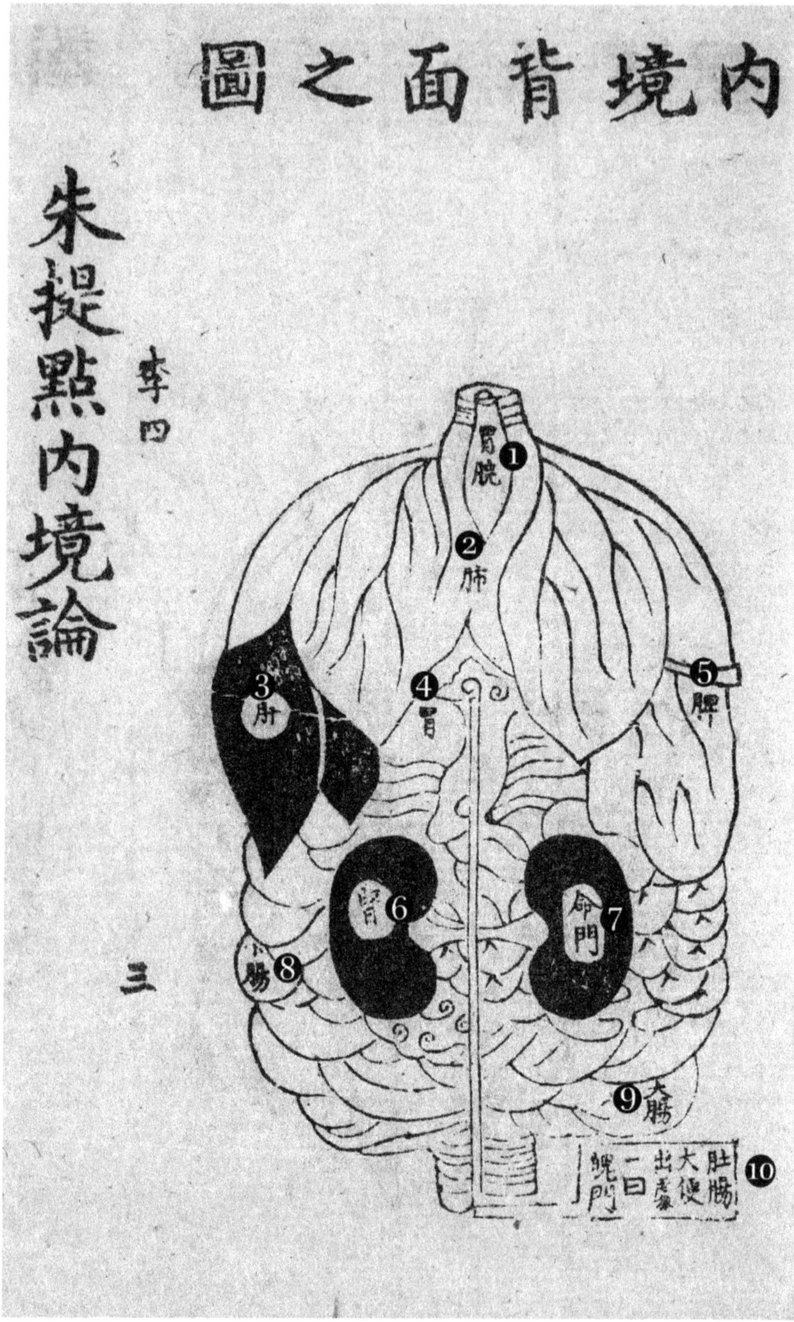


FIGURE 1.6 "Representation of the inner aspect of the body seen from behind [by Yanluozi]". (*Neijing beimian zhi tu* 内境背面之圖). *Xiuzhen shishu* (DZ 263), 18.3b

1. Esophagus (*weiguan* 胃管)
2. Lungs (*fei* 肺)
3. Liver (*gan* 肝)
4. Stomach (*wei* 胃)
5. Spleen (*pi* 脾)
6. Kidneys (*shen* 腎)
7. Gate of the Vital Force (*mingmen* 命門)
8. Small intestine (*xiaochang* 小腸)
9. Large intestine (*dachang* 大腸)
10. Rectum for defecation, also called the Gate of the *Po* [Soul] (*duchang dabian chu yi yue pomen* 肚腸大便出, 一曰魄門)

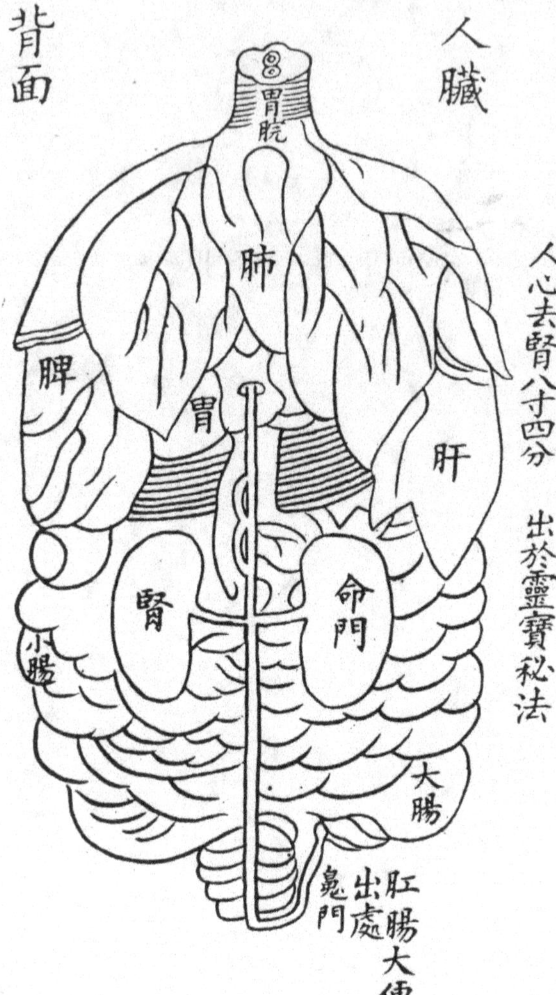


FIGURE 1.7 *Drawings of the Interior of the Body by Hua Tuo* (*Hua Tuo xuanmen neizhao tu* 華佗玄門内照圖), 1.20. Representation of the dorsal side of the trunk; the liver is drawn on the right side of the image

1102–1106, and gave also rise to similar drawings. These were made in Sizhou 泗州 (Jiangsu province) by painters accompanying prefect Li Yixing 李夷行 and physicians who examined the corpses of rebels recently sentenced to death. The membranes were cut off these bodies and the diaphragms removed, after which the painters meticulously drew the curves of the inner body. Afterwards, Yang Jie, the famous doctor of Emperor Huizong (r. 1101–1125), revised these charts. Yang was a native of Sizhou, the place where the dissections occurred, and revised these plates after comparing them with old documents. By Yang's account, he found the Sizhou dissection charts much better than those made by Ou Xifan.[9] These drawings of the viscera revised by Yang Jie were published in 1273 by Sun Huan 孫煥 in a book called *Drawings of the Interior of the Body by Hua Tuo* (fig. 1.7). This document, first written in 1095 by the imperial librarian and archivist Zhu Shen 銖沉, was revised in 1273 by Sun Huan, who published it, adding these drawings to those of Yang Jie. In 1304, Sun's redaction was reproduced in a Japanese text from Kajiwara Seizen 樟原性全.[10]

On these representations, unlike those of Yanluozi, the liver is located on the right. The first part of the text incorporates the illustrations of Ou Xifan's anatomical analysis. There are three significant changes in this text from earlier ones. The first echoes the writing of Shen Gua, a famous rationalist of his day who claimed the throat has only two orifices; the plates by Ou Xifan, by contrast, contained three.[11] Like Shen Gua, the author of this piece justifies this position by reasoning that it is mechanically impossible to separate liquid and foods; therefore, there could only be two different holes. The second criticism concerns the location of the liver. In the *Drawings of the Interior of the Body by Hua Tuo*, the author writes without explanation that the liver is on the right side of the body, in front of the right kidney and beside the stomach.[12] A third point concerns the kidneys that are, according to the plates, higher than the location traditionally described; instead of being located lower down and attached to the sides, they are below the diaphragm in the middle of the spinal column. A membrane with two tubes also surrounds the kidneys: one that connects up to the heart and another lower one that connects the two kidneys.

9 *Junzhai dushu houzhi* 郡齋讀書後志, 2.31a–b; *Siku quanshu*, 674.405–406.

10 This is included in the *Ton'isho* 顿醫钞 [Excerpts on swift medicine] by Kajiwara Seizen 梶原性全. This manuscript is held at Waseda University.

11 *Hua Tuo xuanmen neizhao tu* 華佗玄門內照圖, 7a.

12 *Ibid.*, 8b.

Dissections had far less impact in China than in the West, which nevertheless developed this practice at a later date; the earliest illustrated books on anatomy in the West are of a crude and naïve appearance.[13] It was the School of Padua in Italy that first conducted dissections in the sixteenth century. The Church was often falsely accused of having prevented the development of dissections, but it actually played a great role in the development of anatomical knowledge. Sixtus IV's bull of 1472, for example, recognizes anatomy as a useful discipline for medical and artistic practices. Although teaching through dissection had been tolerated, Pope Clement VII (r. 1523–1534) formally authorized the practice and it was thereafter widely practised.[14] The sixteenth century marks a turning point in Western knowledge of the body through the multiplication of dissections and the finesse of graphic representations such as the drawings of Leonardo da Vinci, whose work reinforced the need for accuracy of observation and the requirement of precision.[15] When we compare the knowledge and the anatomical representations of the twelfth and thirteenth centuries in the West and in China, we realize that in China they were as accurate, if not more so, than in the West.

Some specialists have hypothesized that the drawings by Yanluozi were also performed by observation of the dissected body. The main organs, which were already subject to detailed descriptions in the medical context and in some Taoist texts of the Yellow Court tradition, are as accurate and well done as they were in the West at the same time.[16] However, Yanluozi's drawings, particularly the first four drawings of the head and of the trunk, contain pictorial elements and inscriptions that reflect the Taoist concepts of the body as a space that transforms and sustains the self. The body is inhabited by many forces comprising different breaths, psychic entities or deities (*shen* 神). In fact, these drawings introduce the main symbols of alchemical transmutations that will be discussed in detail in the study of the *Chart for the Cultivation of Perfection*. Yanluozi mixes topographical descriptions, physiological and alchemical

---

13 See Grmek and Barnabeo 1997: 10–11.

14 See Grmek and Barnabeo 1997: 8.

15 *Ibid.*, 11.

16 This tradition appearing at the beginning of the Six Dynasties developed a set of meditative practices in which the Yellow Court is an important place inside the body for actualizing (*cun* 存) the inner gods and by this mean obtain longevity and protection. Two texts expose this system of body deities: the *Huangting neijing yujing zhu* 黃庭內景玉經註 [Commentary on the jade scripture of the Yellow Court's inner landscape (DZ 402) and the *Huangting waijing jing* 黃庭外景經 [Scripture on the yellow court's outer landscape] (DZ 403).

representations. Topographic features also tend to disappear from the later alchemical representations of the body, while later descriptions of alchemical sites of the body reveal a more advanced state of anatomical knowledge.

## 2 The Synthesis of the Yanluozi Diagrams in the Commentary on the *Classic of the Difficulties* (*Nanjing* 難經) (Late Thirteenth Century)

A representation of the inner body is inserted in a commentary of the *Classic of the Difficulties* (fig. 1.8), which also includes a preface by Li Jiong 李駉 dated to 1269,[17] This text is a late thirteenth century commentary on a medical classic attributed to Bian Que 扁鵲 (d. 310 BCE), the semi-legendary physician of ancient China.[18] The introduction of the commentary to this text includes seventeen pages of drawings on the pulses on the forearm, acupuncture points on forearm and legs, as well as full body maps. First, there is a side representation of the body (4a–b), followed by two representations of the front and back (5a–b), and a diagram titled "Drawing of the Beginning and the End of Cycles of Yin and Yang in the Universe" (*Tiandi yinyang shengjiang shizhong tu* 天地陰陽升降始終圖).[19] The side representation (fig. 1.8) is in fact a synthesis of the first four drawings of Yanluozi. His first two drawings of the head with the alchemical sites and of the "Audience with Perfected Deities" are depicted in one drawing with all captions arranged in and around the head. Similarly, the representations of right and left sides of the body by Yanluozi are combined here on the same plate that represents a three-quarter view of the body. Two quatrains of septasyllabic verse appear on the right near the middle of the map. These two quatrains do not appear on the Yanluozi diagrams, but they precede them in the *Ten Books on the Cultivation of Perfection* and are introduced by the

17 *Huangdi bashiyi nanjing zhushi tuxu lun* 黃帝八十一難經注釋圖序論 [Treatise with illustrations and commentaries on the eighty-one difficulties of the *Yellow Emperor's Canon*] (DZ 1024) written by Li Jiong 李駉 in 1269. Li Jiong, social name Zigui 子桂, was a native of Linchuan in Jiangxi. He was nicknamed Xifanzi 晞范子. We now abbreviate in designating this drawing as with the drawing of the commentary on the *Classic of the Difficulties*.

18 See the English translation of this work, its main comments and the introduction by Unschuld 1986.

19 In the outermost part are represented the eight trigrams, then in the first circle going inwards the names of the twenty-four nodal breaths of the year, in the second circle black and white points representing the yin and the yang, in a third circle the four agents and the four cardinal points, characters denoting the heavenly door, the terrestrial, the door of the human world and the door of the demons, and finally in the central circle the character "earth" (*tu* 土). See DZ 1024, 6a.

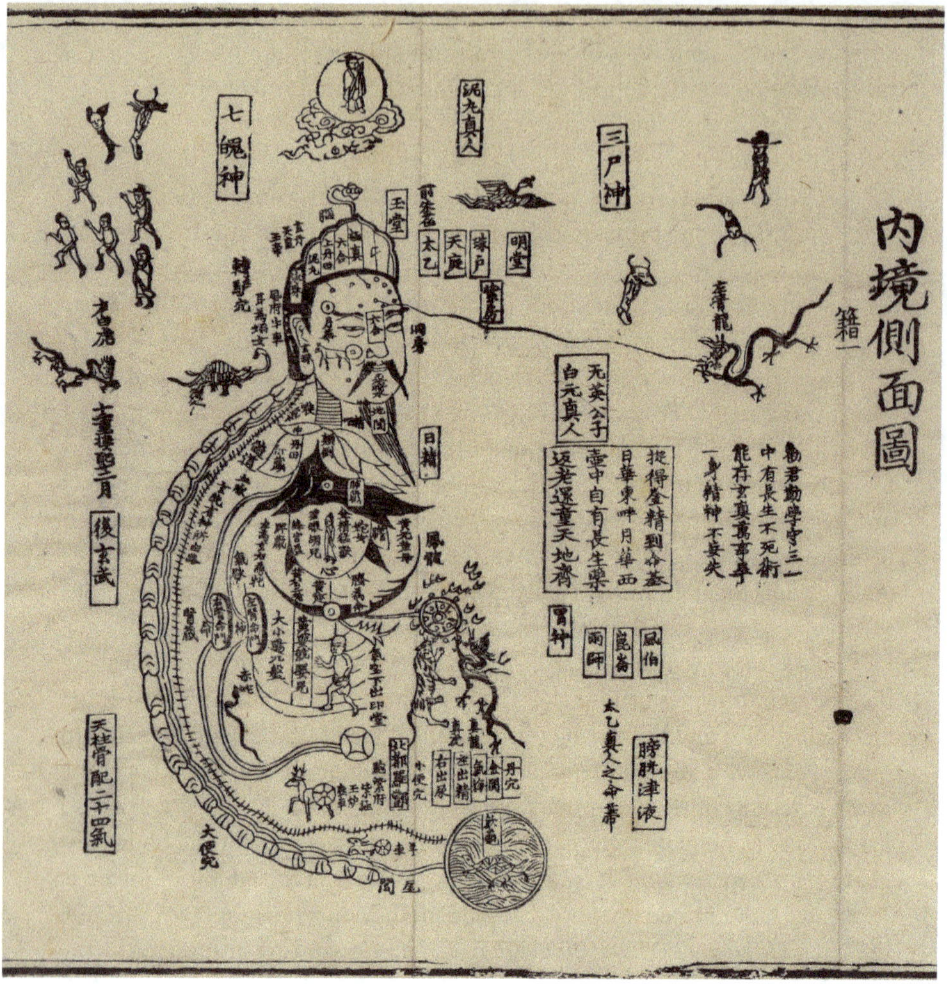


FIGURE 1.8 "Side representation of the inner aspect of the body". (*Neijing cemian tu* 内境側面圖) (1269). *Huangdi bashiyi nanjing zhuyi tu xulun* (DZ 1024), 4a–b

title "Poems on Nourishing Life and Resting the Vital Force". The first one in the cartouche is the following:

> Quick, grasp the Metal Essence to nourish the foundation of the Vital Force;
> The solar flower rises to the eastern shore, the moon flower to the west.
> The pot contains the medicine for long life,
> It rejuvenates you and makes you the equal of heaven and earth.

捉得金精養命基，
日華東畔月華西。
壺中自有長生藥，
返老還童天地齊。

And the second one:
I beseech to you, concentrate assiduously on the triple unity:
Therein lies the art of longevity and immortality.
Visualize the Real Mystery and everything will happen,
Your efforts will not have been in vain.[20]

勸君勤學守三一，
中有長生不死術。
能存玄真萬事畢，
一身精神不妄失

Joseph Needham has published a similar figure which bears some minor variations,[21] taken from a 1478 edition of a book written about 1264–1265 by Chen Yuanqing 陳元靚: the *Guide through the Forest of Events* (fig. 1.9).[22] It is unclear whether Li Jiong, whose text includes a preface written in 1269, has copied from Chen Yuanqing, who finished his work four years earlier in 1265. These two authors may have taken this figure from another source unknown to us. It is also possible that the publisher from 1478 added himself this drawing to the work of Chen Yuanqing, taking it from the work of Li Jiong or another unknown source.

## 3 The Body as a Mountain (Early Thirteenth Century)

A representation of the body as a mountain contains the names of the main parts of the body, as well as the circuit of the breath going from the Control Vessel (*dumai* 督脈) through the middle of the back and onto the Function Vessel (*renmai* 任脈) flowing at the centre of the body front.[23] It is inserted

20 *Yangsheng ximing shi* 養生息命詩 as quoted in *Xiuzhen shishu* (DZ 263), 18. 2a.
21 Needham 1983: 5.117.
22 *Shilin guangji* 事林廣記 by Chen Yuanqing. Chen Yuanqing is also the author of a calendar (*Suishi guangji* 歲時廣記), in *Gezhi congshu* 格致叢書 and *Siku quanshu* 四庫全書.
23 On the body as a mountain, see Despeux 1990: 194–198, and Lagerwey 1991: 127–142.

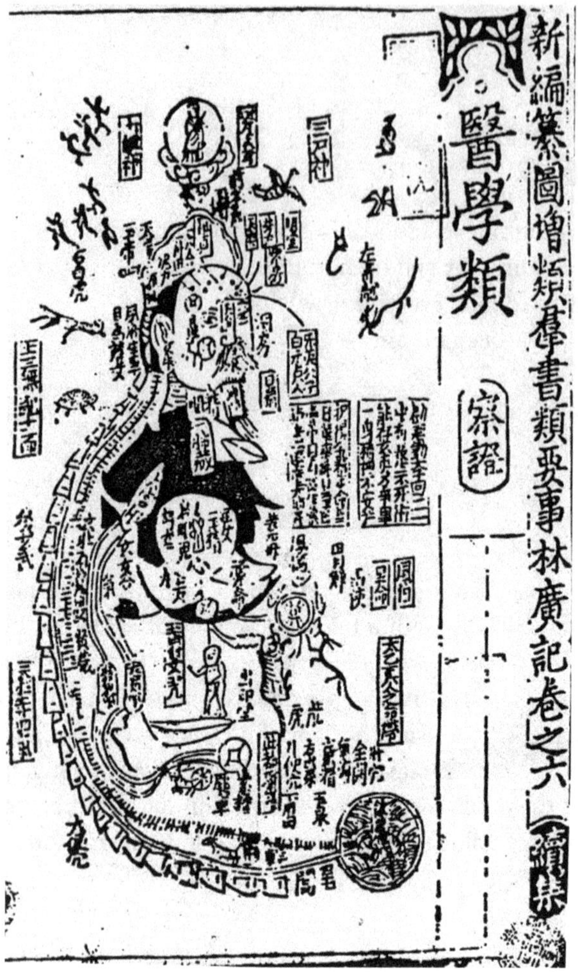


FIGURE 1.9 Side representation of the body in the 1478 CE *Shilin guangji* 事林廣記 [Guide through the forest of events] (Needham 1983: 5.117)

into a commentary on the *Book of Universal Salvation*,[24] with the title "Chart on Increasing and Decreasing Yin and Yang in the Human Body" (fig. 1.10).[25]

24 Short title by which we now refer to this text entitled in the Ming Taoist Canon *Yuanshi wuliang duren shangpin miaojing* 元始無量度人上品妙經. This book belongs to the Numinous Treasure tradition and its first part dates from the fourth or fifth century. But the common edition in Taoist Canon with sixty chapters more is an expansion composed by Taoists of the Divine Empyrean School early in the twelfth century.

25 Xiao Yingsou (fl. 13th cen.), *Yuanshi wuliang duren shangpin miaojing neiyi* 元始無量度人上品妙經內義 [Esoteric interpretation of the *Book of Salvation*] (DZ 90), 8a–b.

This commentary was written by Xiao Yingsou 蕭應叟 that begins with a memorandum that the author presented in 1226 to the Emperor Lizong (r. 1225–1265) along with the entire commentary. He signed as "Master of the three lights methods of the Obscure City of the Great Grotto of the Upper Clarity tradition,"[26] a title that suggests that he was belonging to the Maoshan current. He is elsewhere presented in another work of the Taoist Canon written by Xu Mingdao 許明道 of the Jiangxi province as a master of the Cultivation of Perfection tradition (Xiuzhen), according to the following lineage: Zhang Tiangang 張天罡, Peng Mengqu 彭夢蘧, Xiao Yingsou.[27] This lineage refers to Taoists of the southern alchemical tradition.

This body map as a mountain was used again with some variants and another title "Chart Depicting the Body of Primordial Breath", in a 14th century text, the *Alchemical Diagrams to Master Shangyang's Essentials of the Elixir* by Chen Zhixu 陳致虛 (d. 1331),[28] that combined the northern and southern inner alchemical traditions (fig. 1.11).[29]

26 *Ibid.*, 2b.

27 *Huandan bijue yang chizi shenfang* 還丹秘訣養赤子神方 [Divine recipes for nourishing the infant according to the secret process of returned cinnabar] (DZ 232), 6a–b. The author of this text, Xu Mingdao 許明道, was the disciple of Xiao Yingsou and Peng Mengqu, whom he met at Mount Tongbo 桐柏山 in the Tiantai Mountains (Zhejiang).

28 *Shangyangzi jindan dayao tu* 上陽子金丹大要圖 (DZ 1068), 2b.

29 See also Chen Zhixu's (ob. 1331) *Shangyangzi jindan dayao liexian zhi* 上陽子金丹大要列仙志 [Monograph on the arrayed transcendents of Master Shangyang's essential elixir] (DZ 1069) where there are sixteen short biographies representing this lineage. Li Daochun (ca. 1288–1292) gave to the southern tradition of Inner Alchemy and to the northern school of the Complete Perfection the same status. He said they had a common source and belonged to the same family. In 1331, Chen Zhixu completed the process of integration by subordinating the five patriarchs of the southern tradition to the Patriarchs of the Quanzhen School. The southern tradition disappeared as an independent movement and became part of Quanzhen. See Baldrian-Hussein, in Pregadio 2008: 759–762. In his lineage, Chen Zhixu begins with an invocation to the famous Taoists from Han to Tang, the various Taoist patriarchs until Wang Chongyang 王重陽. Then is given the name of the seven Perfected of the Complete Perfection lineage, the five masters of the "southern lineage": Zhang Boduan 張伯端, Shi Xinglin 石杏林 (ob. 1158), Xue Daoguang 薛道光 (1078–1191), Chen Niwan 陳泥丸 and Bai Yuchan 白玉蟾, as well as Song Defang 宋德方 or Song Piyun 披雲, who went with Qiu Changchun 邱長春 and Genghis Khan to the southwest regions, Li Jue 李珏, Zhang Mu 張模 and Zhao Youqin 趙友欽, and himself, Chen Zhixu, *Shangyang jindan dayao xianpai* 上陽子金丹大要仙派 [Lineage of transcendents with Master Shangyang's Essential Elixir] (DZ 1070), 2b. On Shangyangzi, see Davis and Ch'en 1942–1943: 126–130; Hudson 2008.

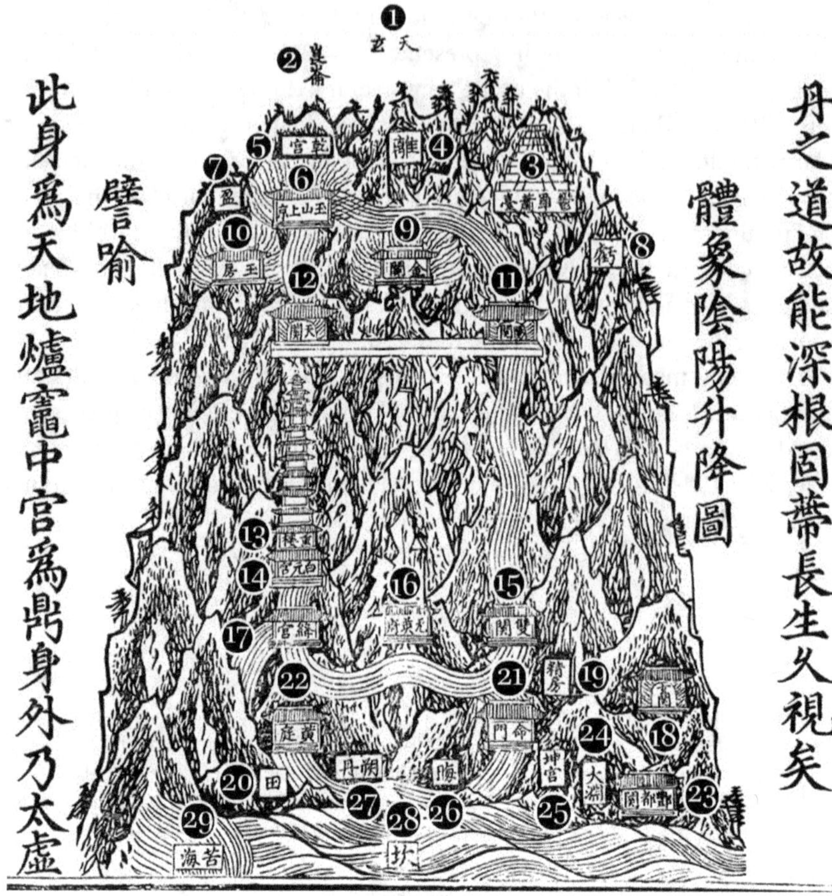


FIGURE 1.10 "Chart on Increasing and Decreasing Yin and Yang in the Human Body" (*Tixiang yinyang shengjiang tu* 體象陰陽升降圖), composed in 1226. Featured in *Yuanshi wuliang duren shangpin miaojing neiyi* 元始無量度人上品妙經內義 (DZ 90), 8a–b

1. Obscure Heaven (*xuantian* 玄天)
2. Mount Kunlun (*Kunlun* 崑崙)
3. Wormwood Terrace of the Yuluo Heaven (*Yuluo Xiaotai* 鬱羅蕭臺)
4. *Li* [Trigram] (*Li* 离)
5. Qian Palace (*Qiangong* 乾宮)
6. Jade Capitol Mountain (*Yujing shan* 玉京山)
7. Full [Moon] (*ying* 盈)
8. Waning [Moon] (*kui* 亏)
9. Golden Porte (*jinque* 金闕)
10. Jade Room (*yufang* 玉房)
11. Yang Pass (*yangguan* 陽關)
12. Heavenly Pass (*tianguan* 天關)
13. Storied Pagoda (*chonglou* 重樓)
14. Palace of the White Origin (*Baiyuangong* 白元宮)
15. Double Pass (*shuangguan* 雙關)
16. Wuying Palace (*Wuying dian* 無英殿)
17. Scarlet Palace (*jianggong* 絳宮)
18. Dark Pass (*xuanguan* 玄關)
19. Essence Room (*jingfang* 精房)
20. Cinnabar Field (*dantian* 丹田)
21. Gate of the Vital Force (*mingmen* 命門)
22. Yellow Court (*Huangting* 黄庭)
23. Fengdu Pass (*Fengdu guan* 酆都關)
24. Great Abyss (*Dayuan* 大淵)
25. Kun Palace (*Kungong* 坤宮)
26. First Quarter Moon (*hui* 晦)
27. New Moon (*shuo* 朔)
28. *Kun* [Trigram] (*Kan* 坎)

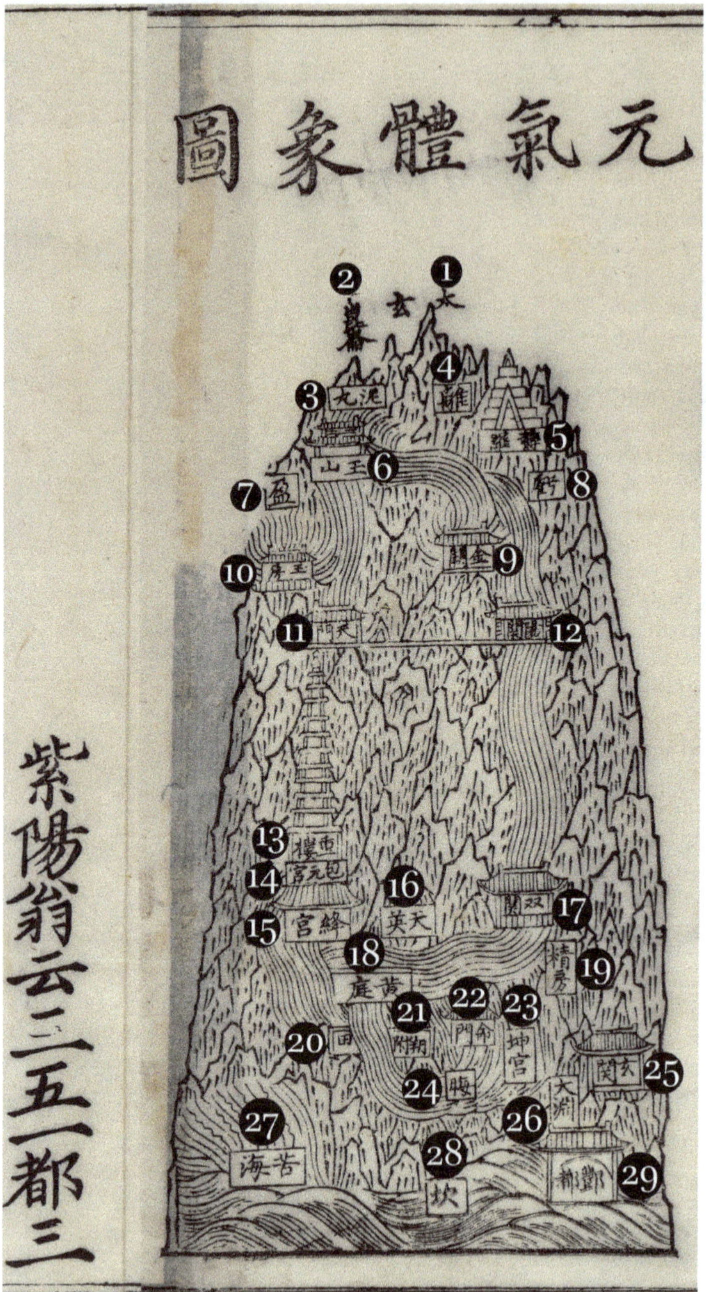


FIGURE 1.11 "Chart Depicting the Body of Primordial Breath" (*Yuanqi tixiang tu* 元氣體象圖) (early 14th century). *Shangyangzi jindan dayao tu* (DZ 1068), 3a–b

1. Supreme Mystery (*taixuan* 太玄)
2. Mount Kunlun (*Kunlun* 崑崙)
3. Muddy Pellet (*Niwan* 泥丸)
4. *Li* [Trigram] (*Li* 离)
5. Yuluo [Heaven] (*Yuluo* 鬱羅)
6. Jade Mountain (Yushan 玉山)
7. Full Moon (*ying* 盈)
8. Waning Moon (*kui* 亏)
9. Golden Porte (*jinque* 金闕)
10. Jade Room (*yufang* 玉房)
11. Heavenly Gate (*tianmen* 天門)
12. Yang Pass (*yangguan* 陽關)
13. Storied Pagoda (*chonglou* 重樓)
14. Embracing the Primordial Palace (*Baoyuan gong* 包元宫)
15. Scarlet Palace (*jianggong* 絳宫)
16. Wuying Palace (*Wuying* 無英)
17. Double Pass (*shuangguan* 雙關)
18. Yellow Court (*Huangting* 黄庭)
19. Essence Room (*jingfang* 精房)
20. Cinnabar Field (*dantian* 丹田)
21. New Moon (*shuo* 朔)
22. Gate of the Vital Force (*mingmen* 命門)
23. Kun Palace (*Kungong* 坤宫)
24. First Quarter Moon (*hui* 晦)
25. Dark Pass (*xuanguan* 玄關)
26. Great Abyss (*dayuan* 大淵)
27. Sea of Sufferings (*kuhai* 苦海)
28. *Kan* [Trigram] (*Kan* 坎)
29. Fengdu (Fengdu 酆都)

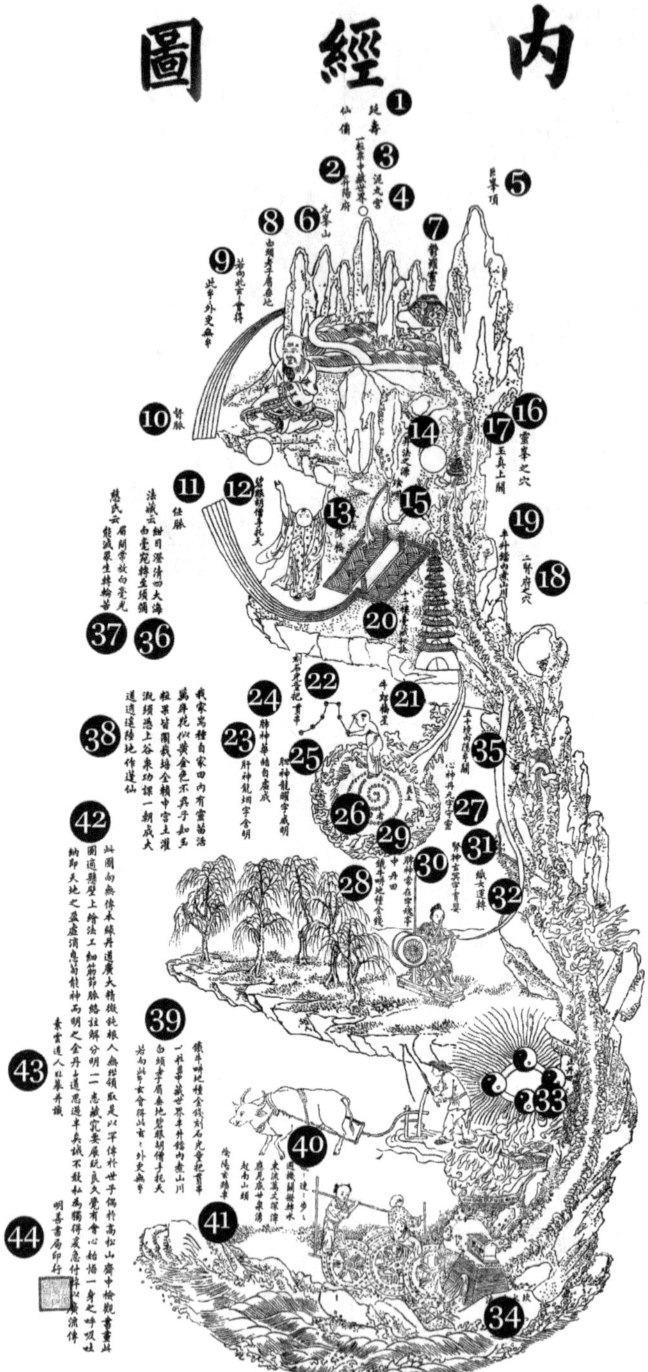


FIGURE 1.12 *Chart of the Inner Landscape of the Body* (*Neijing tu*). White Cloud Temple, Beijing

1. Residence of the Long-lived Transcendent (*Yanshou xianju* 延壽仙居)
2. Palatine of Ascending Yang (*shengyang fu* 升陽府)
3. A Grain of Millet Containing the Universe (*yili su zhong cang shijie* 一粒粟中藏世界)
4. Muddy Pellet Palace (*Niwan gong* 泥丸宫)
5. Summit of the Giant Peak (*jufeng ding* 巨峰頂)
6. Nine Peaks Mountains (Jiufeng shan 九峰山)
7. Numinous Terrace of the Yuluo [Heaven] (*Yuluo Lingtai* 鬱羅靈臺)
8. White-haired Laozi whose Eyebrows Touch the Ground (*Baitou Laozi mei chuidi* 白頭老子眉垂地)
9. "Facing this mystery enables one to grasp it, but there will be no mystery if one is outside it" (*ruoxiang ci xuan xuan huide, ci xuanxuan wai geng wu xuan* 若向此玄玄會得, 此玄玄外更無玄)
10. Control Vessel (*dumai* 督脈)
11. Function Vessel (*renmai* 任脈)
12. Cyan-eyed Foreign Monk Supporting the Sky with His Hands (*biyan huseng shou tuo tian* 碧眼胡僧手托天)
13. Breath Quickly Passing across the Bridge (*qi ji jiang qiao* 氣疾降橋)
14. Source of the Ascending Method (*shengfa zhi yuan* 升法之源)
15. Larynx (*yan* 咽)
16. Cavity of the Numinous Peak (*Lingfeng zhi xue* 靈峰之穴)
17. Upper Pass of the Jade Perfection (*Yuzhen shangguan* 玉真上關)
18. Cavity of the Two Kidneys' Palatine (*er shen fuxue* 二腎府穴)
19. Mountains and Rivers Boil Halfway up the Cookpot (*bansheng chengnei zhu shanchuan* 半升鐺内煮山川)
20. Secret Formula Locked in the Twelve-Storey Pagoda (*shierlou tai cang mijue* 十二樓臺藏秘訣)
21. Star of the Cowherd's Bridge (*niulang qiaoxing* 牛郎橋星)
22. Lithic Child Threading Together (*shike ertong ba guanchuan* 石刻兒童把貫串)
23. Deity of the Liver, Dragon Haze, with the cognomen Enveloping Light (*ganshen Longyan zi Hanming* 肝神龍煙字含明)
24. Deity of the Lungs, Hoary Blossom, with the cognomen Vacuous Achievement (*feishen Haohua zi Xucheng* 肺神皓華字虛成)
25. Deity of the Gallbladder, Dragon Brilliance, with the cognomen Majestic Light (*danshen Longyao zi Weiming* 膽神龍耀字威明)
26. Field with great tilth (*tianzhe liangtu* 田者良土)
27. Deity of the Heart, Cinnabar Origin with the cognomen Protector of Numina (*xinshen Danyuan zi Shouling* 心神丹元字守靈)
28. Planting Gold Coins as the Bronze Buffalo Plows the Land (*tongniu gengdi zhong jinqian* 銅牛耕地種金錢)
29. Median Cinnabar Field (*zhong dantian* 中丹田)
30. Deity of the Spleen, Eternally Present, with the cognomen Pavilion of the Hun [Soul] (*Pishen Changzai zi Hunting* 脾神常在字魂亭)
31. Deity of the Kidneys, Obscure Dimness with the cognomen Procreator of the Child (*shenshen Xuanming zi Yuying* 腎神玄冥字育嬰)
32. Weaving Maid Spinning the Wheel (*zhinü yunzhuan* 織女運轉)
33. Correct Cinnabar Field (*zheng dantian* 正丹田)
34. Water of Kan Flowing in the Opposite Direction (*kanshui niliu* 坎水逆流)
35. Obscure Pass Hidden in the Fifty Areas of Conscience (*wushi jing nei yin xuanguan* 五十境内隐玄關)

36–44. Poems and inscriptions

## 4 The Chart of the Inner Landscape (*Neijing tu* 內景圖) in the White Cloud Temple (1886)

An alchemical representation of the body called "Chart of the Inner Landscape [of the Body]" (*Neijing tu*) and engraved on stone was kept in the White Cloud Temple in Beijing (fig. 1.12).[30] It was engraved in 1886 at the request of Liu Chengyin 劉誠印, a powerful eunuch at the Court, after he saw a similar old silk scroll at the house of Gao Songshan 高崧山[31]. Upon seeing the scroll, Liu exclaimed:

> I have examined this drawing a long time and realized that my consciousness was expanding. I began to perceive that exhalation and inhalation, as well as expelling from and ingesting into the human body waxed and waned just like the cosmic ebb and flow. He who can have a penetrating insight into [these processes] will have progressed more than halfway on the Great Way of the Golden Elixir.

Liu Chengyin, alias the Taoist Master of Simple Clouds (Suyun daoren 素雲道人), was a prominent Taoist in the White Cloud Temple and a patron of several other groups. He made large donations for the reconstruction of temples in and around Beijing or for organizing great ceremonies of ordination. A drawing was engraved on wood and several stamps remain, but the plate itself disappeared according to Wang Yi'e 王宜娥, a specialist of Taoist arts in the White Cloud Temple. A new version on wood was engraved in 1984, it is currently the most common version.

This representation is the oldest known and was introduced into the West by Erwin Rousselle who had presented two copies in an article of 1933.[32] Thereafter, the White Cloud Temple illustration became the most widely disseminated; a colour scroll that was made based on the stele of White Cloud Temple, shows minor changes from this source version.[33] Another example of a similar colour scroll was that of the People's Republic of China at the Museum for the History of Traditional Chinese Medicine (see fig. 1.13). It was painted by

30 On this map, see Komjathy 2008 and 2009.

31 See Konayagi 1934: 158. He mentions a stele written by Xiyou 熙佑 titled "Suyun Liu Daoxing bei" 素雲劉道行碑. According to this text, Liu Suyun 劉素雲 (i.e., Liu Chengyin) repeatedly made collections for the reconstruction of the temple, the ordinations of Taoists and for printing texts. See Yin 2014: 297–301.

32 See Rousselle 1933; Schipper 1982:143; Despeux 1990: 192; Sakade 1991: 45–85; Needham 1983: 115.

33 Rousselle 1933: 209.

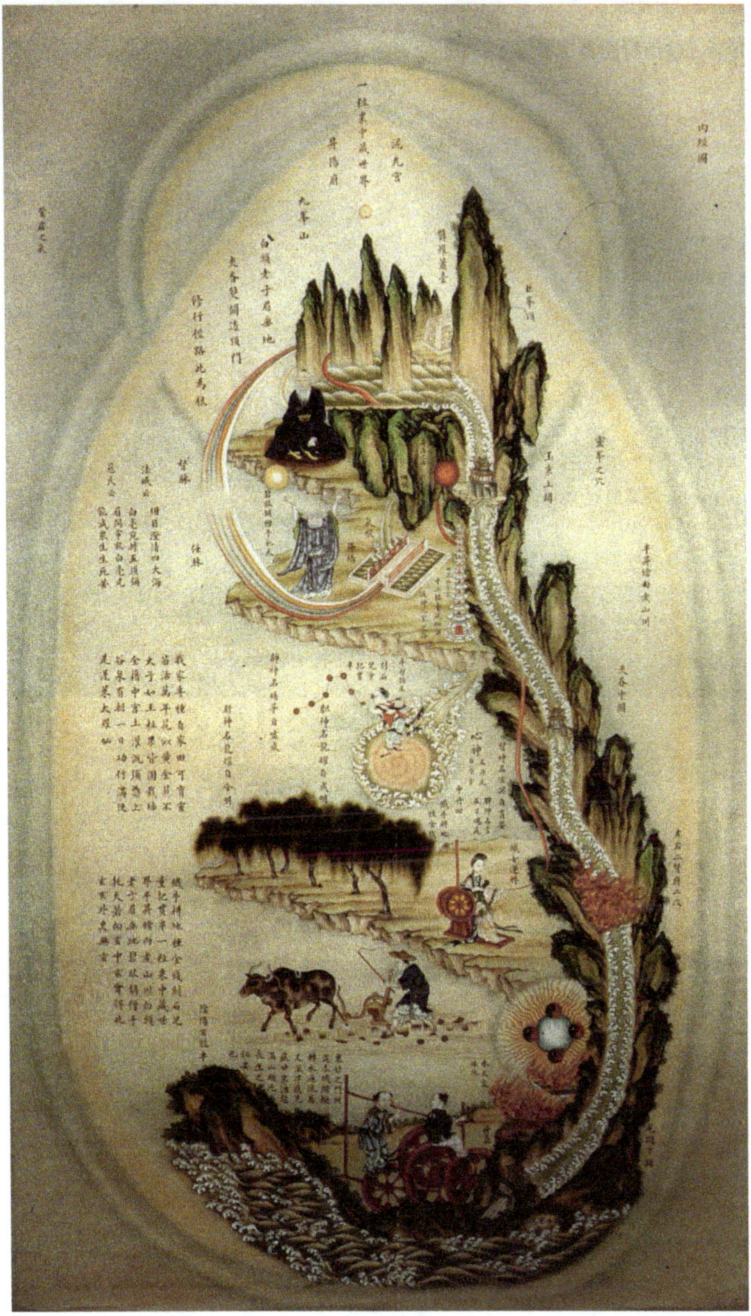

FIGURE 1.13 Representation of the Inner Vision of the Body (*Neijing tu* 內經圖) in colour painted by the Painting Academy of Wishes Fulfilled (Ruyi guan 如意館). In *Zhongguo gudai yishi tulu* 中國古代醫史圖錄, 82

the Academy of Painting of Fulfilled Wishes (Ruyiguan 如意館) at the Imperial Palace, under the Qing dynasty.[34] The academy was founded in 1692 on the desire of the Emperor Kangxi originally to exhibit the technical and scientific findings of the West; then it became a place for exhibitions of paintings offered to the emperor. There resided the best painters, calligraphers and potters of the empire. This scroll has minor variations with the colour scroll published by Erwin Rousselle.

34 See Li et al 1992: 85.

CHAPTER 2

# Different Versions of the *Chart for the Cultivation of Perfection* (*Xiuzhen Tu*)

When I began to study the *Chart for the Cultivation of Perfection* in 1985, little was known about this Taoist representation of the alchemical body. Versions had just begun to resurface in China. By 1994, I had examined six different versions of this chart and featured them in my book *Taoïsme et corps humain: Le Xiuzhen tu*. I have since learned of the existence of other versions, including a booklet belonging to a private collector living in France. This booklet includes two colophons that reveal new information concerning the history and diffusion of this chart in the 19th and 20th centuries. Recently, five more copies of this chart were revealed and discussed by Zheng Hong 鄭洪, a professor at the Zhejiang University of Traditional Medicine.[1]

In total, there are twenty-five versions of the text known from ancient stele monuments, wooden plates, stampings, copies, or by their mention in colophons. All these maps have slightly different titles and not all are dated. There are variations between the different copies. Most of these are errors or copyist mistakes, e.g., variations of characters, additions or summaries concerning the texts. Many of these different copies also contain colophons that have similar and dissimilar views on the dating and circumstances surrounding the reproduction of this chart. Thanks to these colophons, we gain a better idea of the possible origins of this chart and the extent of its diffusion.

The earliest attested version dates from before 1781, the most recent from 1988. They come from places far apart, from Beijing and Tianjin in the north to Guangzhou (Guangdong), Mount Shuangji 雙髻山 (Fujian) and Nanning (Guangxi) in the south, Chengdu (Sichuan) in the west, Mount Wudang in central China (Hubei), and, in the East, Moli 莫厘 and Sheyang 射陽 (Jiangsu), Wenzhou, Taizhou 台州 and Hangzhou 杭州 (Zhejiang) (see fig. 2.12). This large number of regions suggests that this chart was widely circulated in the nineteenth and twentieth centuries.

With the development of Internet, this chart has become the subject of numerous discussions and comments on many sites and has been modernized.

---

1 Zheng 2017, 2.5863. This article is also available on a site specialized in the study of ancient texts and manuscripts, the Shanben guji 善本古籍; cf. https://item.btime.com/m_90ea92c694b833be5. Accessed on April 15, 2018.

 | DOI:10.1163/9789004383456_004

In many cases, the chart now appears in colour versions. Many *qigong* and martial arts practitioners know this chart and most Taoist temples possess and sell rubbings supplied by the National Taoist Association of China, which has its seat in the White Cloud Temple in Beijing. The popularity of the Chart is spreading internationally, given the development of Taoist associations in the United States and Europe and the importance of relations between them and the Taoist associations of various provinces of China.

## 1 The *Chart for the Cultivation of Perfection* (*Xiuzhen tu*) in Guangzhou (1812)

The *Chart for the Cultivation of Perfection* of Guangzhou was engraved in 1812 on a stele erected at the Palace of the Three Origins (Sanyuan gong 三元宮), a Taoist temple in Guangzhou. It is the first dated example that still exists. A photograph of an engraving of this stele was published in 1988 in a book on the history of *qigong*.[2] The Japanese scholar Sakade Yoshinobu reproduced a copy in an article from 1991 about another body map, the *Chart of the Inner Landscape* (*Neijing tu*).[3] The stele, though badly damaged and split in its central part, was still visible when I visited this temple in 1993 (see fig. 2.1). It was located in the left wing of the building, in the courtyard before the hall dedicated to the deities of heaven, earth and water, collectively known as the "Three Offices" (*sanguan* 三官) (see fig. 2.2).

The Palace of the Three Origins is one of the oldest Taoist temples in this area. According to an inscription on a stele erected to the left of the one representing the *Chart for the Cultivation of Perfection*, the temple would have been built around 319 and initially called the Yue Ridge Cloister (Yuegang yuan 越崗院), for Yue was the former name of this region. It was built by the prefect of Nanhai 南海, Bao Qin 鮑靚, whose daughter Baogu 鮑姑 (ca. 309–363) married the famous Taoist scholar Ge Hong 葛洪 (281–341?). Baogu was revered from an early date as a deity with healing powers. In subsequent centuries, she remained well known for her mastery of Chinese pharmacopoeia and moxibustion.[4] This temple was originally a local place of worship for devotees

2 Li 1988, 1. Zheng Hong notes that this version was previously published in Huang 1982, 6; 52–54; see Zheng 2017: 58.

3 Sakade 1991: 54.

4 According to her biography in *Lishi zhenxian tidao tongjian houji* 歷世真仙體道通鑑後記 [Continuation of the comprehensive mirror of transcendents who embodied the Tao through the ages] by Zhao Daoyi 趙道一 (Yuan dynasty), her father obtained middle-ranking rituals (*zhongbu fa* 中部法) and the seals of the Three Sovereigns and the Five Peaks

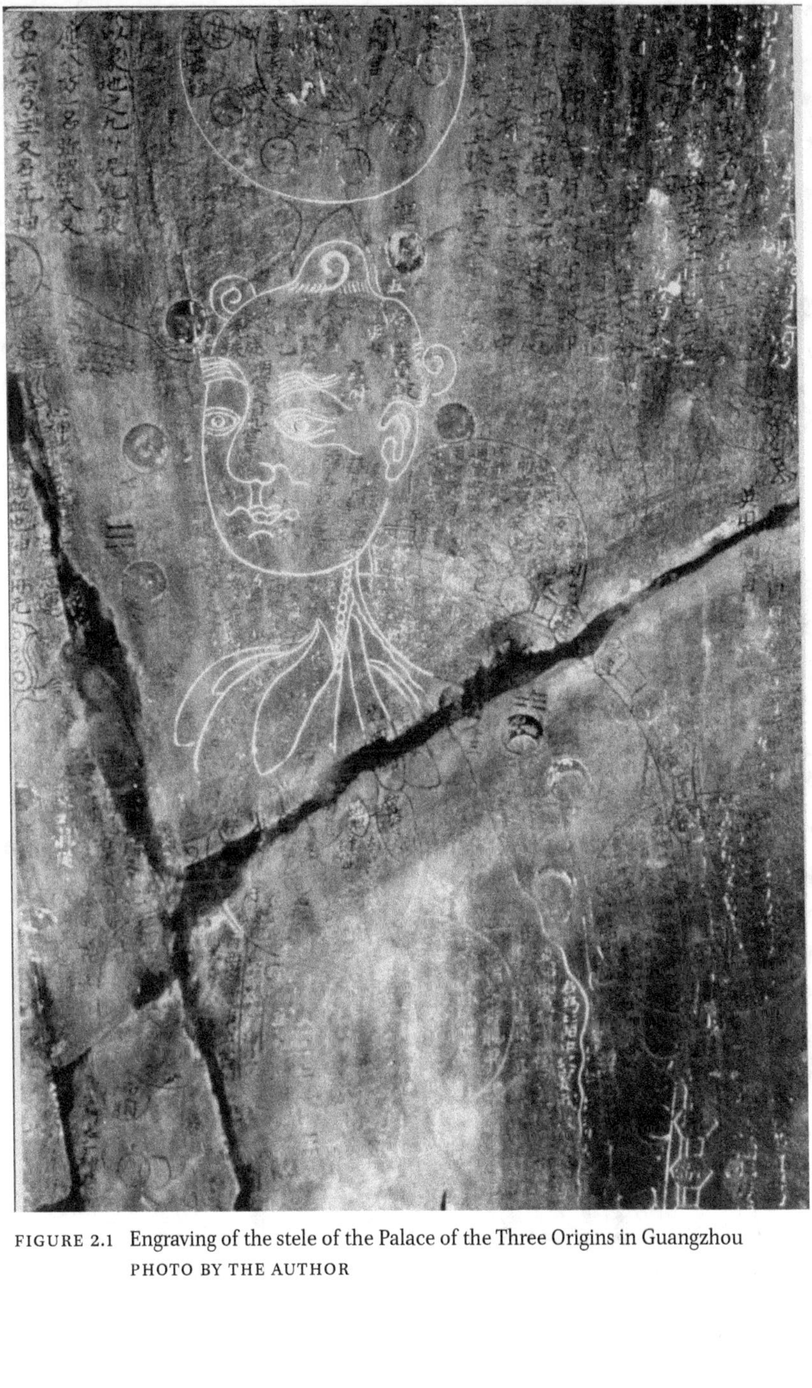

FIGURE 2.1 Engraving of the stele of the Palace of the Three Origins in Guangzhou
PHOTO BY THE AUTHOR

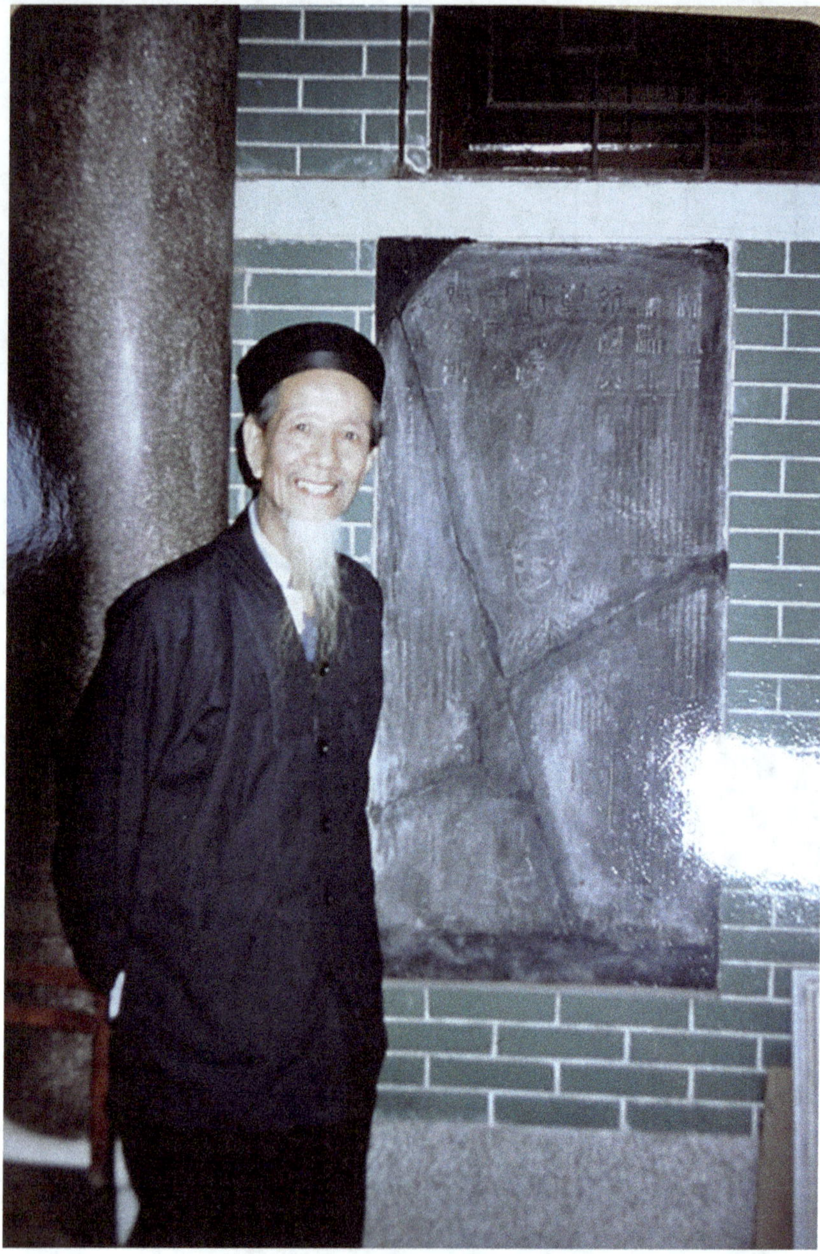

FIGURE 2.2 Stele at the Palace of the Three Origins with in the foreground Su Xinhua 蘇信華, then president of the Guangdong Taoist Association and the superior of the temple
PHOTO BY PAUL JEAN-ORTHIZ (1993)

of Baogu's healing powers. It grew over the centuries and often incorporated allegiance to other deities. In 1643, the temple's name was changed to the Palace of the Three Origins, because the main worship was that of the *sanyuan* 三元 [Three origins, or three offices]. At that time, Du Yangdong 杜陽東, originally from Shandong, became the head of the temple. He belonged to the twelfth generation of the Heart lineage (Xinzong 心宗), a branch of the Dragon Gate lineage (Longmen 龍門) which is usually traced back to Qiu Chuji 邱處機 (Changchun 長春) (1148–1227), one of the seven Perfected of the Complete Perfection school.[5]

The Dragon Gate lineage was established by Wang Changyue 王常月 (ob. 1680), a man who became national master in 1656 and received the precepts in Beijing's White Cloud Temple.[6] In some branches of the Dragon Gate tradition, we can perceive influences of Tantric Buddhism. It is the case for the Heart lineage, which began with Huang Shouzhong 黄守中 from Jizu Mountain (Jizu shan 鷄足山) in Yunnan, under the full name of "Heart Lineage of Western India" (Xizhu xinzong 西竺心宗).[7] Du Yangdong thus introduced it to the Palace of the Three Origins during the early Qing period. This temple in Guangzhou was destroyed and rebuilt many times.

From 1789 to 1837, the temple prospered thanks to the leadership of Taoist masters such as Yu Jiaoning 郁教寧, Li Yongshou 黎永受 and Yang Hejiong 楊賀炯. It is not clear, however, if these individuals were affiliated with the Heart Lineage of Western India like Du Yangdong or another branch of the Dragon Gate tradition. It is during this time that the *Chart for the Cultivation of Perfection* was engraved on the stele of 1812. It is also unknown whether or not one of the aforementioned masters ordered Qiu Fengshan 邱鳳山 to engrave this stele. An anonymous donator, or even Qiu Fengshan himself could have also funded the monument. Until now, the historical information we have does not allow us to say to which current the author of this chart belonged.

from Zuo Yuanfang 左元方 (Zuo Ci 左慈). As such, she had both demons and deities at her service. In 318, her father met Yin Changsheng 陰長生 at Mount Jiang 蔣山; here he received transmission of the ritual to deliver his body by the sword. According to this story, Baogu died after marrying Ge Hong even though she had never been ill. She was buried in the Luofu Mountains 羅浮山 in Guangdong. See DZ 298, 4.8b–10a.

5 On this school and the controverse on its origin, see Esposito 2004: 621–698.

6 Koyanagi 1934: 38.

7 On this current, see Esposito 1993; PDF of the two volumes: http://universitymedia.org/Esposito_PhD.html.

This Cantonese version includes in its upper part a long inscription on the practice of Inner Alchemy. It is written in seal script and arranged in eight columns of three characters each:

| | |
|---|---|
| Forlorn and lost, I must cross the ford at night, | 悲迷夜渡津 |
| Abandoning frivolities, I embody Heavenly Perfection. | 剖紋質天真 |
| As if it were hidden deeper and deeper in darkness, | 似昧層中層 |
| With peace, I perceive a body outside my body. | 寧識身外身 |

The eighth and last column of this text, placed high on the left, has only one character, under which we can see two seals respectively bearing the following inscriptions: "A Man of the Tao who Travels by Boat" (*Xingzhou daoren* 行舟道人) and "Engraved by Qiu Fengshan" (Qiu Fengshan ke 邱鳳山刻). From the front matter of the text, we know that "A Man of the Tao who Travels by Boat" is a nickname of Qiu Fengshan. Qiu's name appears in the upper left corner of the stele: "Stele engraved by Qiu Fengshan, the 'Man Traveling by Boat,' in the *renshen* year of the *jiaqing* reign (1812) and stored at the Palace of the Three Origins in Mount Aoxiu of Jinyang city."[8]

## 2 The Booklet Manuscript of the *Chart for the Cultivation of Perfection* (*Xiuzhen tu*) in a Private Collection (19th Century)

There is a booklet owned by a private collector who has requested anonymity. He contacted me after seeing my previous 1994 study in a bookstore. After reading this study, he understood the identity of the manuscript in his possession, and contacted me to discuss the document further. He explained that he came in possession of the texts when he inherited from his grandfather. At this time, the text was in very poor condition. His grandfather, born in 1861, traveled for business in Asia extensively, especially in Indonesia, Malaysia, China and Japan. He might have bought this document while traveling in Asia. The exact origins of the text are unknown but given the navigator's birthdate, it is unlikely he obtained this manuscript before the 1880s. Even so, the yellow paper of this manuscript has fine grain and is high-quality, which suggests that it old at the time of acquisition.

Although the manuscript has no title, the content corresponds to the *Chart for the Cultivation of Perfection* (*Xiuzhen tu*). This version is special because unlike other versions of the chart (e.g., the stele of Guangzhou) that are carved

8 Mount Aoxiu 奥秀山 or Mount Yuexiu 越秀山 is a hill in the north of Guangzhou.

on one block, this one is spread over ten sheets, including two colophons that provide us with valuable information on the circulation and distribution of this chart.

The current owner has restored the document and has mounted the booklet-shaped leaflets for conservation. The ten sheets of this manuscript are handwritten on a light-yellow paper, the grain of which is rather thin, and which is a manufacturing of average quality. The leaves, measuring 35.5 cm × 24 cm, were pasted during the restoration on a booklet measuring 46.5cm × 33.5cm. The binding is crafted according to traditional Chinese bibliographic conventions, which means it must be read from right to left. They are mounted between two wooden covers covered with an embroidered cloth. Two sheets are torn; for one (sheet 1), it lacks all the upper third part of the inscription and the drawing; for the other (sheet 4), only the upper right corner is missing. Several other sheets contain some minor tears in the paper eaten by worms in places, but it does not deface the drawings and removes only a few characters.

The major difference between this manuscript and the aforementioned version from Guangzhou is that it is split into several sheets. Whereas the other known versions of the charts were mostly produced by taking rubbings from an engraved stele or a wooden plate, the author of this booklet has handwritten and painted directly on these sheets the elements of the chart, probably for private use and not for multiple distributions. We do not know anything else concerning the original document the author copied to make this booklet. The same colophon, however, appears in a copy from Tianjin discovered by Zheng Hong, and it is possible that the owner of the booklet acquired it in Tianjin. At the very least, there is a link between this booklet and the Tianjin plate.[9]

The pages of this manuscript have not been assembled in a logical order. It is possible that the original order of the sections of the chart has been lost, and the later restorer did not know the content of the sheets. It is also possible that the document originally was a single folded sheet, split in two vertical and five horizontal lines, giving two current sheets in width and five pairs height. As every sheet measures 35.5cm × 24cm, the entire sheet measures around 50cm wide × 178cm high.

Following this hypothesis, I reconstructed the order of the ten sheets by comparing with the *Chart*. There are five pairs which are as follows: the two layers of the pages (1 and 4) of the current booklet, the first one for the general chart of the body and ripped in its upper right, the second one with three

9 See the description of this Tianjin version in Zheng 2017: 60.

circles along the spine and torn in the third higher should be the highest part of this great height leaf, because on one hand the form of tears suggests they occurred on one of the edges of the large sheet (upper or lower). Since they are on the upper edge of the two sheets, this suggests that they were originally a pair sharing the upper edge of the large sheet.

Next, I aligned these eight sheets to test the probability that they fit together like a puzzle. First, there are six sheets bearing the six animal forms of the image of the six viscera deities of the body with the accompanying text (liver, heart, spleen, lungs, kidneys, gallbladder). These animals and the texts appear on the different versions of the *Chart for the Cultivation of Perfection*, in the following order: [1] at the head, upper right, the azure dragon corresponding to liver; [2] at the upper left, the vermilion sparrow corresponding to the heart with a colophon inscribed before the drawing; [3] in the middle left, the tiger corresponding to the lungs; [4] on the middle right the turtle and snake matching gallbladder; on the lower part, [5] the kidneys and [6] the spleen, right two heads deer corresponding to the kidneys and left the phoenix corresponding to the spleen. It was assumed that the sheets of the current booklet must be arranged in the order of the versions of the *Chart for the Cultivation of Perfection* and that the six pages bearing six animals should therefore be originally presented in the same order. At the upper level, one should have the dragon (liver) to the right, the vermilion sparrow (heart) to the left; a few tears still visible on the left side of the dragon sheet and right vermilion sparrow leaflet match.

In the middle level, the turtle and the snake (gallbladder) are on the right, the tiger (lungs) to the left; in the lower level, deer (kidney) to the right, and the phoenix (spleen) to the left. In fact, a few tears still visible on the left side of the deer slip and the right edge of the phoenix sheet match. These clues enable us to locate six of the eight sheets of this map.

There are two sheets of this map that are more difficult to place. The first is a detail of the center of the abdomen with texts, which are located within the central part on the *Chart*; the second is a general description of body that usually is located in the spaces around the representation of the body. The most logical way to place these two sheets would be to follow the reading order of the body map from top to bottom. This would mean that these two sheets would be placed among the turtle/snake and tiger. This arrangement would bring the sheet bearing the phoenix and a colophon on the left lower part of the body map where colophons are usually written. This would be the last feature of a chart as this text would be read via the traditional convention of reading right-left, top-bottom. As such, the lower left corner would be at the end of a document.

Here is a recapitulation of the rebuilt order of the different sheets

1. On the right-upper portion, the representation of the spine and three passes and to the left-upper part, the general outline of the body.
2. On the second row, the blue dragon on the right, and the vermilion sparrow on the left.
3. On the third row, the turtle and the snake on the right, and the tiger on the left.
4. On the fourth row, the center of the body on the right and the general text describing the body on the left slip.
5. On the fifth row, the deer on the right, and the phoenix on the left. This is followed at the end by a colophon.

Of course, as it is a copy, it is possible that the original form was a booklet. Even if we cannot verify that this was originally a single sheet, we can at the very least restore the correct pairing for the leaves.

## 3 Diffusion of the *Chart for the Cultivation of Perfection* according to the Colophons of the Booklet and of Two Copies found by Zheng Hong

Two colophons on the booklet provide us with valuable information concerning the history of different prints and on the diffusion of the body map. Zheng Hong studied two copies, titled "Reprint of Yang Laiji (1798)" and "Version of the Palace of the Three Pures of Tianjin (1882)." Both bear the same two colophons (one in the middle of the chart and one on the left lower part of the chart) as the booklet with minor variations. The dates, however, are missing in the colophons from the booklet, and Zheng does not indicate where he saw these copies or where they are kept.

The first colophon on the booklet is handwritten on the sheet containing the drawing of the Vermilion Sparrow (sheet 4, fig. 2.4) and a second on the sheet with the drawing of the phoenix, on the lower left (sheet 10). The following colophon was written under the drawing of the Vermilion Sparrow, the heart deity:

> This was originally engraved at the Altar of Joy in the Dao at Sheyang (Jiangsu). A disciple of the Taoist tradition of the cultivation for perfection, Xuan Huahai of the Resonating with the Tao Temple in Wenzhou, carved it for a second time.
>
> A subsequent engraving was made at the Two Transcendents Abbey at Black Sheep Palace in Chengdu (Sichuan).

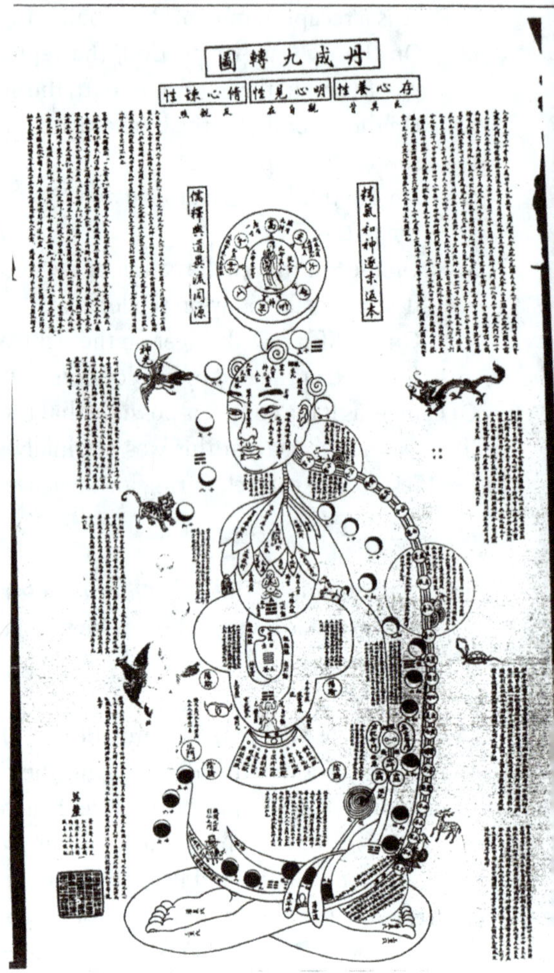


FIGURE 2.3
*Chart for Achieving Cinnabar by the Ninefold Revolution* and a reconstruction of the sheets in the booklet

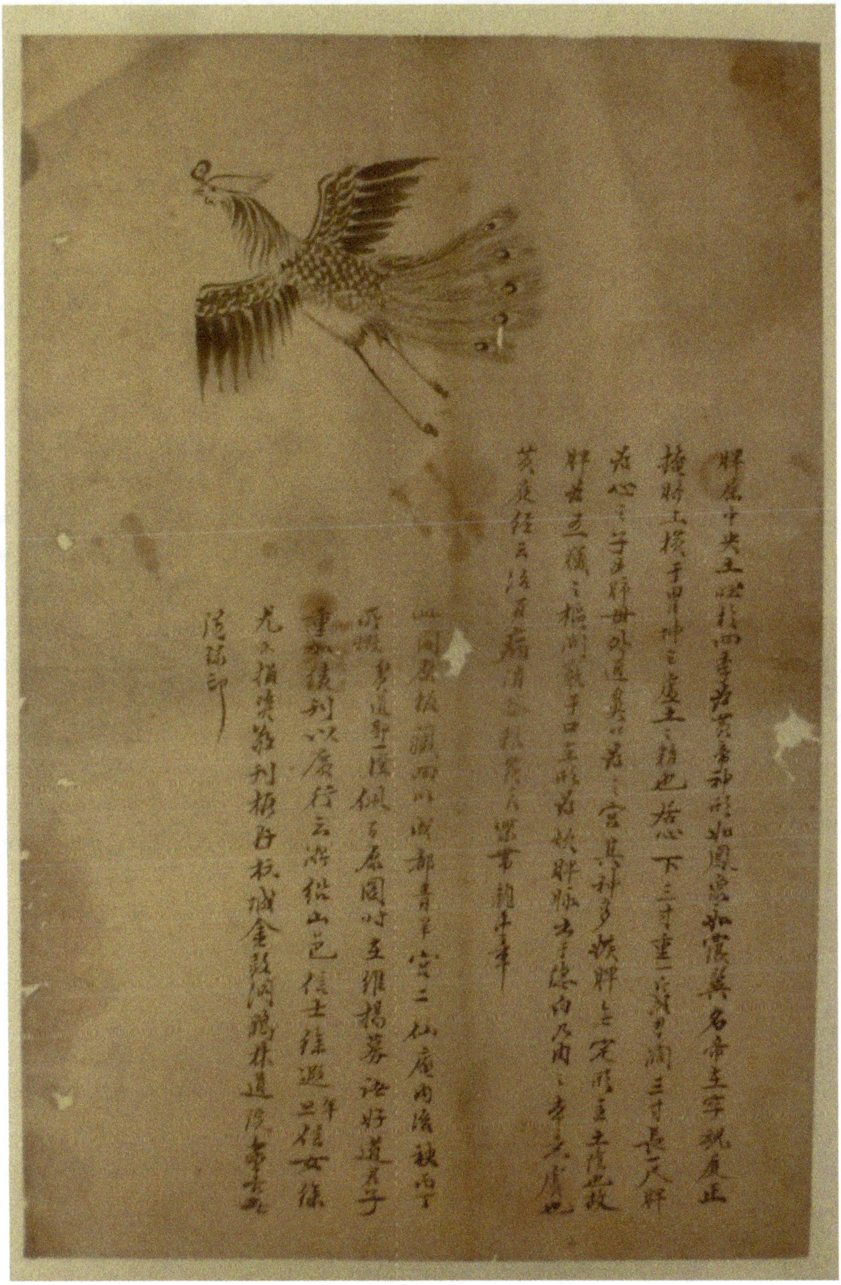

FIGURE 2.4 The page of the booklet bearing a colophon and the representation of the Phoenix, which is the image of the spleen deity

> Yang Laiji of Juyang, abbot at the Grotto of the Vacuous Light in the Weiyu Mountains of Huangyan District (Taizhou, Zhejiang) has once again made a new engraving.
>
> 射陽樂道堂原刻。溫州府應道觀修真之子宣華海重 [刻]。四川成都青羊宮二仙庵復刻。浙江台州黃巖縣委羽山空明洞聚陽楊來基又刻。

According to this colophon, the original version would have been made in Sheyang, a coastal city in Jiangsu Province, not far from Yangzhou (formerly called Weiyang) at the otherwise unknown Altar of Joy in the Dao. The text following the first sentence on the Sheyang engraving poses problems of interpretation. It can be best understood if one considers that the copyist omitted the character "engrave" (*ke* 刻) from the first column. This allows for four times the character "engrave," corresponding to four different locations: a first one in Sheyang (Jiangsu), a second in Wenzhou (Zhejiang), a third in Chengdu (Sichuan) and a fourth in Taizhou (Zhejiang). From Jiangsu and Zhejiang, the chart would have migrated to the west to the Black Sheep Palace in Chengdu which appears from the colophon of Guo Yicheng on the version of the White Cloud Temple to be the main place from where the chart has spread in Beijing.[10]

The author of the second engraved plate, Xuan Huahai of Wenzhou, lived as early as the late eighteenth century. The Wenzhou temple to which he was attached, the Resonating with the Tao Temple, bears this name only from the *jiaqing* reign (1796–1820) and Xuan Huahai became then the abbot of the temple.[11] It was initially built during the *kangxi* reign (1661–1722) as a small structure under the name of temple for Pacifying ancestors (Anzu miao 安祖廟), but was renamed after it was expanded at the turn of the nineteenth century. It belonged, like two other temples of the city, to the Purple Yang lineage (*Ziyang pai* 紫陽派) whose patriarch is Zhang Boduan of the southern lineage of Inner Alchemy, which became an undercurrent of Quanzhen Taoism; most other temples in the area were either under the power of the Dragon Gate lineage or the Orthodox Unity tradition.[12]

According to this colophon, the fourth engraving was done by Yang Laiji. Yang Laiji (fl. late 18th century or early 19th century), a renowned Taoist of Taizhou (Zhejiang), was a Taoist at the Grotto of Vacuous Light of the Weiyu Mountains 委羽山 which since the Jin Dynasty, was a famous Taoist place and was among

10 See above, p. 45.
11 See Zhang Baolin's 张宝琳 *Yongjia xianzhi* 永嘉縣志 in Dai 2010: 1677.
12 See Liu 2013.

the ten largest grotto-heavens, that is to say the top ten sacred sites of Taoism. According to Du Guangting (850–933), the Weiyu Mountains were the second of the ten grotto-heavens.[13] Yang Laiji was from a poor family of farmers in the eastern village of Henglin 横林 in Huangyan 黃巖 District. When his father and mother died, he became a novice at Palace of Great Existence (*Dayou gong* 大有宮) in the Weiyu Mountains near his hometown. He practiced what is called "walking in the clouds" (*yunyou* 雲遊), i.e., he visited major sacred mountain sites of Taoism in search of teachers and teachings. When he arrived in his city, he lived at the Palace of Perching in Auroras (Qixia gong 棲霞宮) and met the abbot Xu Yangming 徐陽明. After becoming Xu's disciple, Yang learned about the *Book of the Way and its Virtue*, the *Zhuangzi* and the *Stanzas on Awakening to Perfection*. He became master of the thirteenth generation of the Dragon Gate lineage according to the following transmission:

> Wang Changyue 王常月 (ob. 1680)—Tan Shoucheng 譚守誠 (ob. 1691)—Yan Tailin 詹太林 (1625–1712)—Sheng Qingxin 盛清新—Lu Binyang 陸賓陽 (Yichun 一纯)—Xu Yangming 徐陽明—Yang Laiji 楊來基.[14]

The transmission of the Dragon Gate on the Weiyu Mountains between 1314 and 1320, especially at Palace of Great Existence, spread quickly throughout the region under Yang Laiji, a master of the thirteenth generation. Yang cultivated the Way in Weiyu Mountains, and became the abbot of the Grotto of the Vacuous Light, the name of a very deep cave behind Palace of Great Existence. His followers became more and more numerous, and on the full moon of the first lunar month of 1796, Yang organized a great initiation rite and transmitted its methods to twelve or fourteen disciples who opened fourteen branches of the Dragon Gate School in the area.[15] In 1814, he expanded the great hall of the Palace of Great Existence. He went on to become one of the main teachers in the Weiyu Mountains, playing a key role in the propagation of Taoism throughout Zhejiang province. The fact that he wanted again to engrave this map shows the importance attached to this representation.

---

13 *Dongtian fudi yuedu mingshan ji* 洞天福地嶽瀆名山記 [Record of the cavern-heavens, auspicious sites, holy mountains, and marshes, and famous mountains] (DZ 599), 4b.

14 Lineage given in the *Zuanxiu Longmen fapai puxu* 簒修龍門法派譜序 (1909). See also Yin 2014: 244–247.

15 Cf. *Zuanxiu Longmen fapai pu* 簒修龍門法派譜; see also Yin 2014: 245.

This first colophon of the booklet thus gives the following four engravings:

1. The Altar of Joy in the Dao engraving at Sheyang near of Weiyang (Jiangsu)
2. The Resonating with the Taoist Temple engraving by Xuan Huahai in Wenzhou (Zhejiang)
3. The Two Transcendents Abbey at Black Sheep Palace engraving in Chengdu (Sichuan)
4. The Vacuous Light in the Weiyu Mountains of Huangyan District (Taizhou) engraving by Yang Laiji (Zhejiang)

Two copies presented by Zheng Hong, "Reprint of Yang Laiji (1798)" and "Version of the Palace of the Three Pures of Tianjin (1882)," have a similar colophon, but half-unreadable on Yang Laiji 1798 reprint, according to Zheng Hong. Here is the text he mentions of the colophon of the Tianjin version of 1882:

> Respectfully engraved at the Altar of Joy in the Dao at Sheyang (Jiangsu).
>
> An engraving kept in the Two Transcendents Abbey at Black Sheep Palace in Chengdu (Sichuan) circulated respectfully. Later on, it was destroyed in a fire and nothing subsisted. Yang Laiji of Juyang, abbot at the Grotto of the Vacuous Light in the Weiyu Mountains of Huangyan district (Taizhou, Zhejiang) has once again made a new engraving.
>
> 射陽樂道堂敬刊。四川成都府青羊宮二仙庵藏板敬行，為後遭丙丁，焚毀無存，浙江台州府黃岩縣委羽山空明洞聚楊來基重刊

This version of the colophon presents variants suggesting that there was a different order of diffusion of the chart. It indicates not the engraving of the Altar of Joy in the Dao as the original and the first one but the version of Chengdu. We note also that this colophon don't mention the engraving by Xuan Huahai in Wenzhou which is mentioned on the second colophon of this plate.

The diffusion of this chart becomes even more complex when one takes account of the second colophon (sheet 10 of the booklet) added after the drawing of the phoenix and the text on the spleen and which is similar on the two versions mentioned by Zheng Hong. On the booklet, we can read:

> The original plate was kept in the Hermitage of the Two Transcendents of the Black Sheep Palace in Chengdu. Later on, it was destroyed in a fire. I, Guo Yicheng, humble follower of Dao, carefully kept a copy of the original. While I was in Weiyang (Yangzhou), I asked all those who love the Way to make their contribution and allow it to be well again published

> and widely disseminated. Two followers of the Shaoshan District[16] in Zhejiang, named Xu Xia and his wife born You, at the beginning of the year,[17] raised funds to respectfully reprint it. The plate is kept in the Crane Grove Daoist Institute of the Metal Drum Grotto near the city of Hangcheng (Hangzhou), so that good people can print it, based on circumstances.[18]
>
> 此圖原板藏四川成都青羊宮二仙庵內。後被丙丁所燬。貧道郭一澄佩有存原圖，時在維揚募諸好道君子重加續(續?)刊，以廣行云。浙紹山邑信士徐遐年旦信女徐尤氏損資敬刊。板存杭城金鼓洞鶴林道院樂善者隨錄印

The version of this colophon on the "Copy of Yang Laiji of 1798" is very similar, but it indicates the dates for the engravings of the plate by Guo Yicheng and Xuan Huahai:

> The original plate was kept in the Hermitage of the Two Transcendents of the Black Sheep Palace in Chengdu (Sichuan). Later on, it was destroyed in a fire and dont exist more. I was able to bring a copy of this chart while I was in Weiyang and thanks to various adepts of the Dao, could have it reprinted so that it spread widely.
>
> Respectfully and sincerely written by Guo Yicheng five days after the full moon, one Zhongchun day of the Xinchou year of Qianlong (1781).
>
> Xuan Huahai, master of the cultivation of perfection of the Resonating with the Tao Temple of Wen Prefecture again carefully arranged and published it in the first year of the Jiaqing era (1796).
>
> 此圖原版藏四川成都府青羊宮二仙庵庵後遭丙丁焚毀無存　貧道　躬帶有原圖時在維揚募諸。。道君子重加續刊以廣行看
> 　乾隆辛丑仲春望後五日郭一澄沐手敬書
> 　嘉慶元年閩郡應道觀修真子宣華海志沐重刊

Given that this plate was reengraved in Weiyang, Jiangsu by Guo Yicheng in 1781, the one that disappeared in the fire of the hermitage of must have been an

16 Shaoshan is near of the Wencheng district in Wenzhou (Zhejiang).

17 The meaning of *niandan* is obscure. It could be for accumulating merits at the anniversary of the death of Xu Xia.

18 See the 1807 *Jingudong zhi* 金鼓洞志 [Monograph on the grotto of the metal drum] in *Zangwai daoshu* 藏外道書 (20. 238), which includes a drawing of the Helin Temple.

earlier version. This hermitage was founded in 1695 by Sichuan Commissioner Zhao Liangbi 趙良璧 asked Chen Qingjue 陳清覺 to become the senior abbot of the hermitage, which he did until his death in 1705. As we do not know the date of the fire of this hermitage, we can only surmise that the Hermitage of the Two Transcendents' plate was engraved between 1695 and 1780. This would be the oldest known copy according to the dates of the different versions available to us. We know also from this colophon that the new engraving was undertaken by Xuan Huahai of Wenzhou in 1796.

Despite all these clues, much about the early diffusion of the chart is unclear. Did it come first from the Black Sheep Palace in Chengdu as is testified by the most part of the colophons or of the Altar of the Joy in the Dao (Jiangsu) as is suggested by one of the two colophons on the booklet? How was Yang Laiji provided with the model of the chart? We know he was "wandering in the clouds," so it is also possible that his steps had brought him to have access to the undated plate of Sheyang, the one of Weiyang (1781) or the plate in Wenzhou (1796).

According to the colophon of the booklet, two followers who were not in Weiyang but in Zhejiang, would have funded a new engraving, whose plate was kept in the Taoist Crane Grove Daoist Institute (Helin daoyuan) of the Grotto of the Metal Drum (Jingu dong),[19] near of Hangzhou. Unfortunately, there is no additional information concerning the link between these followers and the great temple of Hangzhou. In any case, it is the only known colophon indicating the presence of an engraved plate in Hangzhou.

The three copies (the booklet, the copy of 1798 and the copy of 1882) indicate that the chart had been circulated in the following locations:

1. Black Sheep Palace 青羊宮 in Chengdu, Sichuan (before 1781) (lost)
2. Weiyang 維揚 plate engraved by Guo Yicheng 郭一誠 in 1781 (lost)
3. Ledao Hall 樂道堂 in Sheyang 射陽, Jiangsu (undated plate, before 1798) (lost)
4. Resonating with the Tao Temple 應道觀 in Wenzhou (Zhejiang) engraved by Xuan Huahai 宣華海 in 1796 (lost)
5. Vacuous Luminousity Grotto 空明洞 near Taizhou, Zhejiang by Yang Laiji 楊來基 in 1798 (lost)
6. Crane Grove Daoist Institute 鶴林道觀 in Hangzhou, Zhejiang (undated plate) (lost)

19 On this place, which was an important centre of the Jiangnan area during the 19th century, see Yin 2014: 247–248.

## 4 The Engraving at the White Cloud Temple by Meng Zhicai in 1873

In our search for information on Guo Yicheng, we found a colophon listed at the end of a martial arts manuscript, which mentions that the plate engraved at the White Cloud Temple in Beijing was done by Meng Zhicai in the twelfth year of the *tongzhi* era (1873).[20]

The colophon we finded is on the website written by Yang Yanming 楊彥明, a follower of a martial art called "plum flower boxing" (Meihua quan 梅花拳). Yang writes that he uncovered several texts in Houmazhuang Pingxiang 後馬庄平鄉 (Hebei), such as the "Preface to Military Art" ("Xiwu xu" 習武序) written by Yang Bing 楊炳 in 1742. This would have been an interview in 1707 at the time the Emperor Kangxi was searching talented people. One of these manuscripts, found in the family of Mr. Zhang Qiuchang 張秋常, is dated the twelfth year of *tongzhi* reign (1873). However, at the end of this manuscript is the following inscription:

> The original board of this chart was preserved at the Two Transcendents Hermitage of Qinghua Temple[21] from Chengdu in Sichuan; but this temple was destroyed by fire, it was only in the year *yiwei* of *daoguang* reign (1835) that, while I, Cai 才 (Meng Zhicai 孟至才), would receive the precepts in the White Cloud Temple, I obtained this chart from the friend of the Way Zhao of Mount Shuangji (Fujian). His predecessors Guo Yicheng of Weiyang, Xuan Huahai of Wenzhou, Lin Yongmao of Min (Fujian), Wang Lizhong[22] and Du Fengchen of Yan (Beijing), had engraved this chart for distribution. (see fig. 2.5)

> 此圖源版藏四川成都青花宮二仙庵內遭丙丁焚毀無存，才於道光乙未秋來戒白雲觀得此圖，於雙髻趙道友。其先維揚郭一澄溫部宣華海以及閩省林永懋並燕人王理中杜逢辰公俱刻此圖行也。

20 This is also what is mentioned in a colophon of the copy of Tianjin (1882) and the colophons of two copies studied by Zheng Hong, who considers that the year should be 1872 not 1873. He says there is an engraved copy (*keben* 刻本) and a handwritten manuscript (*chaohui ben* 抄繪本), but he does not indicate where he found these texts.

21 The manuscript's Black Blossom Palace (Qinghua gong 青華宮) is read as an error for Black Sheep Palace (Qingyang gong).

22 According to the colophon of the Tianjin version, the name is Wang Lishen 王理申.

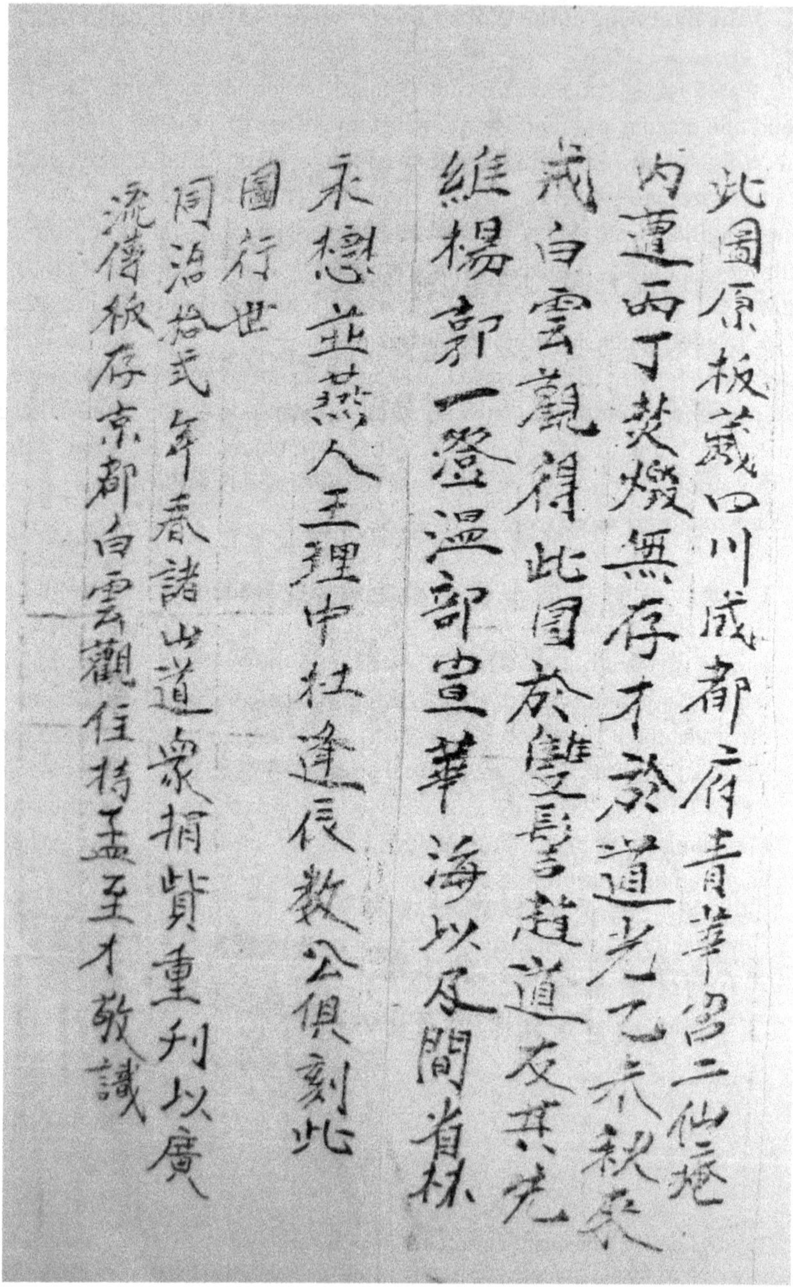
此圖原板藏四川成都府青華宮二仙菴
内遭丙丁焚燬無存才於道光乙未秋冬
我白雲觀得此圖於雙鳳趙道友其先
維揚郭一澄温部宣華海以及閩省林
永懋並燕人王理中杜逢辰数公俱刻此
圖行世
同治拾弍年春諸山道衆捐貲重刊以廣
流傳板存京都白雲觀住持孟至才敬識

FIGURE 2.5 Sheet of the manuscript of the "Xiwu xu" 習武序 found in Houmazhuang 後馬庄

This colophon was followed by another inscription:

> In the spring of the twelfth year of the *tongzhi* reign (1873), the crowd of those who aspire to the Way has raised money for republish it, so that it will spread widely. The board is kept in the White Cloud Temple in Beijing. Noted by the head of the temple (*zhuchi* 主持) Meng Zhicai.[23]
>
> 同志拾貳年春，志山道眾捐資重刊，以廣流傳。版存京都白雲觀。主持孟至才敬識

Meng Zhicai 孟至才 or Meng Yongcai 孟永才 (1813–1881), originally from the prefecture of Zunhua 遵化州 in Zhili 直隸 (Hebei), received his precepts at the White Cloud Temple in 1835. He was responsible for repairing the Taoist Canon held at the White Cloud Temple during his tenure at the capital. During his tenure as abbot, he presided over three consecrations, in 1872, 1873 and 1881.[24]

According to Yang Yanming, this colophon is related to the manuscript of the "Xiwu xu." For us, the connection with the registration of this book makes us think that the chart (*tu* 圖) in question is a version of the *Chart for the Cultivation of Perfection*, which was included in the booklet of the "Xiwu xu" and disappeared from the latter that would be incomplete. The use of the term *tu* 圖 [Chart], instead of *shu* 書 [Book], and the mention of a *ban* 版 [Engraved plate], are two elements that reinforce our belief that it is linked with the body map rather with the book "Xiwu xu." This is confirmed by the existence of both versions studied by Zheng Hong.[25] To the versions already known, this colophon adds four that were made respectively by a certain Taoist Zhao of Mount Shuangji, by Lin Yongmao of Fujian, Wang Lizhong and Du Fengchen from Beijing, which were earlier than that of Meng Zhicai from 1873.

## 5 Copies of the Plate of Tianjin (1882, 1910, 1920)

Tianjin was also an important place for the diffusion of this map. Zheng Hong has seen a copy from a version seen at Guandi Temple in Haixia District,

23 Text found on the blog by Jianyi Furong 劍倚芙蓉, site http://blog.sina.com.cn/s/blog_4abe4f1001000621.html, accessed on March 23, 2014. See also Yang 2004.

24 On Meng Yongcai, see Goossaert 2007: 145, 155, 172.

25 Zheng Hong mentions a plate and a copy bearing similar colophons (Zheng Hong, 2017: 55–56).

Tianjin. The author of the colophon in this copy mentions a plate engraved by Chen Pujing, abbot of a temple:[26]

> The original plate was kept in the Hermitage of the Two Transcendents of the Black Sheep Palace in Chengdu. The plate preserved in the White Cloud Temple of Beijing dating from the 12th year of the *tongzhi* era (1873) was made after. In the *wuyin* year of the *guangxu* era (1878), I was able to see this chart at the Guandi Temple outside the southern gate of the new Haixia City of Tianjin District in Tianjin Prefecture of Zhili. But every time I could not get to see this chart. Fan Daren offered three ounces of silver, as well as the respectable Master Song. Plate printed respectfully by the superior of the temple whose name of Dao is Chen Pujing.
>
> 此图原板藏四川成都府青羊宫二仙庵内，于同治十二年京都白云观见此藏板，后造。光绪戊寅年直隶天津府天津县海下新城南门外关帝庙见此图，每求不得顾此藏板也。范大人施银三两，宋师爷施银三两，住持道号陈普敬刊板

Another copy, kept in the Museum of Traditional Medicine in Canton, contains two colophons indicating impressions or copies made from the plate of Tianjin mentioned above.[27] The first colophon reads:

> This map was originally in the Black Sheep Palace in Chengdu (Sichuan); afterwards it was destroyed in a fire. The friend of Dao Guo Yicheng received it at the Two Transcendents Hermitage and brought it to Weiyang to make stampings and offer them. In 1873, I saw this plate preserved in the Beijing's White Cloud Temple. In the *renwu* year of the *guangxu* era (1882), I saw this chart in the hall of the Assembly of the Humanists of the Three Pures Palace of the New City of Haixia in Tianjin District and made a painted copy to preserve it.

---

26 Zheng Hong considers that the new engraving was made four years after that of 1878, in 1882, according to the colophon of the copy kept in Guangzhou. But this colohon mentions a "copy" (*hui cangben* 繪藏本) and not an engraving and the name of the temple is different.

27 On this copy see the research work by Lin Qinzhen 林沁臻, « Guangzhou zhongyiyao daxue yishi bowuguan cang daojia liangong tu yanjiu » (Research on the Chart for the raffining work in taoism, kept in the History museum of the Chinese traditional Medicine University in Guangzhou) 廣州中醫藥大學醫史博物館藏道家煉功圖研究, published by the Guangzhou Chinese Traditional Medicine University in Guangzhou in 2005.

> 此圖刊自四川成都府青羊宮，後毀于火。郭一澄道友得自二仙庵，携至维扬，仿刻印送。　同治十二年京都白雲觀見此藏版，光绪壬午年天津縣海下新城三清宮集仁堂見此圖繪藏

In the lower left corner of this copy, there are still three inscriptions:

> Dai Wenyuan and Cui Shurong of Yangliuqing township of Tianjin, the 2nd year of the Xuantong era (1910), made five hundred lithographs.[28]
>
> The summer of the year *gengshen* (1920), I obtained this map at the Beijing's White Cloud temple, many characters were damaged. I engraved another plate so that it can be kept long and can have a wide diffusion. Jointly reviewed by the Tianyin Woodcutters Community and the Kunlun Immortals Community in their building at Tianjin.
>
> The plate is kept in the engraving department of Yongcheng Studio of Yangmeizhu byway.

> 宣统二年天津楊柳青鎮戴文淵、崔樹榮石印五百張
>
> 庚申季夏得此圖於京都白雲觀，字多殘毀，爰另鐫镌一整版，以冀持久而廣流傳。天印山樵、崑崙仙館合校于津門寓次。
>
> 板存前門外楊梅竹斜街永盛齋刻字部。

The Yongcheng studio of Yangmeizhu byway is a shop renowned for its engravings and printings in a street near of Liulichang. It is mentioned in a copy of the *Chart for the Cultivation of Perfection* exhibited in a gallery at Beijing's White Cloud Temple that I examined in 1993. It has a text inscribed in the lower left corner detailing its source, which mentions, as the forehead colophon, the conservation of a plate in Yongcheng studio:

> This representation was given by a friend of the Way, Guo Yicheng, at the Hermitage of the Two Transcendents (Erxian'an 二仙庵) of the Black Sheep Palace 青羊宮 in Chengdu (Sichuan). He brought it to Weiyang (Yangzhou), so that I could contemplate it. I had it engraved on a plate, so that it could be widely disseminated. This plate is kept in the engraving shop at Yongsheng Studio on Yangmeizhu byway near Qianmen (Beijing)."

It is likely that the revision of the damaged White Cloud Temple plate was done using stampings made from the Tianjin plate of the Three Pures Palace. Then,

28 This place is very famous for the stamping art, especially the *nianhua* 年畫 or stamps for the new year.

the engraving will have been made in Beijing, in this famous shop. This plate in question would be another engraving, made after that of Meng Zhicai of 1873, by revising the damaged plate comparing it with that of Tianjin.

## 6 The *Complete Chart for the Cultivation of Perfection* (*Xiuzhen Quantu* 修真全图) from Mount Wudang (1888 or 1924)

A chart similar to that of the Palace of the Three Origins is preserved at Mount Wudang, with minor variants (fig. 2.6). Mount Wudang, which is sixty kilometers southeast of Shiyan City 十堰市 in northern Hubei province, has been an important site for Taoists since it was dedicated to the Dark Warrior (*Xuanwu* 玄武) in the thirteenth century.[29] When the Complete Perfection school flourished in the Yuan (1271–1368), it also spread to Mount Wudang, where it mingled with the existing elements of the Divine Empyrean (*Shenxiao* 神霄) tradition and the Correct Method of the Heavenly Heart (*Tianxin zhengfa* 天心正法) which is related to the Heavenly Masters school as well as military rituals and exorcisms.[30] At the end of the Yuan dynasty, a new Taoist current developed and spread in southern China, the Pure Tenuity tradition (Qingwei 清微), which is similar to the Divine Empyrean and Correct Method of the Heavenly Heart traditions. Alongside these traditions, the adepts of the Pure Tenuity developed a new regimen of thunder rites (*leifa* 雷法).[31] This movement is best exemplified by the Taoist Bai Yuchan 白玉蟾 (1194–1229?), who placed the rites associated with the Correct Methods of the Heart of Heaven and those of Divine Empyrean on the same level. He integrated the Pure Tenuity and the Pure Divine Empyrean traditions, but used different talismans, and places greater importance on the Pure Tenuity tradition and

---

29 On the importance of this mountain in Taoism, see Lagerwey 1992: 293–332; De Bruyn 2010. During the reign of Emperor Zhenzong (998–1013) the name of Xuanwu 玄武 was changed to Zhenwu 真武 due to a taboo for the character *xuan* 玄 [dark].

30 The Divine Empyrean tradition arose in the Song dynasty, especially by the prestigious and influential Lin Lingsu 林靈素 (1076–1120). See Li 2003. The term "heavenly heart" (*tianxin* 天心) dates back to an ancient divination system, *dunjia* 遁甲. According to the *Wuxing dayi* 五行大義 [Compendium on the five agents] by Xiao Ji 蕭吉 (530–610), the sixth of nine stars of the Northern Dipper is called "heart of heaven." Xiao cites as authority a *Dunjia jing* 遁甲經. See Boltz 1985: 67, and Kalinowski 1991: 386.

31 One of the longer sources on these Thunder Rites is *Daofa huiyuan* [Taoist Methods, United in Principle] (DZ 1220) of the fourteenth century. This document contains 268 *juan* and is a compilation of thunder rituals and techniques. It combines alchemical processes, inner culture, rituals, talismans and incantations." See Schipper and Verellen, 2004, vol. 2: 1105–1113.

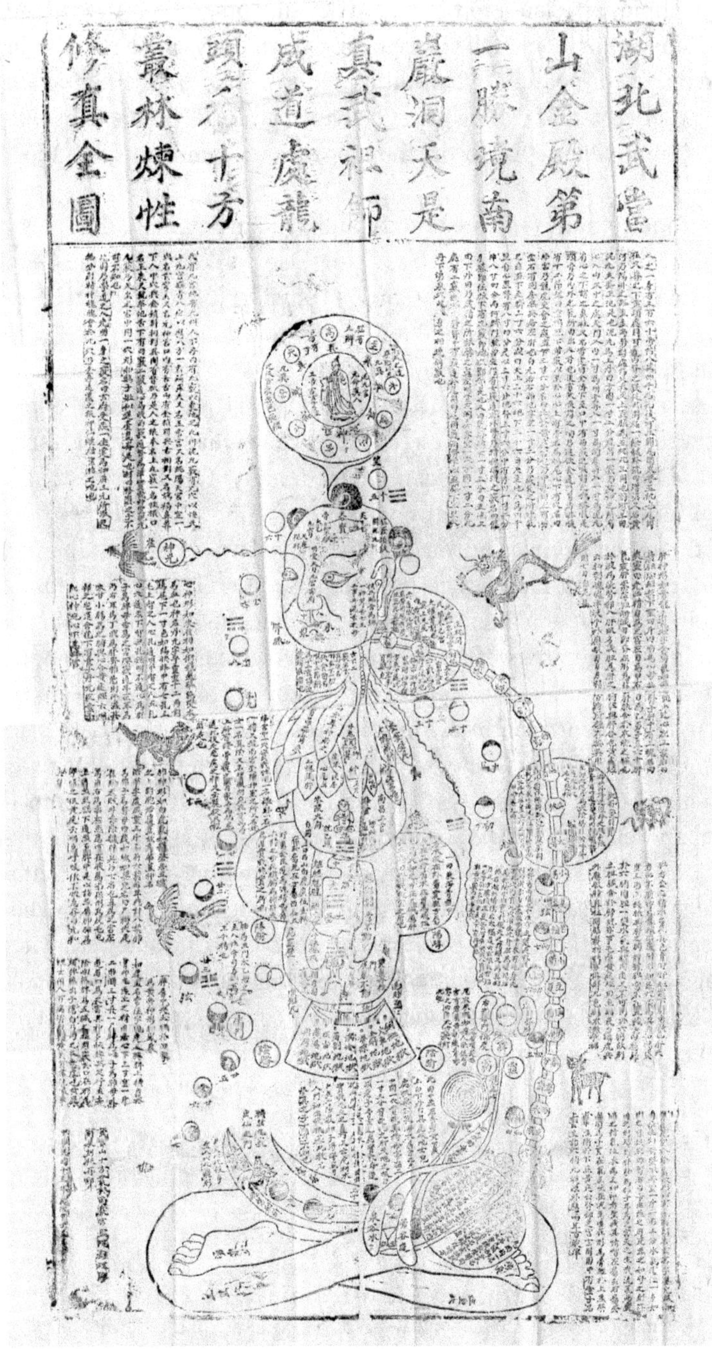


FIGURE 2.6 *Complete Chart for the Cultivation of Perfection* (*Xiuzhen Quantu* 修真全圖) from Mount Wudang

meditative techniques related to the Inner Alchemy practice.[32] According to Bai, any transformation could take place in one's own body, and a practitioner must be prepared to meditate when the thunder comes.[33] With Bai's Inner Alchemical practice, an officiating priest delivered effective rituals to heal the sick, and this curative function of the thunder rites was among its key appeal to adepts.

The Pure Tenuity tradition spread to Mount Wudang through disciples of Huang Shunshen 黄舜申 (b. 1224) such as Zhang Daogui 張道貴 (ca. 1264–1294 in Wudang shan), Liu Daoming 劉道明 and Ye Yunlai 葉雲萊 (b. 1251).[34] Zhang Daogui transmitted methods of the Pure Tenuity to Zhang Shouqing 張守清 (b. 1253) who was originally a Taoist belonging to the Complete Perfection school whose master was Lu Dayou 魯大宥 (ob. 1285) of Mount Wudang. Huang Mingyou 黄明佑 and Peng Tongwei 彭通微, his main disciples, mixed elements of Complete Perfection and Pure Tenuity tradition. Ye Yunlai received the transmission in his native village in Jianning 建寧 (Fujian), but because of the many troubles during the Yuan Dynasty (1271–1368), he took refuge at Mount Wudang. He owes his fame in part to Kubilai Khan because in 1285, Ye received an imperial invitation to court where he prayed for rain and good health for the members of court. The following year, he was promoted to superintendent of the main temple of Mount Wudang. Between the fourteenth and nineteenth centuries, these impressive mountains were a place where a branch of the Dragon Gate tradition developed which had integrated many elements of the Pure Tenuity tradition. The teachers became experts in military arts and exorcism rituals against the demons, especially those that bring diseases. Mount Wudang was finally associated with a local cult, that of Zhang Sanfeng 張三豐, a Taoist master who, according to his hagiography, died during the early years of the Ming Dynasty, but returned to life and was invited by the emperor to the Court. The first emperor Ming Taizu 太祖 (1368–1398) built a temple in his honour in the Mount Wudang. Zhang Sanfeng is one of the immortals who would be involved in the miraculous events that accompanied

---

32 The history of the Thunder Rites of the Divine Empyrean (Shenxiao 神霄) and Pure Tenuity traditions are notably recounted in *Daomen Shigui* 道門十規 [Ten rules for Taoists] (DZ 1232) by Zhang Yuchu 張宇初 (1361–1410).

33 See Judith Boltz 1985 and 1987.

34 On the Pure Tenuity tradition, see Reiter 1988. Liu Daoming is the author of *Wudang fudi zongzhen ji* 武當福地總真記 [Comprehensive perfected record concerning the blissful land of Wudang] (DZ 962). A biography of this author is found in the *Dayue Taihe shan zhi* 大嶽太和山志 [Monograph of the high peaks of the mountain of the supreme harmony] written in 1431 by Ren Ziyuan 任自垣 and published in the *Daojiao wenxian* 道教文獻 [Documents on Taoism].

the foundation of the dynasty.[35] He died in 1393. He was honoured twice during the late 14th and early 15th centuries, and canonized by Ming Emperor Yingzong (r. 1435–1449). In later texts, Zhang Sanfeng appears variously as a god who reveals texts to spirit mediums, a master of alchemy, as well as a master of sexual techniques, although his name was written with a different character, *feng* 峰. His following remained widespread throughout the Qing dynasty; his popularity rivalled the worship of Lü Dongbin 吕洞賓, one of the famous Eight Immortals of China, whose cult is also implanted at Mount Wudang.

The bibliography of the official history of the Ming assigns to two books to Zhang Sanfeng, though both are no longer extant. Some texts attributed to him originate in fact from spirit writing and were published in Leshan 樂山 (Sichuan) by Li Xiyue 李西月 (ca. 1806–1856), who became the patriarch of the western lineage of Inner Alchemy.[36] The revealed maps from Zhang are typically stamped from a wooden plate. Its title is the *Complete Chart for the Cultivation of Perfection* (*Xiuzhen quantu*) and the front matter includes the following inscription: "The bronze palace of Mount Wudang in Hubei is a very beautiful place.[37] The *Chart for the Cultivation of Perfection and the Refinement of the Innate Nature* comes from the Southern Cliff Heaven-Grotto, where the master and patriarch True Warrior achieved the Way; its influence has spread to Taoists of the whole universe."[38] The wooden plate once housed at the Southern Cliff Palace (Nanyan gong 南巖宫) is actually kept at the Purple Empyrean Palace (Zixiao gong 紫霄宫), currently the most important temple of Mount Wudang.

The lower left corner of this version bears an inscription giving the date and the provenance: "The fifth month of the year *jiazi* or the thirteenth year of the Republic (1924). Printed and kept by inspector Liu Liqing 劉理卿." In China, between 1985 and 1988, three articles on this representation were published.[39]

---

35 Seidel 1970: 483–531.

36 Titles attributed by *Mingshi* [Ming history] to Zhang Sanfeng 張三峰: *Jindan zhizhi* 金丹直指 and *Jindan bizhi* 金丹秘旨. Zhang Sanfeng is also credited with the preface to *Taiyi jinhua zongzhi* 太乙金華宗旨 and Zhang Sanfeng's preface in the *Sanfeng zhenren xuantan quanji* 三峰真人玄譚全集. These two texts are featured in the *Daozang xubian* 道藏續編, a 1834 collection edited by Min Yide 閔一得.

37 This building, which sits at the top of the highest peak of Mount Wudang and houses a statue of the True Warrior, was built in the *dade* era (1297–1307). See Lagerwey 1992: 299.

38 According to *Wudang fudi zongzhen ji* by Liu Daoming: "South Cliff is where the True Warrior cultivated perfection. There is a bronze statue of the "Holy Protector" (Lü Dongbin). In 1295, Wang Daoyi 王道一 and Zhu Daoxing 朱道興 collected money among the faithful of Luling and cast the statue." DZ 962, 2.1a.

39 Xiao 1985.1: 35. Shi Weixue 1988.2: 2–3, and 1988–3: 6–7. Peizhen Changsheng 培真長生 1988.4: 8–10.

The authors of these articles diverge in the description of the *Chart*, which suggests that the copy in question is another version than the copy dated to 1924. According to Xiao Xinzhu 蕭新鑄, author of one of these articles, the wooden plate was engraved on the 14th day of the 4th month of the 14th year of the *guangxu* era (1888),[40] at the date of Lü Dongbin's birthday.[41] The author of the engraving was Wu Mingxuan 吳明玄, or Master of Sapiential Light (Huiguang zi 慧光子). Wu is still referred to as the "Taoist of Water and Clouds" (Yunshui daoren 雲水道人) of the Dragon Gate tradition.[42] According to Shi Weixue's 石维學 brief description of this chart, the drawing included the images of a monkey and a horse.[43] This 1924 print of the body map was reproduced by the Research Centre on Martial Arts of Mount Wudang and released on September 1, 1986. Copies of the map were distributed to participants of the third research symposium on the *Classic of Changes* (*Yijing* 易經), which took place the same month near Beijing.[44] Dimensions of the original are indicated in the lower left corner: 114 cm high and 53 cm wide.

## 7 The *Chart for Achieving Cinnabar by the Ninefold Revolution* (*Dancheng jiuzhuan tu* 丹成九轉圖) of Moli 莫厘 (1918)

The *Chart for Achieving Cinnabar by the Ninefold Revolution* (fig. 2.7) was printed in 1918 and inserted in the *Illustrated Principles on Inner and Outer Practices*,[45] a series of illustrated texts compiled by Xi Yukang 席裕康.[46] Xi was originally

40 See Xiao 1985.1: 35.

41 See *Lüzu zhi* 呂祖志 [Monograph on the patriarch Lü Dongbin] where it states that "The fourteenth day of the fourth month, Lü Dongbin 'came down' (i.e., was born) in the world of men." DZ 1484, l.lb. It was common in China that commemorative steles were etched at important religious ceremonies, and these steles have an almost talismanic value.

42 If we consult the Cipai 詞牌 of the Dragon Gate tradition reported in *Hakuunkan shi*, Wu Mingxuan having in his name the character *ming* 明 belonged to the twentieth generation of the officially ordained masters.

43 Shi 1988.3: 6.

44 Shi 1988.2: 2.

45 *Neiwaigong tushuo jiyao* 內外功圖說輯要 [Illustrated principles on inner and outer practices] by Xi Yukang 席裕康, republished in 1990 in a collection of texts on the vital principle and *qigong*, edited by Ma Jiren 馬繼人. The first edition of this book dates from 1920. An edition published in 1962 in Taiwan by Ziyou chubanshe does not include this representation of the body, which is nonetheless mentioned in the preface written by Xi Yukang himself in 1918, and is therefore a part of the work.

46 Zheng Hong reports a version of the chart published after it in 1939 by a certain Chunzhen zi or 純真子 or Lu Shangxiao 陸上孝 of the Cihang xizi Buddhist Association 慈航惜字佛會.

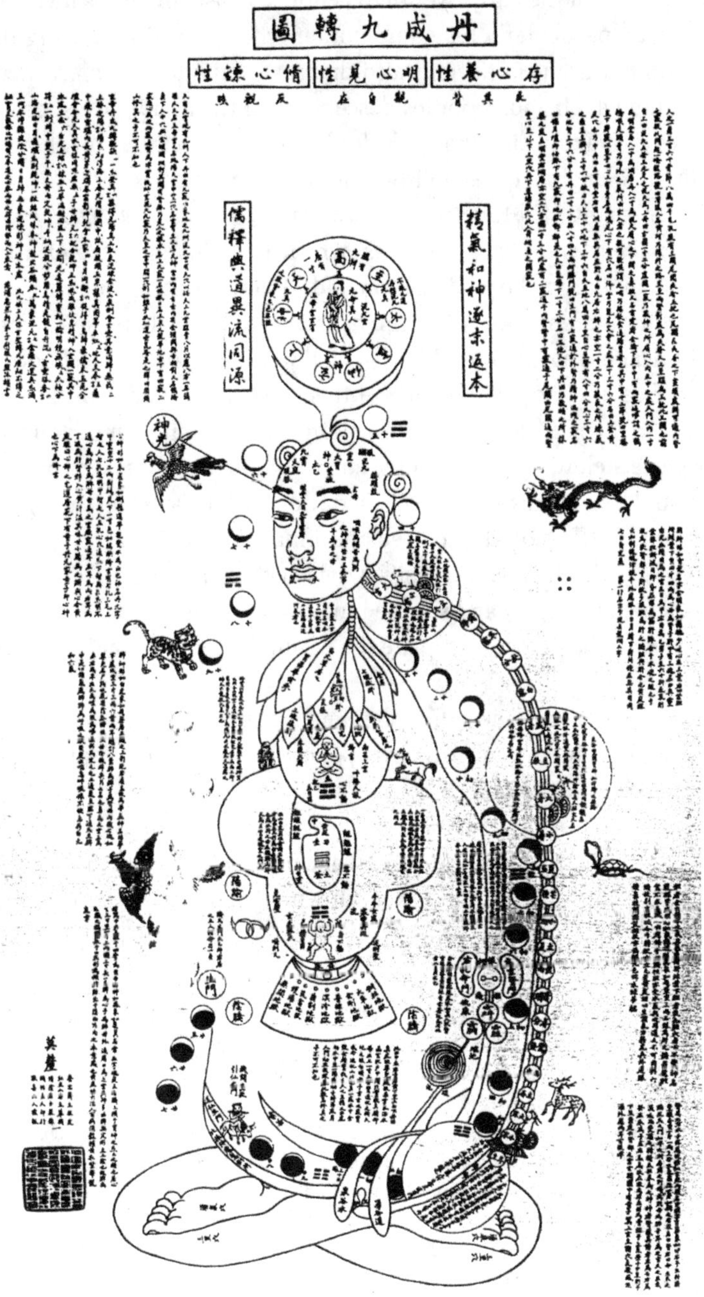


FIGURE 2.7 "Chart for Achieving Cinnabar by the Ninefold Revolution" (*Dancheng jiuzhuan tu* 丹成九轉圖). *Neiwaigong tushuo jiyao* 內外功圖說輯要 [Illustrated principles on inner and outer practices]

from Moli 莫厘, a peninsula of Taihu Lake in the Jiangsu. He was an active trader in Shanghai in the early twentieth century.[47] His family was involved in Taoist practices, particularly his grandmother who enjoyed practicing Inner Alchemy with her friends. It seems also that he often attended spirit-writing sessions during which Taoist deities descended on the altar.[48] He succeeded several times in making cinnabar pills, for healing the members of this small association. In Shanghai, he established from 1910 onwards an "altar" (*tan* 壇) named Huiran xuan 惠然軒. Between 1910 and 1918, he compiled his *Illustrated Principles on Inner and Outer Practices,* which contains at the end a body reproduction similar to those of Canton and Mount Wudang, but with some variants and a different title. With the assistance of an otherwise unknown patron, Gu Liancheng 顧聯承, Xi was finally able to print his book and distribute it free of charge.[49] The title of this version, the *Chart for Achieving Cinnabar by the Ninefold Revolution* is mentioned in a rectangular cartouche on the frontispiece. Below, we can see three entries of four characters inserted into cartouches and below these are three inscriptions, which start on the right:

a) "Concentrate the mind and feed the innate nature" (*cunxin yangxing* 存心養性), with below "immobilize the back" (*gen qibei* 艮其背).[50]
b) "To brighten the mind and see the innate nature" (*mingxin jianxing* 明心見性),[51] with below "contemplate the natural independence" (*guan zizai* 觀自在).[52]
c) "Cultivate the mind and refine the innate nature" (*xiuxin lianxing* 修心鍊性), and below "reverse [the light] to contemplate and illuminate [the inside]" (*fan guanzhao* 反觀照).

These three groups of four characters correspond to common expressions characterizing the main doctrines of Confucianism, Buddhism and Taoism. Moreover, on each side of the circle crowning the head, there are two

47 Moli, Xumushan 胥母山, was the name of an island in Taihu Lake; the island has now become a peninsula called the Eastern Mountains of Dongting 洞庭東山.

48 For more on this kind of spiriting writing, *fuji* 扶乩, see Xu 1961 and Overmeyer 1986.

49 See preface in *Neiwaigong tushuo jiyao* by Xi 1962: 6.

50 Sentence from the hexagram *gen* in the *Yijing* 易經: "He who immobilizes his back, protects not his person. He walks in the yard and does not see others. No blame." This phrase was used by Neoconfucian writers to denote the calm and steadfast leadership of the wise.

51 A classic expression in Chan Buddhism. The mirror is a well-known metaphor for the mind, which, according to the gradualist Chan School of the North, should be polished in order to shine.

52 Guan zizai 觀自在 is one of the Chinese names for the Buddhist bodhisattva of compassion, Guanyin (Avalokiteśvara).

framed inscriptions confirming the underlying syncretism of this example characteristic of these small secular movements:

a) "May the essence, the breath and the spirit expel demons and return a person to their root" (*jing qi he shen zhumo fanben* 精氣和神逐魔反本).
b) "Confucianism, Buddhism and Taoism are three different streams having the same origin" (*ru shi yu dao yiliu tongyuan* 儒釋與道一流同源).[53]

In the lower left corner, a small text indicates the source of this version: "At Moli. Revised by the Master from Nourishing Resolve Studio (*Yangzhi zhai zhu jiaoding* 養志齋主校定). Chart drawn by the Master of the Red Bean Mountain Hermitage (*Hongdou shanfang zhu zuantu* 紅豆山房主纂圖); respectfully noted by the householder Jieyin (Jieyin jushi jinglu 借陰居士敬錄). Printed and distributed by the Master who Preserves his Innate Nature (*Yixing zhuren yinxing* 頤性主人印行). Plate kept by the mountain hermit Jingshan 敬善."

The Master of Red Bean Mountain Hermitage in this inscription is probably Hui Shiqi 惠士奇 (1671–1741) or his son Hui Dong 惠棟 (1687–1758), both scholars of the eighteenth century. The Hui's home was in Suzhou, near Moli, and was named Mount Red Bean Hermitage due to the presence of red bean plants in the front of their house. The Master who Cultivates his Innate Nature was the nickname of Wu Ziding 吳子鼎 (1873–1945), a painter famous for his landscape and portrait paintings, it may be he who is mentioned in the inscription as a printer and distributor of this chart of Moli.

## 8 The *Complete Chart for the Cultivation of Perfection* (*Xiuzhen Quantu* 修真全圖) of Chengdu (1922)

*The Complete Chart for the Cultivation of Perfection* in Chengdu was made by Duan Fu 段甫 in 1922 (fig. 2.8). In 1943, an engraving of Du's text was offered to Joseph Needham by a friend, Mr. Fan Wu 范無.[54] Needham reproduced it in his *Science and Civilization in China* in 1983.[55] This version bears on the frontispiece, and in the left corner at the bottom, the words "plate kept in Flashing Pattern Altar (Huanwen tang 煥文堂) on Donggui Road 東桂街 near the south gate of the provincial capital (Chengdu)." It is similar to the other

53 The syncretism of these three currents during the Ming and Qing was not only prevalent in popular circles, but also among scholars. See Brook 1993: 13–44.

54 An inscription found in the title between the characters *quan* 全 and *zhen* 真 actually says: "This copy was donated by Mr. Fan Wu to the University of Cambridge." This was the institution where Joseph Needham worked.

55 Needham 1983: 117.

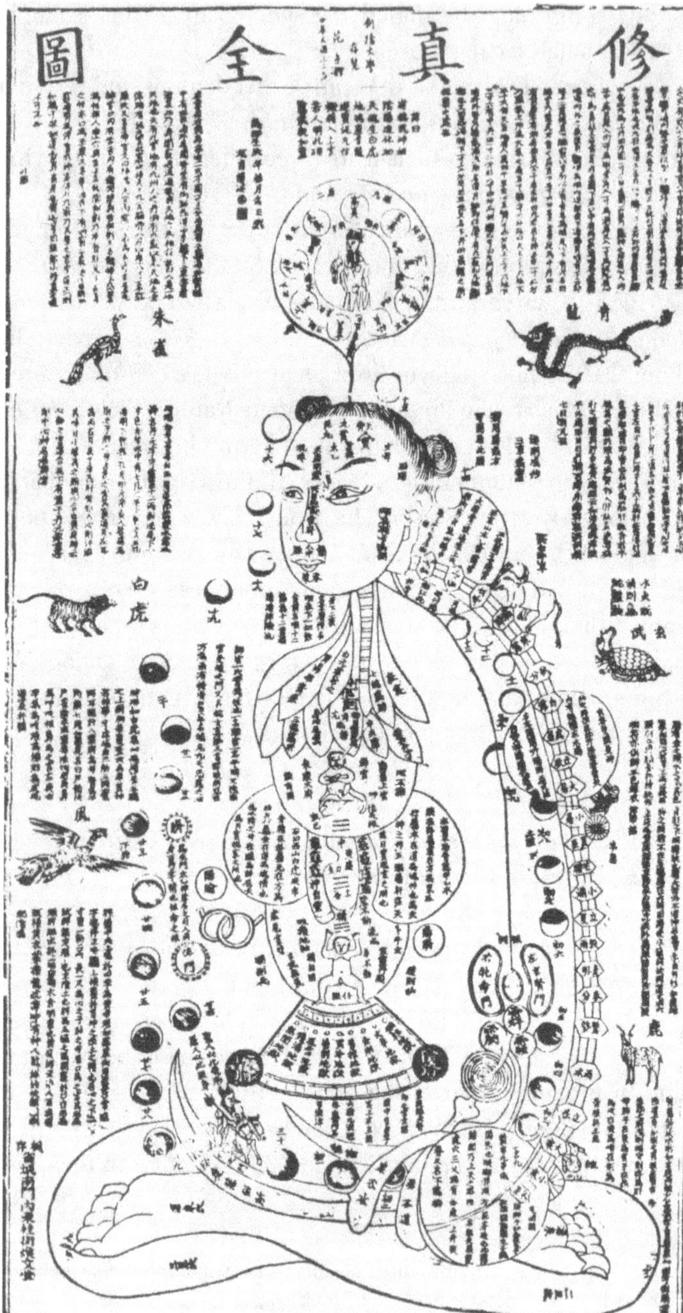


FIGURE 2.8 *Complete Chart for the Cultivation of Perfection* (*Xiuzhen quantu*) by Duan Fu 段甫 (1922). Joseph Needham, *Science and Civilisation in China*, vol. 5, 1983: 117

versions, except for the indication of its origin, most abridged and corrupted texts, and some pictographic variants.

## 9 The Copy of the Hall for the Lengthy Cultivation (Xiuyuan Tang 修远堂) (1936)

This copy, examined by Zheng Hong, measures 106 cm by 50 cm. It bears two colophons, similar to those we have already seen. It is based on the copy of Tianjin. The colophon adds that the copy was offered by Xu Jing 徐敬 of the Hall for the Lenghty Cultivation in Wenren village 温仁村 of the Qingyuan district 清苑县 in Hebei and printed in 1936 in relation with the Baoding Buddhist Society for Universal Salvation of Baoding in Hebei (*Baoding puji Fojiao fenhui zhizhong guanyi xiushen wei ben fangqiu zhiren yanjiuhui* 保定普濟佛教分會執中貫一修身為本訪求至人研究會).

## 10 The *Chart for the Cultivation of Perfection*, Engraved in 1984 at Beijing's White Cloud Temple

There was during the year 1993 a stamp in the left-hand gallery of the White Cloud Temple (fig. 2.9). The inscription on the lower left was simply, "Plate kept in the White Cloud Temple of Beijing."[56] According to the information we were provided with by Wang Yi'e 王宜娥, the Taoist association decided in 1984 to engrave a new plate according to the version of Guo Yicheng, in order to widely disseminate reproductions of this body map.[57] Recently, a new stele was engraved on stone and is exposed in a courtyard of the White Cloud

56 A copy of the stamp was purchased in 1990 by Sakade Yoshinobu. See Sakade 1991: 45–85. The same year, John Lagerwey also bought a copy, of which he gives a brief description in his book *Le continent des esprits*, 1991: 128–130. I myself bought a copy during the summer of 1992, which is much sharper than the previous two: a new board was likely engraved.

57 This version is therefore a print of the 1984 plate, and Sakade Yoshinobu's hypothesis, saying that this reproduction could be similar to the *Daoliu ru ding tu* 道流入定圖 [Chart of Taoists in contemplation], which was in the Hall of the Seven Perfected (Qizhen dian 七真殿) in the White Cloud Temple and is mentioned in a book of 1774, must be considered as unfounded. See Sakade 1991: 51. The title, *Daoliu ru ding tu*, also suggests that this fresco represented eminent Taoist saints, and not the alchemical body. This is what emerges from the brief description given by the book to which Sakade refers: the *Rixia jiuwen kao* 日下舊聞考 [An investigation of old legends that often circulate] by Yu Minzhong 于敏中 of 1774, according to a citation reported by the *Hakuunkan shi*, 26: "The clouds and banners shown in this fresco are innumerable, and they are not portraits of the eighteen disciples of the seven Perfected."

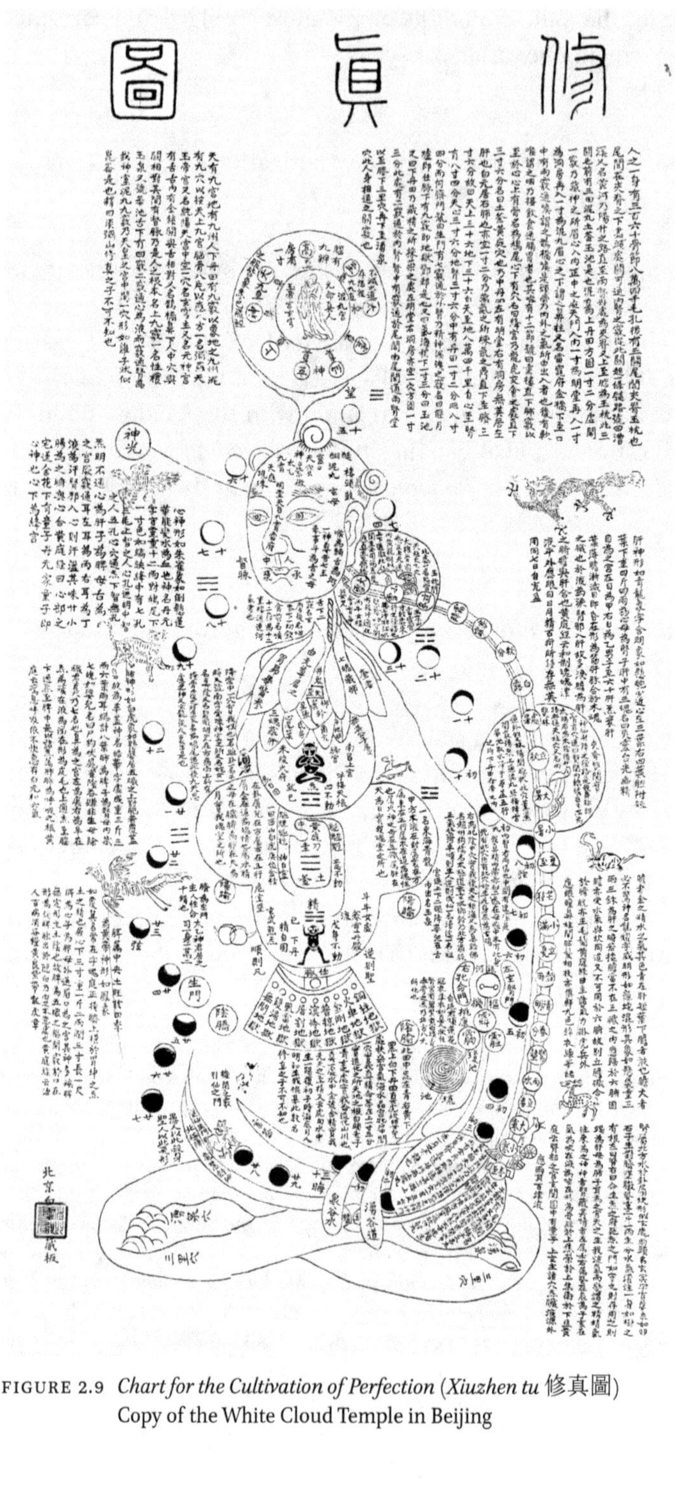


FIGURE 2.9 *Chart for the Cultivation of Perfection* (*Xiuzhen tu* 修真圖)
Copy of the White Cloud Temple in Beijing

Temple with a stele of the *Chart of the Inner Landscape* (*Neijing tu*). A version with colours corresponding to the six viscera, to the animals of the three chariots along the spinal column and to the hydraulic chariot at the bottom of the spine, was printed by Miaochunzi 妙春子, the nickname of Xi Chunsheng 席春生. This is the master of the second generation of the Thousand Peaks lineage (Qianfeng pai 千峰派) that originated with Zhao Bichen 趙壁塵 (1860–1942) in Beijing (fig. 2.10).

## 11 The *Register and Chart on the Cultivation of the True Origin* (*Xiuchi Zhenyuan Tulu* 修持真元圖籙) of the Tiger and Dragon Altar (Longhu Tang 龍虎堂)

There is a version in Nanning Province (Guangxi): the *Register and Chart on the Cultivation of the True Origin* (*Xiuchi zhenyuan tulu*) from the Tiger and Dragon Altar. This map (fig. 2.11) was engraved by Yang Hua 楊華, a disciple of Li Zhaosheng 李兆生, a colour version of this engraving is often featured on websites. This more recent version was given to me by a disciple of its author. While the chart emerged in Nanning, a city in the deep south of China, it is known widely, as is best evidenced by its 1988 engraving in Beijing.

Li Zhaosheng 李兆生, or Li Zhenyang 李真陽, is a leading figure of the world of martial arts. He was born in 1937 in the region of Deqing 德慶 of Guangdong Province (Tongling 同齡 according to another source). Various sites on the Web trace the major stages of his life and list the principal masters he knew. He made several trips to Japan, particularly to present martial arts of Mount Wudang and techniques of Taiji quan. He lived for some time in Beijing, including in 1993 when he was director of the Institute of Chinese Traditional Culture (*Zhongguo wenhua chuantong xueyuan* 中國傳統文化學院). He is himself a famous calligrapher and painter; he has exhibited his works and is the author of books on martial arts and Inner Alchemy. He produced an encyclopaedia of the representative texts of this school—some written by himself—which was published under the title of "Genuine Collection of Texts Housed in the Pavilion of Unified Origin" (*Tongyuanlou cangzhen congdian* 統元樓藏真叢典).

Some of the most important teachers in this lineage include Yan Zhengchang 閻政昌, the venerated master of the twelfth generation, the Iron Pine and Great One of Mount Wudang (*Wudang Taiyi Tiesong shier dai shizun* 武當太乙鐵松十二代師尊), Xiang Gong 恭祥, venerated master of the seventeenth generation of the Precelestial Great Ultimate (*Xiantian Taiji shiqi dai shizun*

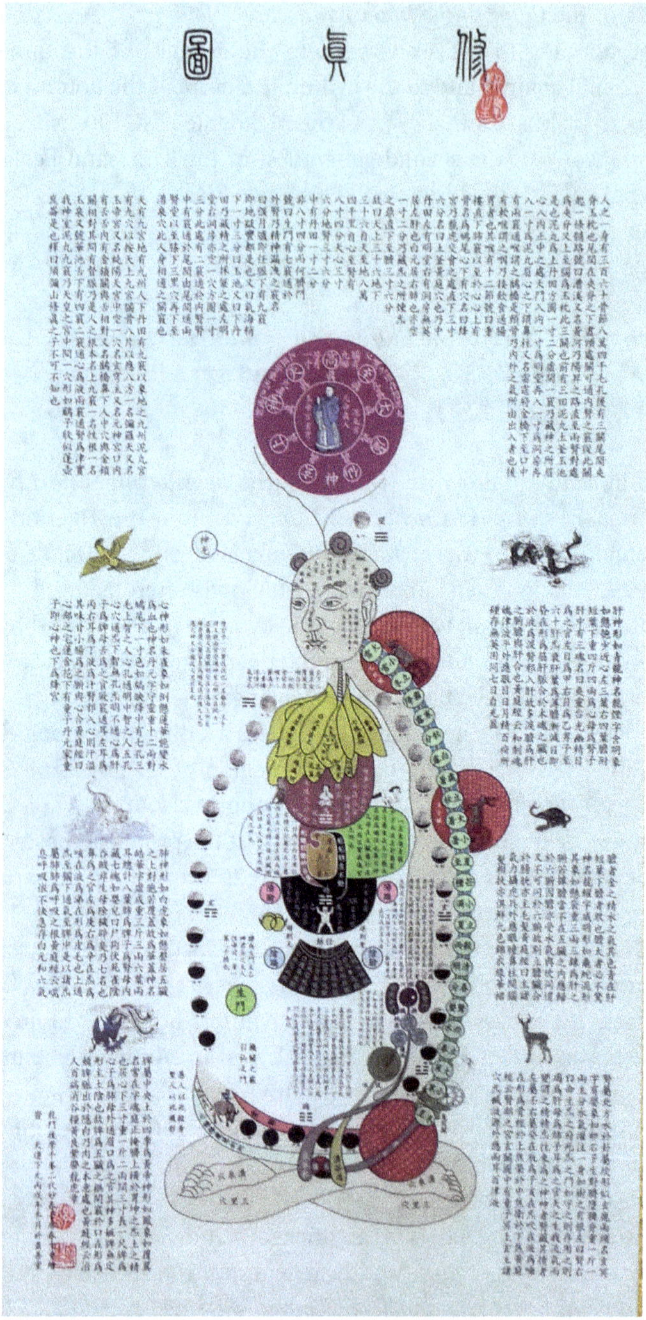


FIGURE 2.10 Reproduction of the coloured *Chart for the Cultivation of Perfection* (*Xiuzhen tu* 修真圖) print from 2006 by Xi Chunsheng 席春生, a second-generation adept of the Thousand Peaks current

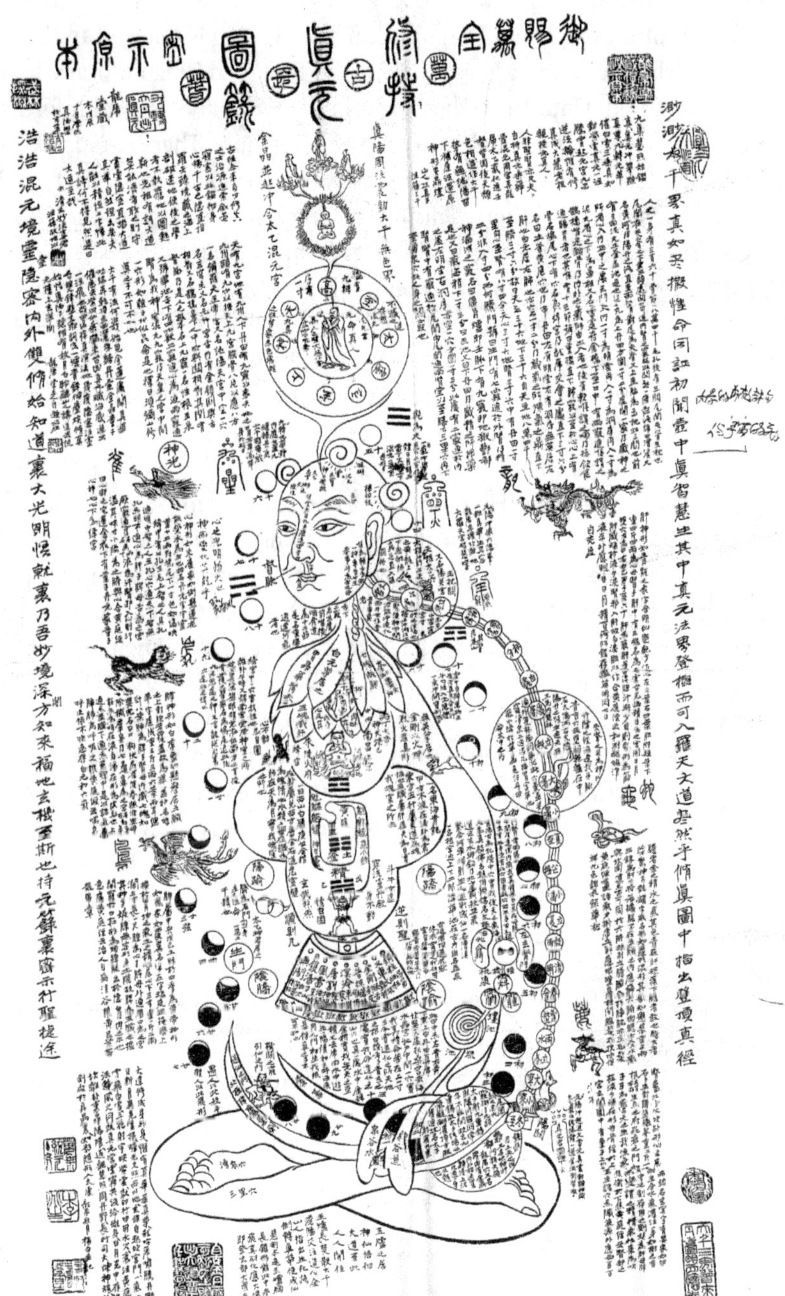

FIGURE 2.11 The *Register and Chart on the Cultivation of the True Origin* (*Xiuchi zhenyuan tulu* 修持真元圖籙) of the Tiger and the Dragon Altar (Longhu tang 龍虎堂) (1988). A stamp belonging to the author

先天太極十七代師尊) and Ma Weiling 馬威令, master of the twenty-second generation of the Tiger and Dragon Altar. Ma Weiling is relevant to the transmission of the charts since he is linked to the Tiger and Dragon Altar where the Chart was stored. Unfortunately, I have not been unable to find information about him, nor have I been able to locate this temple. There is indeed a Tiger and Dragon Mountain close of Nanning city, but we do not know if a temple by this name can be found there. This temple might correspond to the Tiger and Dragon Basilica (*Longhu dian* 龍虎殿) at Mount Wudang.

The title of this chart is written on the top in two lines of three characters. Two readings are possible: the first would be read from top to bottom and from right to left which gives the following meaning: the "Register and Chart on the Cultivation of the True Origin" (*Xiuchi zhenyuan tulu*), the second would be read horizontally, i.e., the three characters of the first row, then those of the second row. Read in this way, the inscription says, "Chart for the Cultivation of Perfection; Register for Holding the Origin" (Xiuzhentu, chiyuan lu 修真圖持元籙). This title, according to the first reading, reminds us that this chart belongs to the lineage of Mount Wudang teaching on the "Unifying Breath of the Perfected Origin" (*zhenyuan yiqi* 真元一氣). To right and left of this central title, still reading from right to left, we can see the following inscription: "Version secretly revealed and offered by the emperor" (*Yuci wan quan mi shi yuanben* 御賜萬全密示原本). According to an oral commentary given by Li Zhaosheng to his disciple Yang Hua, the emperor here is the Perfected Warrior (*Zhenwu*), a fundamental divinity for the exorcist rituals and martial arts, and also the main deity venerated in Mount Wudang, with which Li Zhaosheng maintains a particular link. An inscription on the left indicates the date and the author of this version: "Made at the capital by Li Zhenyang, the tenth month of the year Wuchen (1988). Plate kept at the Tiger and Dragon Altar" (*Longhu tang cangban xuchen shiyue Li shi Zhenyang zhi yu Jinghua* 龍虎堂藏版戊晨十月李氏真陽制于京華). The original map was burned before the Cultural Revolution and the stele disappeared. Li Zhaosheng relied on his memory to engrave this chart. A comparison of the drawings and the inscriptions with the other versions of this body map reveals a great similarity with the Mount Wudang version, according to the version described by Shi Weixue. It includes a monkey and a horse instead of a raven and a toad on the aforementioned chart. However, this Nanning chart contains, in addition to other versions, two texts at the top, respectively right and left, written by two different people: "Annotated Register of the Correct and Perfected Being of the Mountains" (*Shanren zhengzhen zi zhulu* 山人正真子注籙) on the right and on the left: "Annotated Register of the Perfected Lord of the Wonderful Method of the Pure Mystery" (*Qingxuan miaofa zhenjun zhulu* 清玄妙法真君注籙).

When compared with other versions of this body map, it is obvious that several texts have been added. There are the names of eighteen hells instead of nine in the lower part of the body. There is also a text describing the "jade furnace" (*yulu* 玉爐), and in the lower-left there are six columns of text describing the refined spirits that lead to Great Emptiness. Concerning the pictographic representations, the main differences with other versions are the presence of a monkey and a horse instead of the solar raven and the lunar toad, and crowning the head a circle surrounding a child, symbol of the [Original] Breath,[58] and above this circle three figures representing the Three Pure Ones, who are three fundamental Taoist deities abiding in the three upper layers of the cosmic breath: Jade Clarity, Upper Clarity and Supreme Clarity. There are also three "numinous talismans" (*lingfu* 靈符) and seals which are mostly related to characteristic notions of this version, such as "Axe-pivot of the Great Ultimate" (*Taiyi shuji* 太乙樞機), "the great elixir of the ninefold revolution that manifests the Perfected Origin" (*Jiuzhuan dadan chu zhenyuan* 九轉大丹出真元), the "Precious vestige preserved and kept in the Tiger and Dragon Altar" (Longhu tang cangcun zhenji 龍虎堂藏存珍迹), or the "forest of warriors plumbing the depths of the abyss" (*Wulin tan yuan* 武林探淵).

According to the geographical distribution of the *Chart for the Cultivation of Perfection* and its affiliation with temples of the Complete Perfection lineage, it is clear that this chart has a close relationship with Complete Perfection masters, especially those after Wang Changyue. It was housed in great Taoist centres such as the Black Sheep Palace in Chengdu (Sichuan), Mount Wudang (Hubei), The Palace of the Three Origins in Guangzhou (Guangdong), Resonating with the Tao Temple (Yingdao guan) in Wenzhou (Zhejiang), Crane Forest Daoist Abbey (Helin daoyuan) in Hangzhou (Zhejiang), Vacuous Luminousity Grotto (Kongming dong) near Taizhou (Zhejiang), the Three Pures Palace in Tianjin. But it was also used in small popular communities where it was often used

58 For the term *qi*, two different characters are employed in Taoism. One, *qi* 氣, designates the ordinary breath; it can be the breath of ordinary breathing, but also the emanation of things, the breath of the organs and the breath circulating inside the body. This is sometimes called the "postcelestial breath" (*houtian qi* 後天氣). The second character, *qi* 炁, is sometimes explained as the negation *wu* 无 at the upper part of the character and below four points representing fire, meaning the [Original] Breath is without the fire of passions; it is sometimes called the "precelestial breath" (*xiantian qi* 先天炁) and refers to the primordial breath in the cosmos and the breath resulting from the transformation of the energies inside the body which return to the primordial breath.

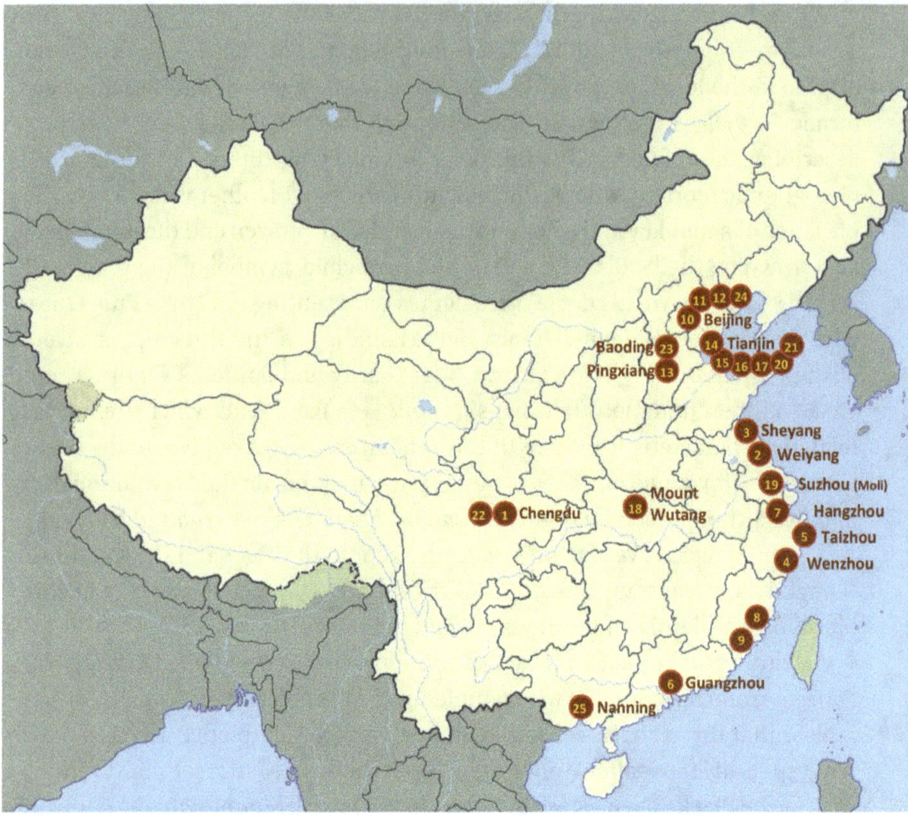


FIGURE 2.12 Map of the diffusion of the *Chart for the Cultivation of Perfection*

in a syncretic fashion; this is evident in the versions of Duan Wu in Chengdu (Sichuan), of Ledao Hall in Sheyang (Jiangsu), of Moli (Jiangsu), of the Hall for the Lenghty Cultivation in Baoding (Hebei) and of Nanning (Guangxi). Based on all available information about the chart and its different versions, the various engraved stelae, plates and copies of the chart we know are as follows (see the map, fig. 2.12):

1. Black Sheep Palace 青羊宮 in Chengdu, Sichuan (before 1781) (plate, lost)
2. Weiyang 維揚 plate engraved by Guo Yicheng 郭一誠 in 1781 (plate, lost)
3. Ledao Hall 樂道堂 in Sheyang 射陽, Jiangsu (undated plate, lost)
4. Resonating with the Tao Temple 應道觀 in Wenzhou (Zhejiang) engraved by Xuan Huahai 宣華海 in 1796 (plate, lost)
5. Vacuous Luminousity Grotto 空明洞 near Taizhou, Zhejiang by Yang Laiji 楊來基 in 1798 (plate, lost). Undated copy seen by Zheng Hong.
6. Palace of the Three Origins 三元宮 in Guangzhou, engraved by Qiu Fengshan 邱鳳善 in 1812 (existing stele)

7. Crane Grove Daoist Institute 鶴林道觀 in Hangzhou, Zhejiang (undated plate) (lost)
8. Plate by the Taoist Zhao of Mount Shuangji (Fujian) (undated plate, before 1882) (lost)
9. Plate by Lin Yongmao 林永懋 of Min (Fujian) (undated plate, before 1873) (lost)
10. Wang Lizhong 王理中 of Yan (Beijing) (undated plate, before 1873) (lost)
11. Du Fengchen 杜逢辰 of Yan (Beijing) (undated plate, before 1873) (lost)
12. White Cloud Temple 白雲觀 in Beijing, engraved by Meng Zhicai 孟至才 in 1873. Copy existing.
13. Manuscript of Houmazhuang (Hebei) (1873)
14. Copy seen at the Guandi Temple 關帝廟 in Tianjin, 1878 (lost)
15. Engraving by the Taoist Chen Pujing 陈普敬 in Guandi temple, after 1878 (lost)
16. Copy seen at the Three Pures palace in Tianjin (1882). Copy existing seen by Zheng Hong
17. Booklet similar to the copies of Tianjin (undated). Copy existing
18. Southern Cliff Palace 南巖宮 in Mount Wudang, Hubei (1888 and 1924 prints). Copy existing
19. Nourishing the Self Studio 養吾齋 near Suzhou, Jiangsu in 1918 (copy). Copy existing
20. Five hundred litographs of the Three Pures Palace made near Tianjin (1910) (lost)
21. Plate engraved by comparing a copy of the White Cloud temple and the copy of the Three Pures palace in 1920 (copy, lost)
22. The Huanwen tang 煥文堂 in Chengdu, Sichuan in 1922. Copy offered to Needham
23. The Hall for the Lenghty Cultivation 修遠堂 in Baoding, Hebei in 1936 (copy). Copy existing
24. The White Cloud Temple 白雲觀 stele in Beijing engraved in 1984 (existing)
25. The Dragon and Tiger Altar 龍虎堂 copy in Nanning, Guangxi, reprint in Beijing in 1988.

The sponsors and individuals associated with this chart are mainly layman, described as "friends of the Way" (*daoyou* 道友) or faithful layman (*xinshi* 信士), or even "man of the Way" (*daoren* 道人), although this last title is rather vague. These indviduals played a vital role in the engraving and die-stamping this chart by donating the funds for its reproduction, and thus contributed to its widespread diffusion. Some great Taoist names are linked to the chart on the booklet version: Yang Laiji, on eminent Taoist of the Weiyu Mountains (Zhejiang) and Meng Zhicai of the famous White Cloud Temple.

The distribution of the different versions reached nearly every corner of China, from Sichuan in the West to Jiangsu and Zhejiang in the East, Guangzhou and Nanning in the South and Beijing in the north. Most of these reproductions were distributed in the nineteenth and early twentieth centuries. Since around 1990, various *qigong* associations have taken an interest in the chart, as well as many martial arts communities and centres of Taoism. It is currently undergoing unprecedented diffusion, partly due to its transmission and explanations posted on the Internet.

In the following chapter, I will use the chart from the White Cloud Temple in Beijing since it is the most commonly used and well-known of these versions. It is similar to the charts in Guangzhou, Nanning and the Chengdu chart recorded by Guo Yicheng. I will supplement these charts with the explanations of the Mount Wudang, but will avoid the 1922 version from Chengdu, which is abbreviated and often contains corrupted or erroneous texts.

CHAPTER 3

# A Description of the *Chart for the Cultivation of Perfection*

The previous chapters examined how the *Chart for the Cultivation of Perfection* grew out of Yanluozi's representations and of the commentary featured in the *Book of the Difficulties*. Nevertheless, the extant charts contain many new pictorial elements and written texts. While the geographical distribution of these representations clearly shows a link with the Complete Perfection lineage and more precisely with a sub-current of it, the Dragon Gate tradition, the intrinsic analysis of the content of this map indicates there was a strong relationship between these maps and Taoist thunder rites (*leifa* 雷法). From the Song dynasty onwards, thunder rites were used by several Taoist schools, most notably the Correct Method of the Heavenly Heart (*Tianxin zhengfa*), the Divine Empyrean lineage (*Shenxiao pai*) and Pure Tenuity lineage (*Qingwei pai*).

This chapter analyses the pictographic elements and the corresponding inscriptions, as well as the texts drawn around the body. The sequence of these elements is determined by its spatial arrangement. It begins with the body, which is oriented in a vertical fashion. The progression starts from the top of the head and descends down the back of the body along the spine to the area of the kidneys and the lower body. The text then moves to the throat and descends the front of the body with its organs in the thorax and abdomen. After studying this representation of the body, I enumerate the texts surrounding the representation of the body and those that are located in certain places inside the body. I highlight the variations between the different versions of the map and pay special attention to passages that diverge from those featured in the first chapter.

For convenience, my description of this map will progress from top to bottom, but in reality, the *Chart* should be read from the bottom to the top. In accordance with the principle of inverting things at the core of alchemical techniques, the bottom is typically correlated with the ordinary world and forms the first steps of Inner Alchemy. The top of the map represents the ultimate accomplishment and ends the chain of images.

 | DOI:10.1163/9789004383456_005

## 1 Pictographic Elements and Inscriptions

### 1.1 *Head Crowned by a Disk*

A disc above the head (fig. 3.1) contains in its centre a drawing of a standing man with a shaved head, flanked on the left by the two inscriptions, the "Jade Emperor Palace" (*Yudi gong* 玉帝宮) and "Mystic Rose-gem" (*Xuanqiong* 玄瓊).[1] These are references to the "Sovereign of the Mystic Rose-gem" (*Xuanqiong zhu* 玄瓊主) mentioned in the text on the left and the top of the chart, and on the right by the inscriptions, "Muddy Pellet Palace" (*Niwan gong* 泥丸宮) and "Perfected of the Original Destiny" (*Yuanming zhenren* 元命眞人). In the Yanluozi diagrams and those related to it, this Taoist is simply called the "Perfected of the Muddy Pellet" (*Niwan zhenren* 泥丸眞). Below the standing Taoist, we can see the character *shen* 神 [Spirit].

The disc itself includes nine encircled characters, each forming a pair with the character *zhen* 眞 [Perfected] written below them.[2] These are the names of the Nine Perfected, deities abiding in nine chambers in the head according to the methods of visualization of the *Yellow Court Scripture*.[3] There are also several inscriptions that cite passages from this scripture, an essential text for the Taoist tradition of the Upper Clarity.

On the head, three spiral loops encircle the top of the head and above the two ears.[4] The Forehead bears three dots arranged in a triangle connected by

1 In the Mount Wudang version, the character resembles a Taoist with a bun on top of his head, while the White Cloud Temple version has a drawing reminiscent of a monk with a shaved head. The version of the Tiger and Dragon Hall has a hairy old man carrying a king's sceptre, a *ruyi* 如意.

2 On the Sichuan version by Duan Fu (1922) the characters *zhen* below nine characters are encompassed by the circles, and we have clearly the name of the Nine Perfected, according to the Yellow Court Tradition. This Sichuan version also includes a text above the disc that we were unable to decipher and, a bit to the left, a date.

3 There are two texts of the Yellow Court: the *Huangting neijing yujing* 黃庭內景玉經 [Precious book on the inner landscape of the yellow court] and the *Huangting waijing yujing* 黃庭外景玉經 [Precious book of the outer landscape of the yellow court]. They were written between the second and fourth centuries CE. Taoist experts have divergent opinions as to which is the older, certain considering the inner vision as being older, others claiming the opposite. Thus, Wang Ming 王明 considers the "inner landscape" (*neijing*) as being the older (1979: 86); Isabelle Robinet is of the same opinion. Schipper (1975) argues that the "outer landscape" (*waijing*) is the older.

4 If the four versions in the White Cloud Temple, the Palace of the Three Origins in Guangzhou, Mount Wudang and of the booklet are identical, the Sichuan version (1922) has only two bun-like loops above the ears, a traditional hairstyle for children in China, which tends to prove that the author of this stele did not know the symbolism of these three loops which we will discuss later.

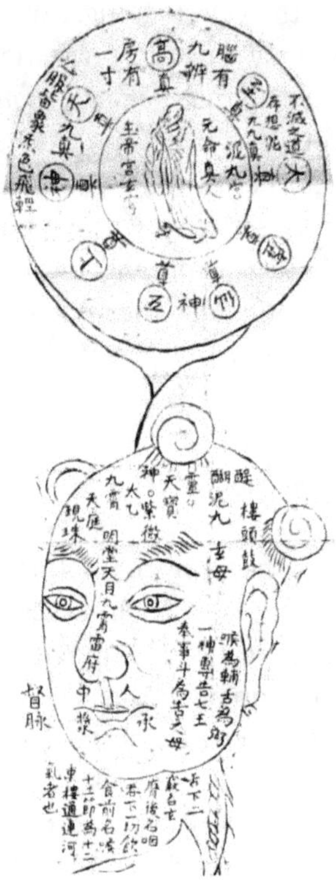

FIGURE 3.1
Detail of the *Chart for the Cultivation of Perfection*: the disk above the head and the head

a line symbolizing the Three Terraces (*santai* 三台) constellation. Inscriptions are engraved on the forehead, the nose, the left cheek, the groove between the nose and the mouth and the chin.[5]

The captions on the forehead arc from left to right: the "apparent pearl" (*xianzhu* 現珠), the "heavenly court" (*tianting* 天庭), the "nine empyreans" (*jiuxiao* 九霄), the "great ultimate" (*Taiyi* 太乙), the "purple tenuity" (*ziwei* 紫微), the "divine treasure" (*shenbao* 神寶), the "celestial treasure" (*tianbao* 天寶), the "numinous treasure" (*lingbao* 靈寶), the "clarified butter" (*tihu* 醍醐), the "muddy pellet" (*niwan* 泥丸), the "mysterious mother" (*xuanmu* 玄母) and the "drum on top of the pavilion" (*loutou gu* 樓頭鼓). These inscriptions evoke heavenly realms.

5 From the three jewels onward, I have included the inscriptions I was able to decipher them in the version of the White Cloud Temple. In the Mount Wudang version, the three jewels is replaced by the three characters *jiu tiangu* 灸天骨 [Make a moxa on the heavenly bone] and below *bao* 寶 [Jewel]. The other inscriptions are illegible, except the Niwan. The Sichuan version has *tiangu* 天骨 [Celestial bone] above three points, and below *bao*, to the right are the characters *xuanmu* 玄母 and *tihu* 醍醐.

The head is the heavenly part of the body and the celestial origin of the individual. In the text, this divine region of the body is called "mysterious mother," a name that often appears alongside "primordial father" (*yuanfu* 元父). These two terms refer to the primordial couple who give birth to the spiritual embryo that the adept conceives on his or her spiritual path. They are mentioned in the writings of the Upper Clarity scriptures: "If we want to cultivate the Way after receiving life, we should begin from the ancestors who have given us life, that is to say the primordial father and the mysterious mother. The primordial father manages transformations of the [Original] Breath and exists prior to the sovereign. The mysterious mother manages the transformations of the vital essence and the forming, by knotting, of the embryo. The vital essence and the breath complete each other in the same way as the yin and the yang create each other.[6] The "drum on top of the pavilion" corresponds to what the ancient texts refer to as the "heavenly drum" (*tiangu* 天鼓). It often refers to a set of bodily exercises named the "eight brocades by Zhongli".[7] According to the drawing accompanying this description, the heavenly drum designates the back of the brain. The origin of this technical term probably comes from the fact that the Taoists believed that the deities in the head lived in buildings and considered as dignitaries, guards manned lookout posts at the entrance to their homes to allow entry only to suitable guests. By hitting the gong and the bell, the adept announces the arrival of the deities in the nine palaces of the upper cinnabar field.[8] It seems that the drum on the top of the pavilion has the same meaning and should be also located at the back of the head, even if it is inscribed above the ear. The first occurrence of this term is found in a fourteenth century text by a Taoist writer affiliated with the Pure Tenuity tradition. It says: "Cover your ears with your hands, hit with your fingers the drum on the top of the pavilion." The commentary adds: "At midnight, cover the ears with both hands, with both fingers hit the back of the brain thirty-six times." Or again: "At the top of the pavilion, the heavenly drum does not resonate, the Kunlun and the Pillar of Heaven are inclined," after which the commentary clarifies: "The drum on top of the pavilion is at

6 *Dongzhen Taiyi dijun taidan yinshu dongzhen xuanjing* 洞真太一帝君太丹隱書洞真玄經 [Mysterious scripture of cavernous perfection and the hidden documents on the supreme elixir according to the Lord Emperor and the Great One] (DZ 1330), 4b.

7 "Embrace with both hands Mount Kunlun. Beat the heavenly drum twenty-four times." In *Xiuzhen shishu* (DZ 263), 19.4a–5b.

8 *Dongzhen Taishang suling dongyuan dayou miaojing* 洞真太上素靈洞元大有妙經 [Marvellous scripture of the unadorned numen and Dayou heavens] (DZ 1314), 17a.

the back of the brain, and the heavenly drum is the gate of the summit of the head."[9]

The inscriptions on the nose are read vertically from top to bottom: the "hall of light" (*mingtang* 明堂), the "celestial eye" (*tianmu* 天目), the "nine empyreans" and the "thunder palace" (*leifu* 雷府). These are also references to Taoist paradises and their corresponding palaces.[10] The inscriptions on the chin begin with "middle of the man" (*renzhong* 人中) and "receiving the prize" (*chengjiang* 承獎), which are the names of two acupuncture points, respectively the name of the 25th point of the "control vessel" (*dumai* 督脈), more commonly known as "water gutter" (*shuigou* 水溝). The final point on the chin is the "function vessel" (*renmai* 任脈). There is an inscription to the left cheek: "The throat is the Fu star; the tongue is the Bi Star. A divinity informs the seven kings, worships the Northern Dipper, which is the mother of the tongue." These seven kings are likely the seven superintendents of the seven stars of the Northern Dipper, which are also called the "stellar sovereigns of the Seven Origins" (*Qiyuan xingjun* 七元星君). Fu and Bi are two invisible stars located on either side of the Pole star. The seven superintendents refer in the human body to the mastery of the seven orifices of the face, that is to say the main sense organs: sight, hearing, smell, taste.[11] The deity who gives orders to this pantheon of gods is likely the one residing in the Pole star, a stationary point in the sky associated to the heart in the body. In other words, the heart controls the seven kings which are the sense organs, and is assisted by the stars Fu and Bi, or in the body by the throat and the tongue. At the level of the mouth is written the inscription "control vessel" (*dumai*). Below that, at the neck are drawn twelve pearls or rings representing the trachea, called in many charts as the "twelve-storey pagoda" (*shier chonglou*).

The version of the Tiger and Dragon Hall also includes a flaming circle surrounding an infant; this is a symbol of the original breath (*yuanqi* 元炁). Above this are three individuals standing on clouds, these represent the breath of the Three Pure Ones (fig. 3.2). On both sides of this group are the following inscriptions: "The true *yang* circulates everywhere and shakes the immense

9 See the third and fourth poems of the *Lingbao guikong jue* 靈寶歸空訣 [Numinous treasure instructions for returning to the void] by Zhao Yizhen 趙宜真 (d. 1382) of the Pure Tenuity tradition. DZ 568, lb.

10 The version of Mount Wudang has "nine palaces" (*jiugong* 九宮) rather than "nine empyreans."

11 The *Huangting neijing yujing* states: "The master of the Seven Origins regulates the harmonization of the breaths." According to the commentary by Liangqiu zi, this is the original breath of the seven orifices, which are associated with the sense organs: eyes, ears, nose and mouth. See *Huangting neijing yujing zhu* (DZ 402), 1.17a.

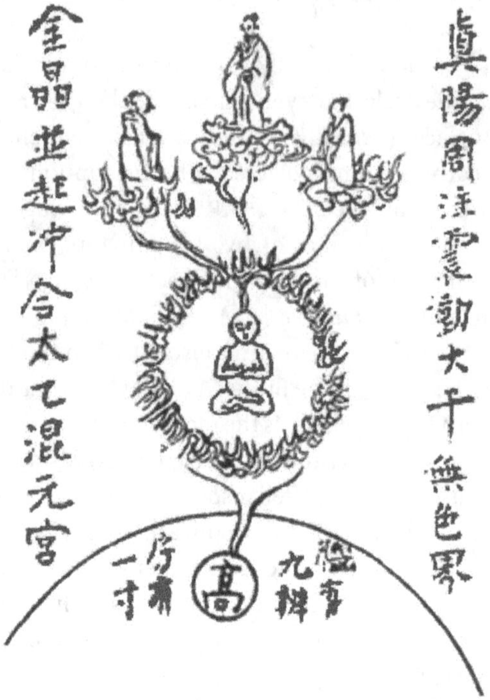


FIGURE 3.2 Detail of the *Chart for the Cultivation of Perfection* of the Tiger and the Dragon Altar: the circle of light with the infant and above, the Three Pure Ones

world of the formless. At the same time the golden crystal ascends and unites with the Great Ultimate in the Chaotic Origin Palace."

### 1.2 *The Spine*

From the lower part of the head, the spine forms an arc to the right (fig. 3.3); it is represented by four lines upon which twenty-four circles representing the vertebra are drawn. These circles are identified with the twenty-four solar nodes (*ershisi jieqi* 二十四節氣). These twenty-four breaths are: winter solstice (*dongzhi* 冬至), "lesser cold" (*xiaohan* 小寒), "greater cold" (*dahan* 大寒), "inception of spring" (*lichun* 立春), "rain and water" (*yushui* 雨水), "insects awakening from hibernation" (*jingzhe*), spring equinox (*chunfen* 春分), "clear and bright" (*qingming* 清明), "grain rain" (*guyu* 穀雨), "inception of summer" (*lixia* 立夏), "initial filling [of the grains]" (*xiaoman* 小滿), "seeding millet" (*mangzhong* 芒種), summer solstice (*xiazhi* 夏至), "lesser heat" (*xiaoshu* 小

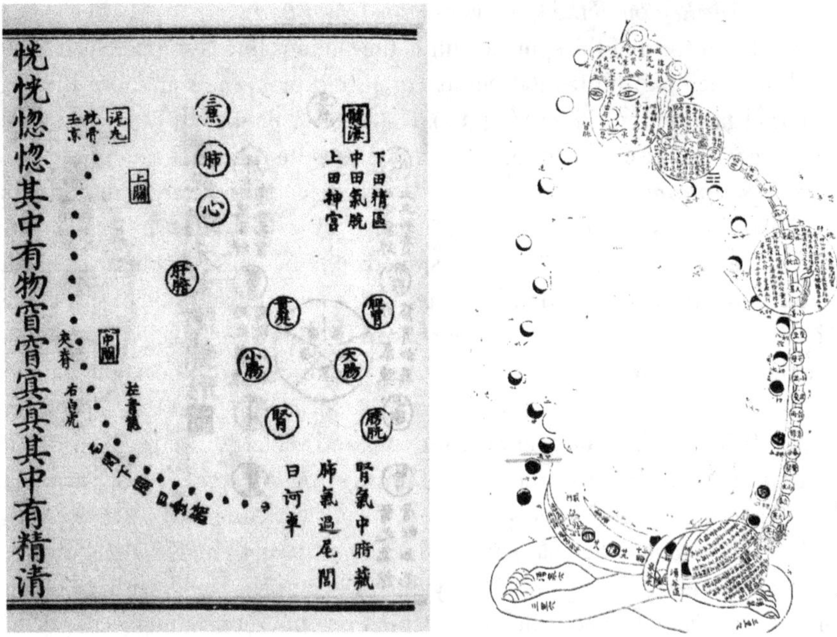


FIGURE 3.3 On the right, detail of the *Chart for the Cultivation of Perfection*; left, "Chart on the Accomplishment by the union of the water and the spirit in the three cinnabar fields" ("Shenshui jiaohe santian jiji tu" 神水交合三田既濟圖). *Dadan zhizhi* (DZ 244), 1.5a

暑), "greater heat" (*dashu* 大暑), "inception of autumn" (*liqiu* 立秋), "cessation of heat" (*chushu* 處暑), "white dew" (*bailu* 白露), "autumn equinox" (*qiufen* 秋分), "cold dew" (*hanlu* 寒露), "frost's descent" (*shuangjiang* 霜降), "beginning of winter" (*lidong* 立冬), "lesser snow" (*xiaoxue* 小雪), and "greater snow" (*daxue* 大雪).

The middle and the lower parts of the spine feature three large circles; each contains a text relating to the Three Passes on the back. These are the points of the three places where the breath rises along the spinal column but often passes with difficulty. At the same level as these circles are three chariots positioned vertically that are pulled by a sheep, a deer and a buffalo; they symbolize the three "hydraulic chariots" (*heche* 河車), the vehicles that assist the upward movement of the energy or breath. Inside the arc of the spine, to the left, a sinuous line bears the inscription "Milky Way" (*yinhe* 銀河), which corresponds to the spinal cord (*suidao* 髓道) of the Yanluozi diagrams, for which the Milky Way is a well-known metaphor.

### 1.3 *The Region of the Kidneys and the Lower Body*

In the lower third of the spinal column, the sinuous line is stopped by a circle within which two horizontal points connected by a line symbolize the two internal gates of the kidneys (fig. 3.4). This circle is flanked by the two kidneys bearing within two inscriptions: "to the right is the maternal gate of the vital force" (*youpin mingmen* 右牝命門) and "to the left is the mystery of the kidneys' gate" (*zuoxuan shenmen* 左玄腎門). There is a one-word inscription beneath the circle, "axis" (*shuji* 樞機).[12] The sinuous line becomes a channel, quickly interrupted by a circle with a character inside and on each side of this circle, forming a triangle, we have two other circles bearing a character within, below the left-hand character an eight turn spiral is drawn, with beside it the two following inscriptions: the "jasper pond" (*qiongchi* 瓊池) and the "lapis lazuli pond" (琉池).[13] Then the channel continues and ends with a bulge bearing the characters the "water from the valley of springs" (*quangu shui* 泉谷水); from the spiral another channel goes down and also ends with an inscription, "swelling valley way" (*yonggu dao* 涌谷道). In this same space, there is a circle divided into sectors representing presumably the lower cinnabar field, with inside the inscription "jade furnace." Below the spiral is a pocket seemingly connected to the circle between the two kidneys; on the Wudang redaction, there is an inscription: "The origin of the embryo is the ocean where I take root" (*Taiyuan zirun, wu suo zhi hai* 胎元滋潤吾所之海).[14] The illustration ends with the legs folded in the sitting lotus position; on the soles of both feet is the inscription the "bubbling spring" (Yongquan 涌泉) and below the knee, "three hamlets" (*sanli* 三里), two names that correspond in acupuncture respectively to the first point of the kidney channel and the 36th point of the stomach channel.

Above the legs on the bottom of the illustration are drawn two sorts of curved blades. The upper blade is marked "bellows" (*tuoyue* 橐籥). The lower double blade carries three inscriptions: "The life gate affording access to immortality" (*songxian shengmen* 送仙生門), the "Northern Culmen where the wisdom sword defeats demons" (*Beiji jiang mohui jiansuo* 北極降魔慧劍所). This wisdom sword is related to the veneration of the True Warrior (Xuanwu or Zhenwu), a deity associated with the northern direction. Ma Yu 馬鈺 (Danyang 丹陽) (1123–1183), one of the seven Perfected of the Complete

---

12 Term absent from the Sichuan version. This term *shuji* is used in *Huangting neijing yujing zhu* (DZ 402), 1.8a: "The double door of the Metal Pass remains sealed thanks the axis; at the dark well, the obscure portico rises high and majestic."

13 This last entry is not included in the Sichuan redaction.

14 This inscription is also on the Guangzhou version, but is not present in the version of Guo Yicheng preserved in the White Cloud Temple, as well as the redactions of Moli and Chengdu.

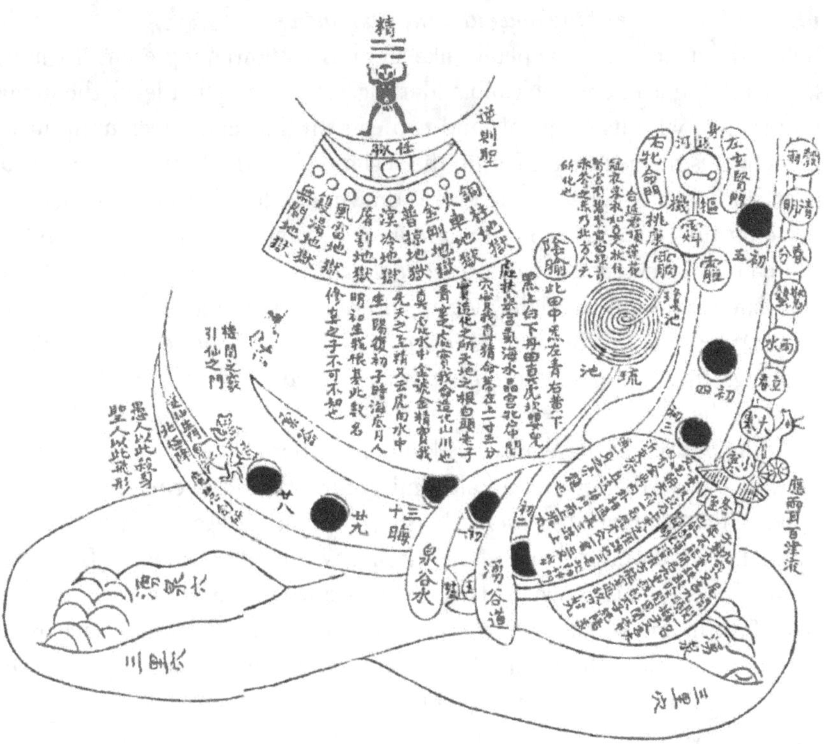


FIGURE 3.4 Detail of the *Chart for the Cultivation of Perfection.* The kidneys area and the lower body

Perfection lineage, writes in a poem: "The Warrior hides the real motive, the true ruler abandons falsehood. Honours, wealth and glory must be abandoned. Take hold of the wisdom sword that kills the three corpses and the unifying breath of the turtle and the snake will welcome you."[15] Between the two blades is the phrase "the gate leading to transcendence, the orifice to the pass of the pivot" (*jiguan zhi qiao, yinxian zhi men* 機關之竅引仙之門).[16] To the left of the double blade is the following dual inscription: "This is where ordinary men meet their death, but where the holy man soars towards transcendence" (*Yuren yici shashen, shengren yici feixing* 愚人以此殺身聖人以此飛行). On the upper blade is drawn a man riding a buffalo. It is replaced by a horse on the Sichuan representation by Duan Fu (1922).

15 "Poem to Taoist Suo from the True Warrior Palace," in *Jianwu ji* 漸悟集 [Anthology on gradual enlightenment] (DZ 1142), 1.12a.

16 This inscription is missing from the Sichuan chart.

### 1.4 *The Centre of the Body and the Abdomen*

Below the trachea, several petals, like an inverted flower, represent the lungs, the heart, the liver and the gallbladder (fig. 3.5). On the first level, the lung is represented with its six petals and two ears. In the centre, like an upturned lotus bud, is the heart with within the seven stars of the Northern Dipper. On each side, slightly below it, the liver is drawn with four leaves on the left and three on the right. Between them, there is a petal with the inscription "the gallbladder is the central earth" (*zhongdi dan* 中地膽). The names of deities correlated to the lungs and the liver are inscribed on several petals: the "Worthy of the White Prime" (*Baiyuan zhenzun* 白元真尊) and the seven *po* souls for the lungs, the "Non-pareil Lordling" (*Wuying gongzi* 無英公子) and three *hun* souls for the liver.

At the bottom of these leaves is kind of cruciferous flower. In its centre, a drawing evokes the form of an alchemical furnace. In the circle forming the upper petal, an infant is represented sitting with crossed legs and with the hands clasped in front of the chest.[17] Below him is written the character "[Original] breath" (*qi* 炁) and is drawn the trigram Li.[18] He symbolises the breath. On each side of the infant, we can see the following inscriptions: the "Fire Palace of the Vermilion Mound" (Zhuling huofu 朱陵火府), the "Scarlet Palace" (*jianggong*), the "Upper Palace of the South Brightness" (*Nanchang Shanggong*), "the heart doesn't move" (*xin budong* 心不動), the "breath strengthens itself" (*qi zigu* 氣自固), "accomplish [the earth] at *ji*" (*jiuji* 就己), and "during exhalation, be connected to the heavenly root" (*hu jie tiangen* 呼接天根).

At the heart level, on each side of the infant drawn in the upper circle, are representations of a monkey and a horse. This alludes to the expression "The mind is like a monkey and the creative thinking like a horse" (*xinyuan yima* 心猿意馬).[19] It refers to the necessity of calming the mind and focusing the thoughts like a man who is taming these restive animals. The monkey and the horse are replaced on the Mount Wudang version by the lunar toad and the solar raven symbolizing the exchange of yin and yang breaths at a certain

17 On the Yanluozi representation and that of the commentary on the *Classic of the Difficulties*, a standing character is represented with the word "maiden" (*chanu*).

18 The Sichuan version has the trigram *qian*.

19 According to the *Hailu suishi* 海錄碎事 [Some crumbs from the oceanic writings], a mid-twelfth century encyclopedia with a one-chapter glossary on Buddhist vocabulary (*xia*, 9a), this expression is derived from the *Chan Master Rong Recordings* 融禪師語: "The horse that is thought, the monkey that is mind." It is frequently found in the writings of Inner Alchemy, including that of Complete Perfection masters. Two examples include the *Zhizhen zi longhu dadan shi* 至真子龍虎大丹詩 [Poems on the great elixir of the dragon and the tiger] by Zhou Fang 周方 (DZ 269, 2b) and *Panxi ji* 磻溪集 [Panxi anthology] by Qiu Chuji (DZ 1159, 4.8b). For this expression, see also Despeux 1980.

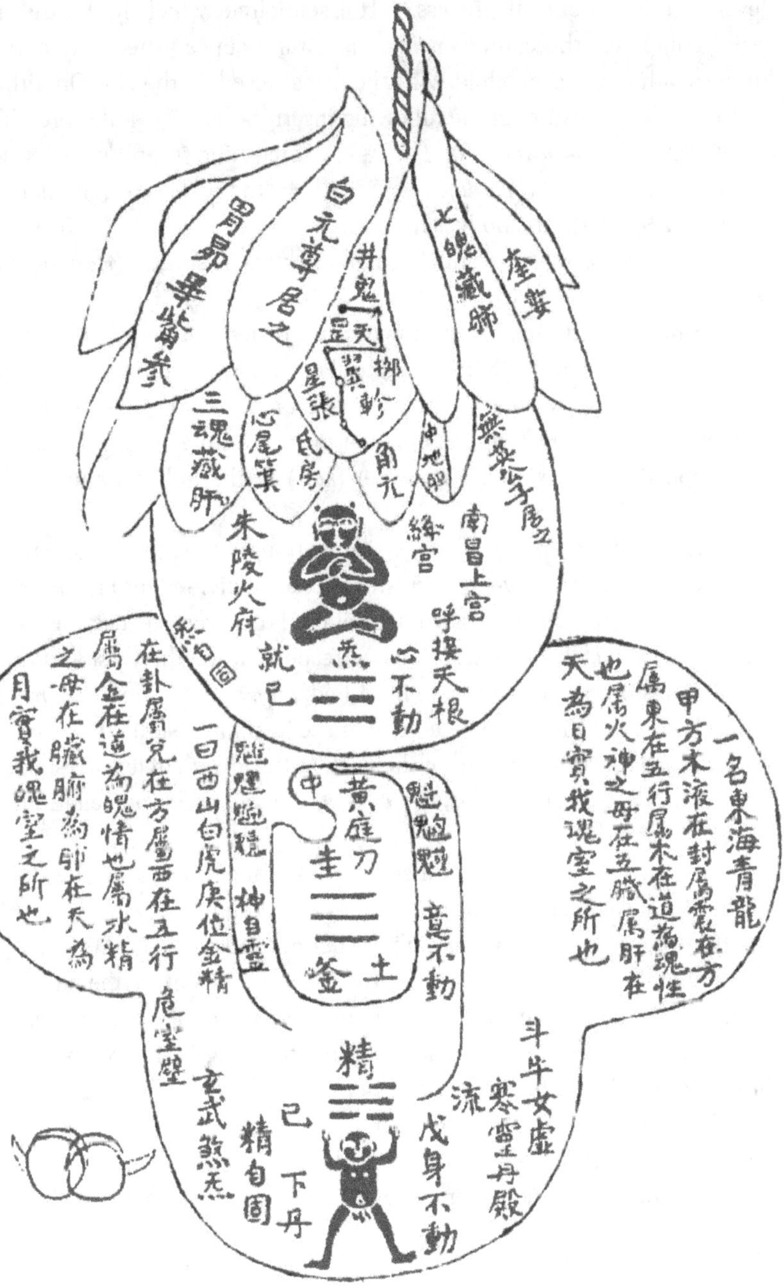


FIGURE 3.5 Detail of the *Chart for the Cultivation of Perfection.* The centre of the body and the abdomen

level of the alchemical process.[20] The semicircle which forms the inferior petal comprises the character *jing* 精, "vital essence," the trigram *kan*, and underneath a standing child with the arms raised to the sky. On either side of this child, we can read the following inscriptions: "The killer breath of the Dark Warrior" (*Xuanwu shaqi* 玄武煞氣), "breathing in and connecting with the terrestrial root" (*xi jie digen* 吸接地根),[21] "the essence strengthens itself" (*jing zigu* 精自固), "the body is motionless" (*shen budong* 身不動), "streaming at Wu" (*liuwu* 流戊), "the cinnabar hall of the cold spirits" (*Hanling dandian* 寒靈丹殿).

Two interlinked circles are drawn more or less at the umbilicus level. It is difficult to ascertain their meaning, because no inscription accompanies them. However, according to the use made of this kind of figure in the Inner Alchemy texts of the Taoist Canon, we may think they express the union of two opposites, for example the water (*kan*) of the kidneys and the fire (*li*) of the heart.

The left and right petals bear texts corresponding to the liver and the lungs. The names of the twenty-eight constellations are divided into the four regions corresponding to four viscera. On two petals of the lungs are inscribed: *wei, ang, bi, jiao, shen, kui, zou*, constellations corresponding to the West and therefore to the lungs. In the heartbud are inscribed: *jing, gui, liu, chou, yi, xing, zhang*, constellations of the South. In a petal of the liver are inscribed: *xin, wei, ji, shi, fang, jiao, kang*, constellations of the East. In the lower circle corresponding to the kidneys are inscribed: *wei, shi, bi, dou, niu, nü, xu*,[22] constellations of the North.

The central element comprises the trigram Qian and the following inscriptions: the "centre" (*zhong* 中), the "yellow court" (*huangting* 黄庭), the "earth furnace" (*tufu* 土釜), the "elixir spoon" (*daogui* 刀圭). We can also see seven characters with the radical of the demon designating the names of the deities of the seven stars of the Northern Dipper: *kui, you, xing, huan, bi, piao, shuo*, and this inscription: "When creative thinking is motionless, the body becomes agile and efficient" (*yi budong, shen ziling* 意不動，身自靈).

Below this flower is a trapezium and in an upper band nine points symbolizing the gates of hells; each name is listed below the points. The ensemble evokes a pot (*hu* 壺) with a trapezoidal foot. We must note that the pot is a

---

20 These animals are not represented on the Sichuan version.

21 The version of Mount Wudang has here "in the end" which is a false reading.

22 The last four names, *dou, niu, nü, xu*, are not legible on the copy of the Mount Wudang we consulted.

metaphor for the body considered as an athanor or a paradise.[23] Between the cruciform flower and the trapeze, we can see the inscription "function vessel" (*renmai*) and a circle.[24]

### 1.5 *Pictographic Elements Placed around the Representation*

Six trigrams are located around different parts of body.[25] The body map is surrounded by thirty small circles representing the thirty phases of the moon: from the coccyx to the top of the head, they are, from the new moon (the term designating the "new moon," *hui* 晦, is inscribed near the first moon), "crescent moon" (the term *xian* 弦 is inscribed next to the first and the last quarter of the moon) and the full moon on the top of the head (the term *wang* 望, "full moon," is inscribed, above). On the front of the body, the moon decreasing from the sixteenth day is drawn from the head just above the crossed legs.[26]

This schematic body map is also surrounded by the drawings of six animals symbolizing the deities of the six viscera according to the Yellow Court tradition.[27] They are from the upper to the lower part and from right to left: the dragon (corresponding to the liver), the turtle and the snake (the gallbladder), the deer with two heads (the kidneys), the vermilion sparrow (the heart), the white tiger (the lungs) and the phoenix (the spleen).

### 1.6 *The Circled Characters*

The Chart includes six circled characters. On the head, a line is drawn from between the eyebrows, which ends with a circle bearing the inscription "light of the spirit" (*shenguang* 神光). Below the left and right petals and at the lower corners of the trapezoid are four circles bearing inscriptions, which

---

23 Jin Yueyan 金月岩, in his *Baoyi hansan bijue* 抱一函三秘訣 [Secret instructions on holding the one and encasing the three], writes, "In the pot is another world." DZ 576, 23b. Huang Gongwang 黃公望 (1269–1354), who transmitted Jin's text, created a "temple of the three religions" while staying in Suzhou. Best known as one of the leading painters of the Yuan, he was also a famous master of the Complete Perfection lineage, having made a syncretism with some elements of the southern alchemical schools. For more on Huang, see Gyss-Vermande 1984.

24 The Mount Wudang version includes the character *hou* 後 [Back] inside the circle.

25 These trigrams are not included in the Sichuan version.

26 If the thirty moons are not drawn on the Yanluozi diagram or on that of the commentary on the *Classic of the Difficulties*, the cycle of thirty moons is evoked by characters designating the new moon, the two quarters of the moon and the full moon.

27 See Hu Yin's 胡愔 *Huangting neijing wuzang liufu buxie tu* 黃庭內景五藏六府補瀉圖 [Chart of the procedures of tonification or purgation of the six receptacles and five viscera according to the inner landscape of the yellow court] (DZ 263), 54.1–24.

are in the top and the left Yangyu,[28] in the top and the right Yangqiao, at the lower left Yinqiao,[29] and lower right Yinyu. These are the names of four of the eight marvellous vessels (*qijing bamai* 奇經八脈). Below these names is a circle with the words "Life Gate" (*shengmen* 生門). Near the umbilicus is a longer inscription: "The navel is the life gate. The Taiyi divinity resides there; it regulates the innate nature and the life force, and is the rector of the twelve thousand essences."[30]

## 2 Pictographic Differences with Other Body Charts in the Taoist Canon

The *Chart for the Cultivation of Perfection* includes almost all the pictographic elements represented in the diagram of the commentary on the *Classic of the Difficulties*. The two texts differ in that the representations of the three corpses, the seven souls around the head, the wheel of fire coming out of the Yellow Court in the centre of the body, the sea turtle at the lower end of the coccyx, the tiger and the dragon facing each other below the diaphragm are removed from the *Chart for the Cultivation of Perfection*. There are also a few pictographic differences such as the omission of the three characters drawn at the location of the three cinnabar fields, as well as a change in position of the lower cinnabar field and the median cinnabar field. Also, in the median cinnabar field, an infant replaces the maiden, and the four animals of the four directions of the commentary on the *Classic of the Difficulties* are replaced by six animals of the six viscera from the Yellow Court tradition. The elements specific to the *Chart* are mainly those that symbolize the fire phasing used for alchemical practices at different stages, such as the thirty phases of the moon around the body, the trigrams and the twenty-eight constellation names. There are also names for the seven stars of the Northern Dipper, the buffalo at the lower part of the body, the monkey and the horse or the solar raven and the lunar toad in the median level, a double linked circle near the navel.[31]

28 On the Mount Wudang version, the character *yu* is written with the radical of the flesh instead of the radical of the foot.

29 On the version of the White Cloud Temple, the character *qiao* is written with the radical of the flesh instead of the foot, and there has therefore been reversed with the character *yu* in Yangyu.

30 The Mount Wudang version has the number thirteen thousand.

31 If these two elements are not present on the representation of the commentary on the *Classic of the Difficulties*, they are however on the *Chart of the Inner Landscape* (1886) of Beijing's White Cloud Temple.

If the *Chart of the Inner Landscape* appears as a map essentially involved with the individual practices of the inner vision of the body as a landscape, with the vision of inner gods and the cultivation of the basic alchemical methods, the *Chart for the Cultivation of Perfection* is more in the continuity of the Yanluozi's diagrams and that of the commentary on the *Classic of the Difficulties*.

The most striking difference between the *Chart* and other texts are those passages describing Thunder Rites. These include the spiral in the kidneys, the nine orifices of hells in the trapezium, the three characters above the spiral in the kidneys area related to the thunder rites, the three loops of the crown representing the three essential breaths according to the Correct Method of the Heavenly Heart, the representation on the forehead of the Three Terraces Constellation, the circle drawn between the two kidneys containing two points connected by a line, and the seven characters at the body centre designating the seven spirits of the seven stars of the Northern Dipper destroying the underworld.

## 3 The Main Texts (fig. 3.6)

### 3.1 *Two Documents on the General Description of the Essential Body Sites (Texts 1 and 2)*

Two texts at the upper part of the chart, respectively on either side of the disk crowning the head, describe the main orifices and crossing sites of the body:

1: The text to the left establishes a correspondence between the macrocosm and the body, detailing the main orifices (translated pp. 114–116);

2: The text on the upper right represents the most important places in the body for the alchemical practices: the three passes, the three cinnabar fields, the stoves and the cauldrons (translated pp. 117–120).

### 3.2 *Six Texts on Six Viscera (Texts 3–8)*

Six texts describing the six viscera according to the Yellow Court tradition are aligned below the representations of six animals and outside the pictographic representation of the body itself:

3: On the upper right level, a text about the liver, topped with the dragon (translated p. 177);

4: On the middle right level, a text concerning the gallbladder framed by a turtle entwined by a serpent (translated pp. 177–78);

5: On the lower right level, a text describing the kidneys with an image of a deer (translated pp. 178–179);

6: On the upper left level, a text on the heart with a vermilion sparrow (translated pp. 179–180);
7: On the middle left level, a text on the lungs topped with the tiger (translated pp. 180–181);
8: On the lower left level, a text on the spleen framed by a phoenix (translated pp. 181–182).

### 3.3 *Three Texts on the Three Passes (Texts 9–11)*

There are inscriptions for the three passes on three circles located at the three levels of the spine:
9: On the upper level of the spine, there is a circle with text about the Jade Pillow Pass (translated p. 134);
10: On the median level of the spine is a circle with the text on the "pass surrounding the spine" (translated pp. 131–132);
11: On the lower level of the spine is a circle with an inscription about the "Caudal Pass" (translated p. 130).

### 3.4 *A Text on the Throat (Text 12)*

12: Below the head to the left of the trachea is an inscription about the throat (translated p. 138).

### 3.5 *Five Texts on the Five Viscera (Texts 13–17)*

13: To the left of the centre of the body, outside the circle containing an infant and near the lungs petals, is a text on the Scarlet Palace, i.e., the heart region (translated p. 210);
14: On the left petal of the central cruciform flower is a text on the metaphor of the white tiger, i.e., the lungs (translated p. 163);
15: On the right petal of the central cruciform flower is a text on the metaphor of the azure dragon, i.e., the liver (translated p. 161);
16: Above the pictographic representation of the kidneys as a bean and near the lower third of the spine is a text on the internal kidneys (translated pp. 210–211);
17: Below the kidneys is a text on Taokang 桃康, the deity governing the kidneys (translated p. 186).[32]

32 Both texts are omitted from the Sichuan version.

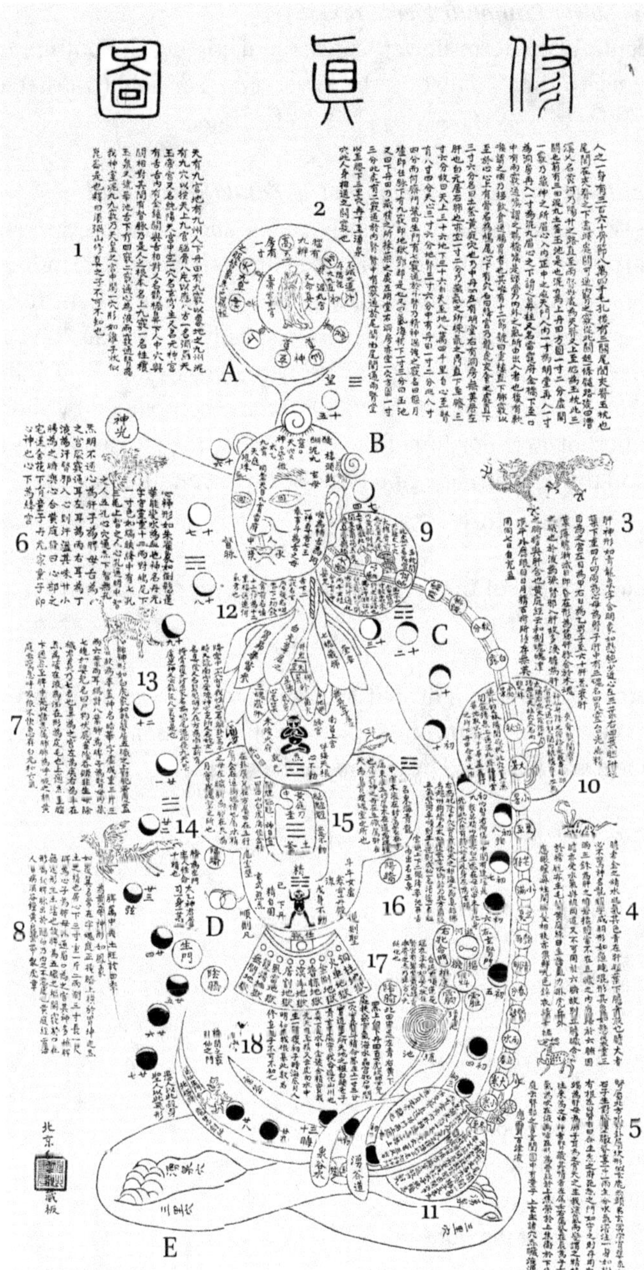


FIGURE 3.6 The *Chart for the Cultivation of Perfection* with numbers corresponding to the explanatory texts and letters on the pictographic body

### 3.6 *Text on the Lower Cinnabar Field (Text 18)*

18: Under the central cruciform flower is a shape depicting the bottom of a pot, and beneath this is a text on the lower cinnabar field (translated pp. 125–126).[33]

### 3.7 *Additional Texts on the Version of the Tiger and Dragon Hall*

The version of the Tiger and Dragon Altar Hall has some additional inscriptions or texts. First of all, on both sides of the chart are columns bearing inscriptions mixing Buddhist and Taoist conceptions. Then, over the left and right texts above the head, are two added texts signed respectively by the Master Zhengzhen and the "Perfected Sovereign of the Wonderful Process of Pure Mystery." Around the head, are drawn three talismans accompanied by short explanatory texts. In the lower portion of the chart below the crossed legs is a text on the stove and the jade furnace, and beside the feet, another text.

## 4 List and Localisation of the terms on the *Chart for the Cultivation of Perfection* (*See Fig. 3.6*)

The references to the terms are indicated according to the texts numbered from 1 to 18 and to the different parts of the pictographic representation of the body divided into five and indicated by letters on the fig. 4.2:

A: disc above the head
B: head
C: upper part of the trunk
D: abdomen
E: lower abdomen and legs

*Baiguang* 白光 [White light]: text 3
*Baihu* 白虎 [White tiger]: text 7, 14
*Bailu* 白露 [White dew]: C (vertebra)
*Baitou Laozi* 白頭老子 [Laozi with white hair]: text 18
*Baiyuan* 白元 [White origin]: text 2
*Baiyuan zun* 白元尊 [Worthy of the white prime]: C, text 7
*Bao* 胞 [Bladder]: text 7
*Batian* 八天 [Eight heavens]: text 17
*Beiji* 北極 [Northern culmen]: E

33 The text is shorter on the Sichuan version.

*Bi* 鼻 [Nose]: text 1, 7
*Bichou* 辟臭 [Stink hunter]: text 7
*Biyan huseng* 碧眼胡僧 [Cyan-eyed foreign monk]: text 13
*Bizhu* 鼻柱 [Nose pillar]: text 2, 4
*Caoxi* 曹溪 [Cao stream]: text 2, 16
*Chang* 腸 [Intestines]: text 2
*Changzai* 常在 [Eternal residence]: text 8
*Chanü* 姹女 [Maiden]: text 13
*Chaotian ling* 朝天嶺 [Summit for an heavenly audience]: text 11
*Chengjiang* 承漿 [Receiving the prize]: B
*Chonglou* 重樓 [Storied pagoda]: text 2, 12
*Chuhui* 除穢 [Eradicator of dirt]: text 7
*Chunfen* 春分 [Spring equinox]: D, vertebra
*Chunyang qi* 純陽炁 [Breath of the pure yang]: text 11
*Chunyang tiangong* 純陽天宮 [Heavenly palace of pure yang]: text 1
*Chushu* 處暑 [End of heat]: C, vertebra
*Cunxiang* 存想 [Visualization]: A
*Dahan* 大寒 [Greater cold]: E, vertebra
*Dan* 膽 [Gallbladder]: C, text 3, 4
*Danyuan* 丹元 [Origin of cinnabar]: text 6
*Daogui* 刀圭 [Elixir spoon]: D
*Dashu* 大暑 ([Greater heat]: C, vertebra
*Daxue* 大雪 [Greater snow]: B, vertebra
*Dazhui gu* 大椎骨 [Seventh dorsal]: text 9
*Ding* 鼎 [Cauldron]: text 2
*Diyu* 地獄 [Hell]: text 2
*Dizhou* 地軸 [Earthly axis]: text 11
*Dongfang* 洞房 [Cavern chamber]: text 2
*Donghai* 東海 [Eastern sea]: text 15
*Dongzhi* 冬至 [Winter solstice]: E, vertebra
*Dui* 兑: text 14
*Dumai* 督脈 [Control vessel]: B, text 1
*Er* 耳 [Ears]: text 5, 6
*Fei* 肺 [Lungs]: C, text 2, 5, 7, 8, 14
*Feidu* 飛毒 [Flying poison]: in text 7, it is *fei sheng mu* (非生母)
*Feng* 鳳 [Phoenix]: text 8
*Fengdu* 豐都: text 2
*Fenglei diyu* 風雷地獄 [Wind and thunder hell]: D
*Fu* 府 [Palace]: C
*Fu* 腑 [Receptacle]: text 3, 4, 6

*Fu* 腹 [Abdomen]: text 16
*Fu* 復 [Return]: text 18
*Fu Bi* 輔弼 [Stars Fu and Bi]: B
*Fusang gong* 扶桑宮 [Palace of the mulberry tree]: text 18
*Fushi* 伏屍[(Buried cadaver]: text 7
*Fuyi* 覆翼 [Protective wings]: text 8
*Gan* 肝 [Liver]: text 3, 4, 5, 6, 15
*Ganshen* 肝神 [Spirit of the liver]: text 3
*Gaohuang xue* 膏肓穴 [Gaohuang point]: text 10
*Gaozhen* 高真 [High perfected]: A
*Gu* 骨 [Bones]: text 5
*Guishe* 龜蛇 [Turtle and snake]: text 4
*Gujie* 骨節 [Articulation of the bones]: text 2
*Gusui* 骨髓 [Bone marrow]: text 11
*Guyu* 穀雨 [Grain rain]: D, vertebra
*Haidi* 海底 [Bottom of the sea]: text 18
*Han* 汗 [Sweat]: text 6
*Hanling dandian* 寒靈丹殿 [Cinnabar hall of the spirits of the cold]: D
*Hanlu* 寒露 [Cold dew]: B, vertebra
*Hanming* 含明 [Containing illumination]: text 3
*Haohua* 皓華 [Hoary flower]: text 7
*Heyan* 合延 [Union to longevity]: text 17
*Hou* 喉 [Larynx]: text 2, 12
*Houtian zhi jing* 後天之精 [Postcelestial essence]: text 16
*Hu* 虎 [Tiger]: text 18
*Huachi* 華池 [Flowery pond]: text 1, 10, 16
*Huagai* 華蓋 [Flowery canopy]: text 7, 10
*Huangdi* 黃帝 [Yellow Emperor]: text 8
*Huanghe* 黃河 [Yellow River]: text 2, 9
*Huanglong* 黃龍 [Yellow dragon]: text 9
*Huangting* 黃庭 [Yellow court]:D
*Huangting jing* 黃庭經 [Book of the yellow court]: text 3, 4, 5, 6, 7, 8
*Huangting xue* 黃庭穴 [Cavity of the yellow court]: text 2
*Hubing* 虎兵 [Army of tigers]: text 4
*Huijian* 慧劍 [Sword of wisdom]: E
*Hun* 魂 [*Hun* soul]: text 3, 15
*Hunshi* 魂室 [Residence of the *hun*]: text 15
*Hunting* 魂庭 [Court of the *hun* souls]: text 8
*Huo* 火 [Fire]: text 15
*Huoche diyu* 火車地獄 [Fiery chariots hell]: D

*Huotang diyu* 火湯地獄 [Boiling cauldrons hell]: D
*Jia* 頰 [Cheeks]: text 8
*Jiaji* 夾脊 [Spinal ridge]: text 10, 11
*Jiaji shuangguan* 夾脊雙關 [Double spinal pass]: text 2, 10, 11
*Jiang* 江 [River]: text 9
*Jianggong* 絳宮 [Scarlet palace]: C, text 2, 6, 10, 13
*Jiguan zhi qiao* 機關之竅 [Orifice of the pass of the pivot]: E
*Jin* 津 [Yang secretions]: text 1, 3, 5
*Jin* 金 [Metal]: text 4, 14, 18
*Jin* 筋 [Tendons]: text 3
*Jinding* 金鼎 [Metal cauldron]: text 11
*Jing* 精 [Essence]: D, text 2, 3, 4, 5, 8
*Jinjing* 金精 [Metal essence]: text 18
*Jin zhi jing* 金之精 [Essence of the metal]:
*Jingang diyu* 金剛地獄 [Vajra hell]: D
*Jinggu* 頸骨 [Neck]: text 2
*Jingshen* 精神 [Essence and spirit]: text 2
*Jingzhi* 驚蟄 [Insects awakening from hibernation]: E, vertebra
*Jinjing* 金精 [Essence of metal]: text 14, 18
*Jinqiao* 金橋 [Golden bridge]: text 2
*Jinsuo guan* 金鎖關 [Golden lock pass]: text 1
*Jiuchong tiegu* 九重鐵鼓 [Nine-tier bronze drums]: text 11
*Jlugong* 九宮 [Nine palaces]: text 1
*Jiuqiao* 九竅 [Nine orifices]: text 1, 2, 11
*Jiutian* 九天 [Nine heavens]: text 13
*Jiutou shizi* 九頭獅子 [Lion with nine heads]: text 11
*Jiuwei* 鳩尾 [Dove's tail]: text 2, 6, 13
*Jiuxiao* 九霄 [Nine empyreans]: B
*Jiuxue* 九穴 [Nine cavities]: text 1
*Jiuzhen* 九真 [Nine perfected]: A
*Jiuzhou* 九州 [Nine continents]: text 1
*Kan* 坎 [Kan trigram]: text 4, 5, 18
*Kou* 口 [Mouth]: text 2, 8
*Kun* 坤 [Kun trigram]: text 8
*Kunlun* 崑崙 [Mount Kunlun]: text 1
*Laozi* 老子: text 18
*Lei* 淚 [Tears]: text 3
*Leifu* 雷府 [Thunder palace]: B
*Leiting fu* 雷霆府 [Bureau of thunder and lightning]: text 2
*Leiting gong* 雷霆宮 [Palace of the thunder and lightning]: text 9

*Li* 離 [Li trigram]: text 13
*Lian* 蓮 [Lotus]: text 6
*Lianhua* 蓮花 [Lotus flower]: text 6
*Lianhua guan* 蓮花冠 [Lotus flower crown]: text 17
*Lianqi* 煉氣 [Refining the breath]: text 2
*Lichun* 立春 [Inception of spring]: E, vertebra
*Lidong* 立冬 [Inception of winter]: B, vertebra
*Lingbao* 靈寶 [Numinous treasure]: B
*Ling'er* 靈兒 [Numinous infant]: text 5
*Liqiu* 立秋 [Inception of autumn]: C, vertebra
*Liuchi* 琉池 [Lapis lazuli pond]: E
*Liufu* 六腑 [Six receptacles]: text 4
*Liuqi* 六氣 [Six breaths]: text 7
*Lixia* 立夏 [Inception of summer]: D, vertebra
*Long* 龍 [Dragon]: text 13
*Longhu xue* 龍虎穴 [Cavity of the dragon and the tiger]: text 11
*Longyan* 龍煙 [Vapours of the dragon]: text 3
*Longyao* 龍耀 [Dragonlight]: text 4
*Loutou gu* 樓頭鼓 [Drum on top of the pavilion]: B
*Lulu xue* 轆轤穴 [Cavity of the Winches]: text 10
*Mai* 脈 [Channel]: text 3, 8
*Mangzhong* 芒種 [Beard of grain]: D, vertebra
*Mao* 毛 [Hair]: text 6
*Maofa* 毛髮 [Hairs]: text 4
*Maokong* 毛孔 [Pore]: text 2
*Mei* 眉 [Eyebrow]: text 8
*Meixin* 眉心 [Middle of the eyebrow]: text 2
*Miluo tian* 彌羅天 [Heaven of the cosmic net]: text 1
*Ming* 命 [Vital force, destiny]: text 5, 18
*Mingdi* 命蒂 [Peduncle of the vital force]: text 10, 18
*Mingleng diyu* 冥冷地獄 [Icy hell]: D
*Mingmen* 命門 [Gate of the vital force]: D
*Mingtang* 明堂 [Hall of light]: B, text 2
*Mu* 木 [Wood]: text 3, 15
*Nanchang shanggong* 南昌上宮 [Upper palace of the southern brightness]: C
*Nangong* 南宮 [Southern palace]: text 13
*Nao* 腦 [Brain]: text 2, 7
*Naofa* 腦髮 [Brain and hair]: text 4
*Neishen* 內腎 [Inner kidneys]: text 2
*Nei shuanglin* 內雙林 [Dual internal forest]: text 10

*Niunü* 牛女 [Cowherd and weaver: text 9
*Niwan* 泥丸 [Muddy pellet]: A, B, text 1, 2, 10, 11
*Niwan gong* 泥丸宮 [Muddy Pellet Palace]: A, text 1
*Pangguang* 膀胱 [Bladder]: text 4
*Penghu* 蓬壺 [Peng pot]: text 1
*Pi* 脾 [Spleen]: Text 6, 7, 8
*Pimao* 皮毛 [Skin and hairs]: text 7
*Po* 魄 [*Po* soul]: text 3, 14
*Poshi* 魄室 [Residence of the *po* souls]: text 14
*Pulüe diyu* 普掠地獄 [Eradication of hell]: D
*Qi* 氣 [Breath]: text 2, 4, 5, 12
*Qi* 炁 [Original breath]: A, C, text 2, 3, 5, 6, 7, 8, 9, 16, 17, 18
*Qi* 臍 [Umbilicus]: D, text 2, 5, 8
*Qiao* 竅 [Orifice]: text 1, 2, 6, 8, 12
*Qihai* 氣海 [Sea of breath]: text 2, 18
*qimen* 臍門 [Gate of the umbilicus]: text 2
*qing* 情 [Passions]: text 5, 14
*Qinglong* 青龍 [Azure dragon]: text 3, 15
*Qingming* 清明 [Pure clarity]: D, vertebra
*Qiongchi* 瓊池 [Jasper pond]: E
*Qipo* 七魄 [Seven *po* souls]: 7, text 7
*Qiqiao* 七竅 [Seven orifices]: text 2
*Qiufen* 秋分 [Autumnal equinox]: C, vertebra
*Quangu shui* 泉谷水 [Water of the valley of fonts]: E
*Queyin* 雀陰 [Sparrow demon]: text 7
*Renmai* 任脈 [Function vessel]: D, text 2
*Renzhong* 人中 [Middle of the human body]: B, text 1
*Ri* 日 [Sun]: text 15
*Rou* 肉 [Flesh]: text 8
*Ruanhou* 軟喉 [Glottis]: text 2
*Sanbao* 三寶 [Three treasures]: B
*Sancha* 三叉 [Triple fork]: text 11
*Sanguan* 三關 [Three passes]: text 2
*Sanhun* 三魂 [Three *hun* souls]: C, text 3
*Sanli xue* 三里穴 [Three hamlets point]: E, text 2
*Santian* 三天 [Three heavens]: text 2
*Shang dantian* 上丹田 [Upper cinnabar field]: text 2
*Shangjiao* 上焦 [Upper heater]: text 5
*Shang jiuqiao* 上九竅 [Upper nine orifices]: text 1
*Shangzhen* 上真 [Superior perfected]: A

*Shaqi* 煞炁 [Killer breath]: D
*She* 舌 [Tongue]: text 1, 6, 12, 16
*Shen* 神 [Spirit]: A, D, text 2, 3, 4, 5, 6, 8, 15
*Shen* 腎[Kidneys]: text 1, 2, 5, 7, 16
*Shenbao* 神寶 [Divine treasure]: B
*Shengmen* 生門 [Life gate]: D, E, text 2
*Shengqi* 生炁 [Life breath]: text 5
*Shengong* 腎宮 [Palace of the kidneys]: text 17
*Shengren* 聖人 [Holy man]: E
*Shenmai* 身脈 [Channels of the body]: text 10
*Shenmen* 神門 [Gate of the spirit]: text 11
*Shenmen* 腎門 [Gate of the kidneys]: D
*Shenshi* 神室 [Divine chamber]: text 1, 13
*Shentang* 腎堂 [Hall of the kidneys]: text 2
*Shenxian* 神仙 [Divine transcendents]: text 10
*Shenzhen* 神真 [Divine perfected]: A
*Shigou* 尸狗 [Corpse dog]: text 7
*Shouling* 守靈 [Guardian of numina]: text 6
*Shuangguan* 雙關 [Double pass]: text 10
*Shuangjiang* 霜降 [Frost's descent]: B, vertebra
*Shuanglin* 雙林 [Dual forest]: text 10
*Shuangling* 爽靈 [Shining numen]: text 3
*Shui* 水 [Water]: text 4, 5, 6, 9, 10, 18
*Shuijing* 水精 [Water essence]: text 14
*Shuijing gong* 水晶宮 [Crystal palace]: text 18
*Shuiqi* 水氣 [Breath of the water]: text 4
*Shuji* 樞機 [Axe-pivot]: D
*Siqi* 死炁 [Breath of death]: text 5
*Taiguang* 台光 [Terrace light]: text 3
*Taiji* 太極 [Great ultimate]: D, text 16
*Taiyang* 太陽 [Supreme *yang*]: text 10
*Taiyi shen* 太乙神 [Spirit of the great one]: D
*Taiyi xue* 太乙穴 [Cavity of the great one]: text 9
*Taiyi* 太乙 [Great one]: B
*Taiyin* 太陰 [Supreme *yin*]: text 10
*Taizhen* 太真 [Supreme perfected]: A
*Taokang* 桃康 [Vigour of peach]: D, text 17
*Ti* 涕 [Mucous]: text 7
*Tianbao* 天寶 [Celestial treasure]: B
*Tiandi zhi gen* 天地之根 [Root of the universe]: text 18

*Tiangang* 天罡 [Celestial net]: C
*Tiangen* 天根 [Celestial root]: C
*Tianhuang zhi gong* 天皇之宮 [Palace of the heavenly sovereign]: text 1
*Tianmen* 天門 [Heavenly gate]: text 2
*Tianmu* 天目 [Celestial eye]: B
*Tianting* 天庭 [Heavenly court]: B
*Tianzhen* 天真 [Celestial perfected]: A
*Tianzhu* 天柱 [Pillar of heaven]: text 9
*Tianzhu xue* 天柱穴 [Cavity of the pillar of heaven]: text 10
*Tihu* 醍醐 [Clarified butter]: B, text 11
*Tongzhu diyu* 銅柱地獄 [Bronze pillar hell]: D
*Tu* 土 [Earth]: text 8
*Tufu* 土釜 [Earth furnace]: D, text 2
*Tuge diyu* 屠割地獄 [Butchers hell]: D
*Tunzei* 吞賊 [Devouring robber]: text 7
*Tuoyue* 橐籥 [Forge bellows]: E
*Waishen* 外腎 [Outer kidneys]: text 2
*Wai shuanglin* 外雙林 [Outer dual grove]: text 10
*Wei* 胃 [Stomach]: text 2, 8
*Weilü* 尾閭 [Caudal pass]: text 2
*Weilü guan* 尾閭關 [Caudal pass]: E, text 2, 11
*Weiming* 威明 [Majestic brightness]: text 4
*Weishen* 胃神 [Spirit of the stomach]: text 8
*Wujian diyu* 無間地獄 [Endless hell]: D
*Wuxing* 五行 [Five agents]: text 10
*Wuying* 無英 [Non-pareil): text 2, 3
*Wuying gongzi* 無英公子 [Non-pareil lordling]: C
*Wuzang* 五臟 [Five viscera]: text 4, 7, 8, 15
*Xi* 膝 [knee]: text 2
*Xia dantian* 下丹田 [Lower cinnabar field]: text 1, 2, 18
*Xiadan* 下丹 [Lower cinnabar]: D, text 10
*Xiajiao* 下焦 [Lower heater]: text 5
*Xiang* 湘 [Xiang river]: E
*Xiantian zhi jing* 先天之精 [Precelestial essence]: text 18
*Xianzhen* 仙真 [Transcendent perfected]: A
*Xianzhu* 現珠 [Apparent pearl]: B
*Xiaohan* 小寒 [Lesser cold]: E, vertebra
*Xiaoman* 小滿 [Lesser fullness of grain]: D, vertebra
*Xiaoshu* 小暑 [Lesser heat]: D, vertebra
*Xiaoxue* 小雪 [Lesser snow]: B, vertebra

*Xiazhi* 夏至 [Summer solstice]: D, vertebra
*Xin* 心 [Heart/mind]: C, text 1, 2, 3, 6, 8
*Xing* 性 [Innate nature]: text 13, 15
*Xinggen* 性根 [Root of the innate nature]: text 1
*Xingming* 性命 [Innate nature and vital force]: D
*Xinshen* 心神 [Spirit of the heart]: text 6
*Xiqiao* 鵲橋 [Bridge of the magpies]: text 1, 2, 9
*Xishan* 西山 [Western mountain]: text 14
*Xuandai* 玄袋 [Mysterious bag]: text 4
*Xuanlu* 玄鹿 [Black deer]: text 5
*Xuanguan* 玄關 [Obscure pass]: text 5
*Xuanlian* 玄蓮 [Obscure lotus]: text 6
*Xuanming* 玄冥 [Obscured darkness]: text 5
*Xuanmu* 玄母 [Mysterious mother]: B
*Xuanpao* 懸匏 [Hanging calabash: text 3
*Xuanpin* 玄牝 [Obscure female]: D, text 16
*Xuanqiong* 玄穹 [Obscure firmament]: A
*Xuanqiong zhu* 玄穹主 [Sovereign of the Obscure firmament]: text 1
*Xuanshui xiang* 玄水鄉 [Village of the dark water]: text 16
*Xuanwu shaqi* 玄武煞氣 [Death pneuma of the Dark Warrior]: D
*Xuanqing* 玄磬 [Mysterious chimestone]: text 7
*Xuanyang* 玄陽 [Mystic *yang*]: text 16
*Xuanying* 玄膺 [Mystic support]: text 12
*Xuanzhen* 玄真 [Mystic perfected]: A
*Xucheng* 虛成 [Attainment of emptiness]: text 7
*Xue* 穴 [Cavity]: text 2, 5, 6, 9, 10, 13, 16, 18
*Xue* 血 [Blood]: text 6, 10
*Xumi shan* 須彌山 [Mount Sumeru]: text 1
*Xuzhen* 虛真 [Vacuous perfected]: A
*Yan* 咽 [Pharynx]: text 2, 12
*Yan* 眼 [Eyes]: text 3, 16
*Yang* 陽: text 2, 9
*Yanggong* 陽宮 [*Yang* palace]: text 9
*Yangguan* 陽關 [*Yang* pass]: text 10
*Yangqi* 陽炁 [*Yang* breath]: text 9
*Yangqiao* 陽蹻: D
*Yangyu* 陽俞: D
*Yantong* 眼瞳 [Pupils]: text 4
*Yanyue lu* 偃月爐 [Furnace of the crescent moon]: text 2
*Yaoji* 腰脊 [Waist and spine]: text 5

*Ye* 液 [Secretions]: text 1, 3, 5, 6, 7, 15
*Yin* 陰: text 8, 16
*Yinbai* 陰白 [Hidden white]: text 8
*Ying'er* 嬰兒 [Infant]: text 7, 9, 18
*Yinguan* 陰關 [*Yin* pass]: text 11
*Yinhe* 銀河 [Milky way]: D
*Yinqiao* 陰蹻 [*Yin* stilts]: D
*Yinshen* 陰神 [*Yin* spirit]: text 9
*Yinyu* 陰俞: D
*Yonggu dao* 湧谷道 [Way of the swelling valley]: E
*Yongquan* 湧泉 [Bubbling spring]: E, text 10
*Yongquan xue* 湧泉穴 [Bubbling spring cavity]: E, text 2
*Youjing* 幽精 [Obscure essence]: text 3
*Yuanming zhenren* 元命真人 [Perfected of the primordial destiny]: A
*Yuanshen gong* 元神宮 [Palace of the primordial spirit]: text 1
*Yuchi* 玉池 [Jade pond]: text 2
*Yudi gong* 玉帝宮 [Jade Emperor palace]: A, text 1
*Yue* 月 [Moon]: text 14
*Yujing shan* 玉京山 [Jade capitoline mountain]: text 9
*Yulu* 玉爐 [Jade furnace]: E
*Yuquan* 玉泉 [Jade spring]: text 1, 16
*Yushui* 雨水 [Rain and water]: E, vertebra
*Yuzhen* 玉枕 [Jade pillow]: text 2
*Yuzhen guan* 玉枕關 [Jade pillow pass]: text 2, 9
*Zhaozhou gou* 趙州狗 [Dog of Zhaozhou]: text 16
*Zhen* 震 [Zhen trigram]: text 15
*Zhengqi* 正氣 [Correct breath]: text 6
*Zhenhu* 真虎 [Perfected tiger]: text 18
*Zhenjing* 真精 [Perfected essence]: text 16, 18
*Zhenqi* 真炁 [True original breath]: text 9
*Zhenqian* 真鉛 [Perfected lead]: text 16
*Zhenyi* 真一 [Perfected one]: text 18
*Zhenyin* 真陰 [True *yin*]: text 13
*Zhijing* 至精 [Ultimate essence]:
*Zhizhen* 至真 [Ultimate perfected]: A
*Zhong dantian* 中丹田 [Median cinnabar field]: text 2
*Zhongdi* 中地 [Central earth]: C
*Zhongjiao* 中焦 [Central heater]: text 5
*Zhuling huofu* 朱陵火府 [Fire palace of the vermilion mound]: C
*Zhuque* 朱雀 [Vermilion sparrow]: text 6

*Zi heche* 紫河車 [Purple hydraulic chariot]: text 16
*Zishi* 子時 [Period of *zi*]: text 18
*Ziwei* 紫微 [Purple tenuity]: B
*Zugong* 祖宮 [Ancestral palace]: text

CHAPTER 4

# The Main Alchemical Loci Inscribed in the *Chart for the Cultivation of Perfection*

From the physical layout of the map, we now analyze its contents. My principal aim is to regroup the information to make comprehensible the processes and methods which are involved in this representation. I will also determine the Taoist context this Chart was elaborated. To this end, I focus on four aspects of the drawings, the texts and inscriptions: body sites specific to Internal Alchemy, divinities located in the body, alchemical methods, and processes of thunder evoked. This chapter focuses on the principal sites of the body which bear specific names in Taoism and internal alchemy, such as the cinnabar fields, the three passes of the back and the "obscure pearl" designating the meeting place of yin and yang.

This chapter also looks at the resonance between the map and conceptions of the body common in Chinese medicine such as the eight marvellous vessels and the twelve meridians. My reason for addressing them here is two-fold: on the one hand, they play an essential role in the process of self-transformation. On the other hand, this conception of the body receives a different interpretation in the Taoist context than is given in Chinese medicine. I will not present all the alchemical places (it would represent a task beyond the scope of this study of the map), but the main loci useful for understanding the processes of Inner Alchemy for the cultivation of the self. Some other loci will be discussed in coordination with the thunder rites; we have left aside, for example, the different lakes or ponds which will be discussed in the last chapter in connection with the thunder rites.

I will study the alchemical sites of the body by first making a brief historical reconstruction of the origin of its terminology, their evolution in the different Taoist contexts and the various currents until the appearance of the Internal alchemy where they have become predominant, have been reinterpreted, or even more detailed. Thus it is possible to retrace the evolution of the main concepts associated with this chart and to specify the context in which this card appeared. It will help us to have a better understanding of the text on these loci inscribed on the *Chart for the Cultivation of Perfection*.

The main sites are as follows: the orifices of the body on which the Southern alchemical tradition coming from Zhang Boduan more emphasizes; the three

 DOI:10.1163/9789004383456_006

cinnabar fields, for which an obvious kinship was detected with the *Rushi wowen* 如是我聞 [Thus I have heard], an anonymous and undated text included in the *Daozang Xubian* [Sequel to the Taoist canon] compiled by Min Yide (1834) of the Dragon Gate tradition from Mount Jin'gai (Jin'gai shan 金蓋山); the three passes of the back; the throat; the gate of the vital force (*mingmen* 命門); the area of the kidneys; and the eight marvellous vessels.

## 1 The Microcosmic Body Becomes an Athanor

The transformation processes in the body occur in a closed circuit, just like the athanor of the alchemist, hence the need to establish a circuit and to close all openings of the body. In other words, nothing was supposed to escape from the body from its lower orifices, nor through the pores of the skin, much less through the orifices of the face, which correspond to the main sense organs. Most of the alchemical transformations take place in the head and in the trunk, while the limbs are accessories. During a cycle in the circulation in breath/energy (*qi* 氣) in the closed circuit (this is shown on the maps representing the body as a mountain, see figs. 1.10 and 1.11), there would be an increase of the breath from the genitals at the top of the head. This is followed by a decrease from the head into the abdomen. This circuit constitutes a key element of these transformations. Sitting in the lotus position in which the legs and arms are folded facilitates the implementation of this closed circuit.

Among the names of ingredients mentioned is a fairly wide range of minerals used in operative alchemy: cinnabar, lead, mercury or silver liquid, metal essence and yellow gold. These terms refer in inner alchemy to physiological and psychic "ingredients" of the person, such as bodily fluids, spermatic energy, the circulating breaths within the body, thoughts, emotions, inner light, innate nature, and so on. Certain metaphors become the alchemical allegory of three elements which are commonly referred to in Taoism as the "vital essence" (*jing* 精), the "breath/energy," and the "spirit" or "spiritual force" (*shen* 神). In addition to these ingredients are the breaths of the five agents (earth, metal, water, wood, fire) that correspond to the energy of the five viscera of the body (the liver, the heart, the spleen, the lungs, the kidneys), as well as the receptacles coupled to these (the gallbladder, the small intestine, the stomach, the large intestine and the bladder). In general, texts on internal alchemy develop in particular the use of two of these elements, water and fire, in a continuous cycle of the rise of internal heat from the abdomen to the top of the head and of the fall of watery discharge from the head into the abdomen. The circulation and the exchanges between the two are at the core of the psychophysiological transformations.

The body becomes an alchemical laboratory or athanor. But it is also a microcosm, a true internal landscape, in which the eyes become the sun and the moon, the head, the Mount Kunlun, the hair, the vegetation, and so on. This image of the body as a microcosm was not unknown in the West. In his *Elucidarium*, Honorius d'Autun (twelfth century) writes: "Man is a reduced world. His flesh corresponds to earth, his blood to water, his breath to air, his vital heat to fire; his head is round like the celestial sphere, the two eyes shine like the sun and the moon, the seven openings in the face correspond to the seven spheres of harmony."[1]

The analogy between the universe and the body that developed in China as early as the third century BCE was used in the medical context as well as in scholastic writings. One of the greatest scholars of the Han dynasty, Dong Zhongshu 董仲舒 (179–104 BCE), details the connections between the macrocosm and the microcosm as follows:

> Man has 360 joints because the macrocosmic orbit has 360 degrees. The body with bones and flesh corresponds to the earth with its thickness. On the upper part, the ears and the eyes correspond to the sun and the moon. The body has channels and orifices, like the earth has valleys and rivers. The person experiences grief, pleasure, joy, anger, which are similar to the vital spirits and the breaths in the cosmos. The head is above the body, round like the sky. The hair is similar to the stars and constellations. The ears and the eyes, quick in their perceptions, are like the moon and the sun. The breath of the nostrils and the mouth are similar to wind and air. In the chest, the penetrating knowledge of the mind corresponds to the celestial and terrestrial spirits of the world. The abdomen and the bowels sometimes full and sometimes empty, are similar to the growth and the decay of all things. As these things are close to the earth, the portion of the body below the waist corresponds to the earth, and the waist is like a belt. The majestic and spiritual part above the neck manifests the characteristics and the nature of heaven. The part below the neck is full and humble, like the earth. The feet are spread, flat, like the earth. It follows that, when the scholar wears his belt adorned with the ceremonial pendants, his neck should be straight to be distinguished from the heart. The part above the waist is yang, below is

1 Gilson 1988–1: 327.

> yin, and each part plays its own role. Yang is the breath of heaven, the yin, that of the earth. When yin and yang become active, maybe the individual will suffer from a pain in the feet or a constriction in the throat; thus, the breath of the earth rises and becomes clouds and rain.
>
> The harmony of heaven and earth and the correspondence between the yin and yang are forever established in the human body. The body is like heaven. Their numerical categories are in mutual correspondence, and their lives are closely bound. The sky perfects the human body by the number of days in a full year. 366 small joints of the body correspond to the number of days in the year and the twelve major joints to the number of months in a year. The body contains five viscera corresponding to the five agents. Outside, it has four members corresponding to the four seasons. The alternating opening and closing of the eyes is like day and night. The alternation of strength and weakness corresponds to summer and winter. The alternation of sorrow and pleasure corresponds to yin and yang. The mind evolves in correspondence with the degrees of revolution. The conduct of man adapts to the correspondences between heaven and earth. All this, either clear or hidden in the body, is born with man. When the being is in resonance with heaven and earth, the correspondences are established. For everything that can be counted, we can establish numerical correlations. Those things that cannot be counted have correlations that are established according to categories. There is identity and correspondence with heaven. Heaven and man are one. This is the reason why I expose that which has shape to make manifest that which does not, and embrace what can be counted to make manifest what cannot be.[2]

This microcosm/macrocosm correlation is, needless to say, heavily developed in Upper Clarity Taoist circles, and later by the various traditions of Inner Alchemy that appear as early as the tenth century. The meditative techniques of these writers make great use of the above symbolism, which is also found on the *Chart*, as well as the world of plants. The search for immortality has been associated with the tradition of metallurgy workers whose patron saint was the mythical Yellow Emperor, and with the tradition of farmers and specialists of the pharmacopeia whose patron saint was another mythical sovereign, the Divine Ploughman (Shennong 神農). They used various plants, either alone or

2 See Dong Zhongshu's 董仲舒 *Chunqiu fanlu* 春秋繁露 [Luxuriant gems of the spring and autumn] 13.2a–3b.

associated with minerals, to produce immortality drugs or provide strict diets as a substitute for ordinary food until the complete cessation of ingesting solid food, replaced by the absorption of breaths. These techniques of breathing and the progressive fast are similar to those of some yoga techniques. They were interpreted and expressed in the Inner Alchemy with symbols referring not only to the chemistry of minerals but also to the register of plants and agricultural techniques.

In Inner Alchemy, the analogy serves as an internalization of the world, whether its mythical history with its legends, or the world with its organised space, with the sun, the moon, the earth, water, or then again, the mechanism of the universe with its references to the fire phasing in alchemy and to time. This internalization is an appropriation and an integration of the outside world within the body. The vocabulary designating different parts of the body and its organs is not developed; the texts mention only a few basic terms of the physiology also used in Chinese medicine. These terms designate elements of the body that are not completely equivalent in Western anatomy and physiology. These include the five viscera, the vital essence, the breath and the spirit. This internalization and integration concludes with a dismantling of the barriers between inner and outer or between the body and the cosmos.

Of course, this transformation process would not be possible without the dynamic imagination or creative thinking (*yi* 意), which emanates from the mind (*xin* 心) and presides at any transformation. Only a peaceful mind ensures the success of the alchemical transformations. The adept progressively becomes the master of his body and mind, the master of the world and of the transformations before, in a final stage, dissolving himself into emptiness and letting the marvellous mechanism of creations and transformations unfold.

The importance of intention (or creative thinking) and the use of analogy were not specific to Chinese alchemists. Some Westerners have also focused on these two elements, as mentioned by the anonymous author of the *Rosaire des philosophes*, who writes:

> The philosophers have said, in all their words, the truth about the stone. They talked about the power of words to hide the truth from the unworthy. Regarding the power of intention, they spoke to those who were worthy, always revealing truth, and philosophers know that such material must be delivered in mystery, as poetry proceeds in fables and parables.[3]

3 *Rosaire des philosophes* 2008: 110.

The correspondence between the body/microcosm and the universe, the description of the body as inner landscape and mythical heaven as well as the main alchemical loci are described in the texts inscribed on the upper left and right of the *Chart for the Cultivation of Perfection.*

## 2 The Main Body Orifices and Places of Transmutations

### 2.1 *The Main Body Orifices* (*the Upper Left Text*)

The upper left text explains the symbolism of heaven and earth in the body with the nine areas of heaven (i.e., nine chambers in the head) and the nine provinces on earth (i.e., nine cavities of the lower cinnabar field). The nine palaces are situated in the head: to the south the Upper Heavenly Palace (*shang tiangong*), to the south-west the Obscure Spiral Palace (*xuanwei gong*), to the west Blue-green Fruit Palace (*Cangguo gong*), to the northwest the New Net Palace (*Xinluo gong*), to the north the Scorpion Sheet Palace (*Yechi gong*), to the northeast the Heavenly Abode Palace (*Tianliu gong*), to the east the Blue-green Gate Palace (*Cangmen gong*) and to the southeast the Luoyin Palace (*Luoyin gong*). The Great One (*Taiyi*), both star and invisible deity, walks, according to the seasons, in each of these palaces. The *Pivot of Numinous Spirits*, a medical text compiled around the first century, includes a chapter titled "The Eight Winds and the Nine Palaces," which is one of the oldest extant documents describing the Nine Palaces.[4] They are aligned according to the eight-wind compass, a divination technique common in ancient China, a copy of which has been found during archaeological excavations.[5] This is what justifies the presence of such a chapter in a medical source, as in antiquity, divining, diagnostic and therapeutic methods were closely related. In this text, the nine celestial palaces cavities in the head correspond in the body to nine heavenly palaces; the head is symbolically the heaven in the human body.

The nine continents are the nine provinces determined by Yu the Great, who oversaw great water and land management projects. The names of the continents are: Jizhou, Yuezhou, Qingzhou, Xuzhou, Yangzhou, Jingzhou,

4 *Lingshu jing* 靈樞經 [Pivot of the spirits], *juan* 11, fascicle 77.

5 See Kalinowski 1983: 318n4: "The Taiyi table was used in the context of a semantic system called 'the circulation of the Great One (Taiyi) in the nine palaces' (*Taiyi jiugong* 太一九宮)" (Yan 1982: 86–90). The earliest references to the method of implementation of this system are described in the *Yiwei qianzuo du* 易緯乾鑿度, in *Jūshū Isho Shusei*, eds. Shohachi Nakamura 中村璋八 and Yasui Kosan 安居香山, 1.1: 41–42 and *Huangdi neijing Lingshu jing* 黃帝內經靈樞經, fascicle 77. Through archaeological discoveries, there is now an almost intact copy from the early Han." This compass is described in *Wenwu* (1978, issue 8): 16, 25.

Yuzhou, Yongzhou and Liangzhou.[6] In the human body, they are, according to the *Chart for the Cultivation of Perfection*, nine orifices in the lower cinnabar field. This is an original interpretation we have not found elsewhere. Some divination scriptures on physiognomy established correspondences between the nine provinces and parts of the face or areas of the body. Writings on Inner Alchemy preserved in the Taoist Canon associated the nine provinces with organs. For example, Xiao Daocun 蕭道存 (ca. 13th cen.) draws the following correspondences: the kidneys correspond to Jizhou, the bladder to Xuzhou, the liver to Qingzhou, the gallbladder to Yuezhou, the heart to Yangzhou, the small intestine to Jingzhou, the lungs to Liangzhou, the large intestine to Yongzhou.[7] The ninth, Yuzhou, is missing; it corresponds to the spleen according to another text, which matches Yuezhou with the gallbladder (instead of Xuzhou) and Xuzhou, with the bladder.[8] While it may be common in China to match the nine regions of ancient China with parts of the body, the association made by the *Chart for the Cultivation of Perfection* between these nine provinces and the lower cinnabar field appears to be an original one. It is further explained that the lower cinnabar field is the earthly part of the human body, while the head corresponds to the heavens. It is a good example of how the analogy works and changes depending on the Taoist schools. It doesn't matter that the correspondences are not always the same; the essential is to establish heaven and earth in the body.

The upper left of the text lists the other main orifices of the head. The orifices play an essential role in Inner Alchemy. A text attributed to Zhang Boduan 張伯端 (987–1082), but more probably written by a disciple, emphasizes the importance of these openings, called "breath palaces":

> The orifices of body hair are the 84,000 breath palaces. Of these, 384 hair holes let the breath escape. The breath cavity in the centre of the navel is the principal of these 384 palaces. Underneath this is the peak of the yang essence. The heart is the Median Cinnabar Field, the top of the head is the Upper Cinnabar Field. Under the tongue is the Xuanying 玄膺 point. There are also openings in the eye called the "silver sea" (*yinhai* 銀海), an orifice between the eyebrows, the bit between the mouth and the nose,

6 See "The Tributes of Yu" (Yugong 禹貢), *Shangshu zhengyi* 尚書正義, in *Shisan jing zhushu* 十三經注疏, 1979: 6.34–42 [pp. 146–153].

7 Xiao Daocun, *Xiuzhen Taiji hunyuan tu* (DZ 149), 13.

8 See the chapter "Revelation of the mystery in the Cultivation of Perfection," in *Daoshu* (DZ 1017), 19.11b. See Baldrian-Hussein 1984: 153.

> openings beside the eyes and ears, along the sides of the pharynx and larynx, and between the ribs.[9]

Some of these orifices are mentioned in the *Chart for the Cultivation of the Perfection* citing, for example the orifices of the mouth and the tongue, the bit between the base of the nose and the upper lip, the "middle of man" (*renzhong* 人中).

The translation of the upper-left text (fig. 3.6, text 1) is as follows:

> Heaven has nine palaces and earth has nine provinces. In the human body, the lower cinnabar field comprises nine orifices,[10] which are the image of the nine provinces on earth. The Muddy Pellet Palace (in the head) has nine cavities corresponding to the nine heavenly palaces. The brain bones form eight sectors corresponding to the eight directions. They constitute the Cosmic Net Heaven (*Miluo tian* 彌羅天), the Jade Emperor Palace (*Yudi gong*)[11] or the Heavenly Palace of Pure Yang (*Chunyang tiangong* 純陽天宮).[12] The centre is a cavity called Primordial Spirit Palace (*Yuanshen gong* 元神宮) or [Heaven] of the Obscure Firmament (*Xuanqiong* 玄瓊).[13] The mouth contains the tongue underneath which is the Golden Lock (*jinsuo guan* 金鎖關) which is also called the Bridge of the Magpies.[14] Under the nose the point "middle of man"[15] is located

9 *Yuqing jinsi qinghua biwen jinbao neilian danjue* [Alchemical formula for the inner purification of the gold treasure; secret writings from the golden box of the Jade Purity heaven, transmitted by the immortal Qinghua] (DZ 240), 1.14b–15a.

10 These nine orifices establish the communication with the outside and lead, according to this commentary, to the nine hells.

11 The chapter "Tianzhong zhang" 天中章 in the *Book of the Yellow Court* reads: "When the numinous residence is purified, the Jade Emperor walks within." See DZ 402, 1.10b.

12 This is probably an allusion to Lü Dongbin 吕洞賓, one of the most famous eight immortals and one of the most revered deities in Taoism during the Ming and Qing dynasties. This divinity is indeed also known as Lü Chunyang 吕純陽 or "Lü of the Pure Yang." Furthermore, in Chinese medicine, the head is considered as the meeting place of all the yang breaths; it corresponds to heaven.

13 The Heaven of the Obscure Firmament (*Xuanqiong*) is equivalent to the "Obscure Heaven" (*xuantian* 玄天), it designates the Northern Heaven. See *Gaoshang Yuhuang benxing jijing* 高上玉皇本行集經 [Combined scriptures of the founding acts of the Jade Emperor on high] (DZ 10), a text of the Southern Song or Yuan. The text is associated with the Jade Emperor, who lives in this Heaven of the Obscure Firmament.

14 The word "mouth" is absent from the version of the White Cloud Temple.

15 It is the name of an acupuncture point on the Control Vessel (*dumai*), more commonly known as the "water rivulet" (*shuigou* 水溝).

at the Gold Lock, between the two are the Control Vessel, basis and root of man, the upper nine orifices or root of the innate nature. The mouth[16] is called the Jade Spring (*yuquan* 玉泉)[17] or the Flowery Pond (*huachi* 華池).[18] Four orifices are open under the tongue. Two of them communicate with the heart and produce yin fluids (*ye* 液), while the other two communicate with the kidneys and produce yang fluids (*jin* 津).[19] In reality, the divine chamber and the nine orifices of the Muddy Pellet Palace are collectively called the Heavenly Sovereign Palace.[20] In the centre are found a cavity that has the shape of a hen's egg,[21]

---

16 This term is present on the Mount Wudang version, but missing on that of the White Cloud Temple.

17 Term already used in the Tang commentary by Liangqiu zi of the *Book of the Yellow Court* in *Yunji qiqian* (DZ 1032, 11.17a): "At the obscure spring, the dark porticos stands, majestic"; Liangqiu zi comments: "The obscure spring designates the liquor of the mouth which is also called the Jade Spring (*yuquan*) or the Nectar Spring (*liquan* 醴泉), or the Jade Secretions (*yujin* 玉津) or the Jade Stock (*yujiang* 玉漿). In *Yangxing yanming lu* 養性延命錄 [Records on preserving one's nature and lengthening life], a text attributed to Tao Hongjing 陶弘景, but most likely dating from the Tang Dynasty, although written from fragments of *Yangsheng yaoji* 養生要集 by Zhang Zhan 張湛 of the Jin Dynasty, it is said: "Drinking at the Jade Spring, we can live longer and eliminate disease" (DZ 1032, 32.16a) or "Grind one's teeth, rinse the mouth with the Jade Spring, and swallow it three times" (DZ 1032, 32. 21a).

18 This term is already used in the commentary by Liangqiu zi of the *Book of the Yellow Court*. See *Yunji qiqian* (DZ 1032, 11.18a): "Within the central pond, the deity wears red pearls"; Liangqiu zi comments: "The gallbladder is the central pond, below the tongue is the Flowery Pond, the womb and the lower abdomen are the Jade Pond." DZ 1032, 12. 20a: "The mouth is called the Jade Pond or the Flowery Pond" (commentary by Liangqiu zi). DZ 1032, 81.11b contains a text on Gengshen 庚申: "Under the tongue is the Flowery Pond, which communicates with the kidneys pond and must never dry out."

19 This term is present on the Mount Wudang version, but missing on that of the White Cloud Temple.

20 Nine holes of the upper cinnabar field are mentioned in *Shangqing dadong zhenjing* 上清大洞真經 [Perfected scripture of the great cavern of Upper Clarity]: "First, keep the gates of the nine holes of the Muddy Pellet and the doors of the deadly breath constantly closed. This will strengthen the Muddy Pellet so that it will harden like jade and the brilliance of gold, illuminating the true body and giving rise to the precious light, so that the nine orifices receive the magical efficiency and that the seven generations of ancestors starting from our parents obtain a lasting peace, are delivered from the karmic faults (of past lives) and have access to the Upper Clarity." (DZ 6, 2.8b).

21 It was the dominant conception of the universe under the Han. Zhang Heng 張衡 said in his commentary on the armillary sphere: "The sky is like a hen's egg, the earth as the egg yolk in its centre." Similarly, in the West in the Middle Ages, a mystic of the Rhineland, Hildegard of Bingen (1098–1179), compared the world to an egg.

> the Lotus Terrace[22] and Mount Kunlun[23] that Buddhists call Mount Sumeru.[24] Those who cultivate the perfection should be aware of this.

If the White Cloud Temple version stops here, the Mount Wudang version has an additional paragraph:

> This representation of the body highlights body orifices for those searching for the Way. It is said that the Obscure Palace receives the breath; it causes lightning and is the Palace of the Spirit, where the three sources meet. Here there is no distinction between the vital essence, the *hun* souls, the *po* souls, and the principal spirit (*shen*) that meet in this cavity. This is the root of Returning to the Origin in the making of the golden elixir; it is the place where the holy embryo is perfected.

The version of Moli near the Taihu Lake also adds a long paragraph to the end of the text as it is found on the White Cloud Temple version. This paragraph is entitled "Formulas and Song on the accomplishment of cinnabar by the

22 I could not find mention of the term "lotus terrace" in Taoist texts. There is a phrase in the *Yuanshi wuliang duren shangpin miaojing neiyi* that mentions a "Wormwood Terrace" (*Xiaotai* 蕭臺): "The sky in the heaven of the great cosmic breath, the upper capital of the Jade Mountain and the wormwood of the Yuluo heaven." Commentary by Xiao Yingsou: "Above the Daluo heaven is the Jade Mount on which is built a city of seven jewels with the Obscure Terrace of seven gems in the Palace of the Jade Clarity, home of the eminent Jade Emperor." (DZ 90, 10a). According to the *Yuanshi wuliang duren shangpin miaojing tongyi*, a commentary by Zhang Yuchu, "the Wormwood Terrace of the Yuluo Heaven, is in the human body on the edges of the brain (*naoji* 腦際). The upper capital of Jade Mountain is the Niwan, which is the heavenly abode of the ten thousand deities." (DZ 89, 2.6a–b). In Buddhism, the lotus terrace or throne is the throne upon which the Buddhas and Bodhisattvas take their place. The version of the White Cloud Temple does not have this term "Lotus Terrace."

23 Mount Kunlun, located to the west or to the northwest of the world, is often considered to be the paradise of the Queen Mother of the West (Xi wangmu 西王母). All body maps preceding our Chart also designate the head as Mount Kunlun. The *Huangting neijing yujing zhu*, for example, reads: "The rolling pearls of the Great One calm the Kunlun"; Liangqiu zi comments: "The rolling pearls of the Great One are the epitome of the heart." It is said in the *Dongshenjing* 洞神經 [Scripture on the cavern spirit]: "The head is the Lord of the Three Terraces, and the Kunlun is the Upper Cinnabar Field." The author further writes: 'The navel is the Lord of Taiyi and Kunlun, it indicates the lower cinnabar field." See DZ 402, 2.14a.

24 The Mount Wudang version does not have the last part "The Buddhists call it Mount Sumeru."

ninefold revolution, according to the Emperor of Darkness (Xuandi 玄帝)," that is to say Zhenwu 真武, the True Warrior, also known as the "Upper Sovereign of Obscure Heaven" (Xuantian Shangdi 玄天上帝). It includes the following new lines:

1) Ascension to perfection by the breath of the One.
2) The earth ship welcomes yang.
3) The exchange between heaven and earth form the hexagram *tai* [Stability].
4) The sun and the moon perform their revolution together.
5) Mother and child return to the Origin.
6) The light of the Three Terraces illuminates the interior.
7) The Great Ultimate divides and creates the great coincidence.
8) A millet pearl glows in the pot of darkness.
9) The ten thousand phenomena are united at the Origin.

### 2.2 *The Main Passage Sites and Places of Alchemical Transmutations (Upper Right Text)*

While the upper left text mostly concerns the head, the upper right text describes the principal alchemical locations of the whole body. It details the two aspects of the body as a microcosm and as a sacred place with heavens and hells. It includes descriptions of the places involved in the three main phases of the transmutations in Inner Alchemy, with the three passes in the back that are difficult to pass, as well as three cinnabar fields in the front which are discussed in detail below. Here is the translation of the upper right text (fig. 3.6, text 2):

> The human body has 360 joints[25] and 84,000 pores.[26] In the rear part are the three passes: the Caudal Pass (*Weilü* 尾閭), the Spinal Handle Pass (*Jiaji* 夹脊) and the Jade Pillow Pass (*Yuzhen* 玉枕). The Caudal Pass is located at the bottom of the spinal column and communicates with the internal orifice of the kidneys; it is the starting point of the spinal cord,

25 See *Chunqiu fanlu*, 13.2a–3b: "The man has 360 joints, which corresponds to the celestial degrees of the macrocosmic orbit."

26 The number 84,000 is common in Buddhist texts. It is used in a text by a disciple of Zhang Boduan (987–1082), quoted above: *Yuqing jinsi qinghua biwen jinbao neilian danjue* (DZ 240), 14b–15a.

called Cao Stream,[27] or Yellow River,[28] and that is the path where yang ascends. The yang passes between the two kidneys, the Spinal Handle Pass, ascends to the Jade Pillow Pass and continues up to the brain. These are the three passes in the back. In the front part of the body are the three cinnabar fields: the Muddy Pellet (*Niwan*), the Earth Furnace (*tufu* 土釜) and the Jade Pond (*yuchi* 玉池). The Muddy Pellet is the upper cinnabar field. It measures 1.2 inches on its side. This port is the Empty Pass (*xuguan* 虛關); this is where the spirit lives (*shen* 神). It is located right in the centre of the head, in the space between the eyebrows. At an inch past the Heavenly Gate (*tianmen* 天門)[29] inside the head is the Hall of Light (Mingtang 明堂); an inch further is the Cavern Chamber (*dongfang* 洞房), and one inch more, is the Muddy Pellet.[30] Below the gap between the two eyebrows is the bridge of the nose; this place is also called the Palace of Thunder and Lightning. Inside the space between the eyebrows is the Golden Bridge (*jinqiao* 金橋).[31] Further down, in the mouth, are two orifices connected to the throat and called the Bridge of the Magpies (*xiqiao*). The larynx is at the level of the heart; this is the place where external and internal breaths enter and exit. To the rear of the pharynx is the place where liquid and solid foods enter and exit; this communicates with the upper orifice of the stomach, the Gate of the Stomach. From

27 Cao Stream (Caoxi 曹溪) is the name of the place where the sixth patriarch of Chan Buddhism, Huineng 慧能, would have experienced enlightenment on hearing the reading of the *Diamond Sutra*. In Inner Alchemy, Cao Stream is a metaphor used relatively late to indicate the spinal cord, which therefore becomes the path to enlightenment. The earliest occurrence we found is in Jin Yueyan's 金月巖 *Baoyi zi Sanfeng laoren danjue* 抱一子三峰老人丹訣 [Alchemical instructions of the old man of the three peaks, the Master who Holds the One] (DZ 281), 15b. Caoxi is also mentioned in the *Xingming guizhi* 性命圭旨 [Principles of the tablets on the innate nature and the vital force] by Yin zhenren 尹真人 (fl. 17th cen.): "Unite heaven and man, pick the remedy and enclose it in the pot." According to the *Rushi wowen* 如是我聞 [Thus I have heard], a 19th-century text included in *Daozang xubian* of 1834 at Mount Jin'gai (Zhejiang) by Min Yide, Caoxi corresponds to the Caudal Pass (Weilü). This collection is mainly devoted to the teachings and practices of Internal Alchemy; cf. Esposito 2005 (2): 347–350.

28 This text is fully incorporated in the *Rushi wowen*, lb.

29 That is to say, the vertex on the top of the head.

30 Text similar in the *Rushi wowen*, 1b–2a.

31 One of the earliest occurrences of this term "Golden Bridge" is in the *Leiting mochao neiyin* 雷霆默朝内音, *Daofa huiyuan* (DZ 1220), 72.1a. The Golden Bridge is also mentioned in the *Rushi wowen*, 2a: "Below the space between the eyebrows is the ridge of the nose, with inside the Golden Bridge. Two orifices lead down to the mouth and communicate with the throat." But this text (published in 1834) does not mention the Palace of Thunder and Lightning.

the larynx rise twelve-storey rings: this is the twelve-storey pagoda that rises to the lung orifice and the heart.[32] The bone called the Dove's Tail (xiphoid tip of the sternum) protects the heart. Below the heart, there is a cavity called the Scarlet Palace (*Jianggong*); this is where the tiger and the dragon meet and join together.[33] Heading down 3.6 inches, one reaches the furnace or Palace of the Yellow Court; this corresponds to the median cinnabar field. It is flanked on the left by the Hall of Light and on the right by the Cavern Chamber. On the left, at the level of the liver, abides the Nonpareil Lordling (*Wuying*).[34] At the right is the lung, residence of the White Prime (*Baiyuan*).[35] This place is a cavity of 1.2 inches, and it is the abode of the breath and is the chamber from which it is refined.[36] If we continue further down 3.6 inches, we arrive at the navel. This is why it is said: "The extent of the heaven is thirty-six, that of land, thirty-six; heaven and earth are separated by 84,000."[37] The heart and the kidneys are separated by 8.4 inches.[38] The heart, which corresponds to heaven, measures 3.6 inches, the kidneys, which correspond to the earth, measure 3.6 inches. Between the two, the median cinnabar field measures 1.2 inches. In all, this is 8.4 inches.[39] The door of the navel is called the Life Gate (*shengmen* 生門). There are seven orifices which communicate with the external kidneys from where flows the vital essence and the vital spirits, and that is called the Furnace of the Bowl-shaped Crescent Moon (*yanyue lu*

32 The *Huangting neijing yujing zhu* reads: "The pagoda consists of twelve rings" (*chongchong louge shier huan* 重重樓閣十二環). The Tang commentary by Liangqiu zi says: "This denotes the pharynx, the larynx, and the twelve rings (of the trachea) which pile-up over the heart." See DZ 402, 19.14b.

33 The location of the meeting place below the heart is common in the Southern School, most notably in Zhang Boduan's *Yuqing jinsi qinghua jinbuo neilian danjue* where it is said: "The orifice below the heart is the place where the meeting and the union take place." See DZ 240, 2.6b.

34 Name of the deity of the liver, according to the *Book of the Yellow Court*.

35 Name of the deity of the lungs, according to the *Book of the Yellow Court*.

36 Text similar to that of the *Rushi wowen*, 2a.

37 See the chapter "Union of Yin and Yang" in *Bichuan Zhengyang zhenren lingbao bifa* 秘傳正陽真人靈寶秘法 [Secret transmission of Master Zhengyang's complete method of the numinous treasure]: "Heaven and earth are distant from each other by 84,000 *li*." See DZ 1191, 1a.

38 See *Bichuan Zhengyang zhenren lingbao bifa* (DZ 1191) translated by Baldrian-Hussein 1984: 203: "The heart and the kidneys are distant each other from 8.4 inches. This corresponds to the distance between the sheltering sky and the supporting earth.

39 The text is similar in *Rushi wowen*, 2a.

> 偃月爐).[40] At the bottom of the Function Vessel are nine orifices which are the gates of hells and the City of Darkness (Fengdu); this place is also called the Sea of Breath (*qihai* 氣海). If we continue down about 1.3 inches, we arrive at the Jade Pond (*yuchi*), i.e., the lower cinnabar field, which houses the essence, and is where the medicine is accumulated. It is flanked on the right and left by the Hall of Light and the Cavern Chamber, and measures 1.2 inches. At this point, there are two orifices that communicate with the internal kidneys.[41] In the kidneys, there are ports that communicate with the Caudal Pass, then from the Caudal Pass to the two external kidneys (gonads), descending under the knees to the Three Lanes,[42] then to the Bubbling Spring under the soles of the feet.[43] These are the main orifices, crossing and connection points of the body.

This second text gives a more detailed description of cinnabar fields than all previous nineteenth century sources we could find; it is quite similar to a fragment of the *Rushi wowen* 如是我聞 [Thus I have heard], an anonymous text of the Dragon Gate tradition included in the *Complement to the Taoist Canon* by Min Yide 閔一得 (1834). Some use terms, such as the Palace of Thunder and Lightning, the hells, the City of Darkness, and the kidney orifices that communicate with the Caudal Pass. The presence of these terms indicates a close relationship between the *Chart for the Cultivation of Perfection* and the Thunder Rites that will be examined latter.

## 3 The Cinnabar Fields

Since the beginnings of Taoism, the cinnabar fields in the abdomen, the heart and the brain have been the main areas in which the adept concentrates during his sexual practices and in his breathing or visualizing exercises. It is the same for the Internal Alchemy practices. The name "cinnabar field" (*dantian* 丹田) evokes both the tradition of farmers by the term "field" and of the alchemists

40 *Rushi wowen*, 2b. This crescent moon, shaped like a furnace, designates the yin furnace of the abdomen. When yang is born within the yin, Jade Stamen would appear in the furnace. This metaphor is used in the *Wuzhen pian zhushi* 悟真篇註釋 [Explanation of the stanzas for awakening Perfection] by Zhang Boduan: "The jade elixir is created in the furnace shaped like the crescent moon." DZ 145, 2.8b.

41 *Rushi wowen*, 2b.

42 In acupuncture, Three Lanes is the 36th point on the stomach channel.

43 In acupuncture, Bubbling Spring is the first point on the kidney channel.

by the term "cinnabar." The cinnabar is red, like blood or sunlight.[44] It is a sulphide of mercury, basis of alchemical transmutations, the prima materia for the philosopher's stone.

In China, the term cinnabar dates no later than 165 where there is a reference to the "cinnabar furnace" (*danlu* 丹爐) on the "Inscription on Laozi."[45] The *locus classicus* for the term "cinnabar field" is in Ge Hong's (281–341?), the *Master who Embraces Simplicity*.[46] Ge, who practised the operative alchemy, writes about a single place in the body: "The breath enters from the hut [nose] to the cinnabar field."[47] The group of three cinnabar fields appears a century or two later in the *Book of the Yellow Court*: "In the three fields, the quintessence of the breath is subtle." Liangqiu zi's 梁丘子 commentary from the Tang Dynasty adds:

> This expression is a metaphor for the interior of the body. The cinnabar field encloses the divine breath, which is in resonance with the heart and transforms itself. It is neither existing nor non-existing, we cannot assign it any colour or any appearance, it is the obligatory passage when one leaves the field of coarse elements to enter that of subtle elements. The breath, ruled by the heart, takes different forms according to the orders given by the master. It is refined, subtle, and cannot be searched for repeatedly.[48]

The descriptions and the texts on cinnabar fields used on the *Chart for the Cultivation of Perfection* are almost word for word the same as in the *Thus I Have Heard*. Without the precise date of the first copy of the *Chart for the Cultivation of Perfection* and of *Thus I Have Heard* of the 1834 Taoist Canon, it is difficult to determine which text predates the other, or if both texts have a common ur-source. But the close relationship between the two is obvious.

---

44 See Pregadio 1991: 543–639.

45 See *Laozi ming* 老子銘, translated by Anna Seidel 1969: 47–48. Seidel translated as "hut" (*lu* 廬), but this character was also a borrowed term for *lu* 爐 [Furnace], the reading which seems preferable here.

46 *Baopu zi neipian jiaoshi* 抱朴子內篇校釋, 18.296.

47 *Taishang huangting waijing yujing* [Precious book on the outer landscape of the Yellow Court] (DZ 332), 1.1a.

48 *Huanting neijing yujing zhu* (DZ 402), 1.8b.

### 3.1 *The Lower Cinnabar Field*

The location of the lower cinnabar field varies in different sources and in different eras. It has been located 2.4 inches,[49] 3 inches or 1.3 inches below the navel.[50] In early writings, its most frequent location is three inches. Gradually, from the Song dynasty onwards, its position was usually placed at 1.3 inches; this is the one adopted by most sources during the Qing dynasty (1644–1911).[51] One of the oldest sources, the *Most High Lord Lao's Book of the Centre*, dated from the Later Han, gives the following description:

> The cinnabar field is the root of man, where his vital spirit remains and where the five breaths originate. There abides the embryo. In this place, men keep their seminal essence, and women, their menstrual blood. It is present at birth, and is the gate of the union of yin and yang. It is three inches below the navel, near to the spinal cord and is the root of the genitals. It is red in the centre, blue on the left, yellow on the right, white on the upper part, and black on the bottom. It is square and round and measures four inches. It is located three inches below the navel, as it follows the pattern of heaven, earth and man. It measures four inches because the air corresponds to one, land to two, man to three and the seasons to four. It is of five colours because it follows the pattern of the five agents.[52]

In these ancient sources, the cinnabar field is described alone, without mention of chambers or secondary palaces, unlike later descriptions, including those of the Ming (1368–1644) and Qing (1644–1911), who added to the left the Hall of Light (Mingtang) and to the right the Cavern-Chamber (Dongfang). On

49 *Baopu zi neipian jiaoshi*, 18.296.

50 The location is given at three inches in *Taishang Laojun zhongjing* 太上老君中經 [The most high Lord Lao's book of the center] (DZ 1168), 1.11b–12a. Cf. *Dadong yujing* 大洞玉經 (DZ 7), 1.8b. It is re-used by *Taixijing zhu* 胎息經註 (DZ 130), 1a, and *Xiuzhen shishu* (DZ 263), 18.9ab, in the text accompanying the Yanluozi diagrams. The location is 1.3 inches in *Huangdi yinfujing zhu* 黃帝陰符經註 (DZ 121), 3.3a; *Baoyi zi Sanfeng laoren danjue* (DZ 281), 3b; *Zhuzhen shengtai shenyong jue* 諸真聖胎神用訣 (DZ 826), 8b. One text, the *Qingwei danjue* 清微丹訣, says that it is transmitted that this location is at 1.3 inches under the navel, but in fact, it is at the level of the nostril, at 1.3 inches under the skin. See DZ 278, 2b.

51 See also Zheng Sixiao 鄭思肖, *Taiji jilian neifa* 太極祭煉內法 [Inner method of Taiji for sacrificing to and sublimating the spirits of the deceased] (DZ 548), 2.30b–31a, giving several different descriptions of the lower cinnabar field.

52 *Taishang Laojun zhongjing* (DZ 1168), 1.12b–13a.

the *Chart for the Cultivation of Perfection*, the text overview of the body to the upper right above the head describes the lower cinnabar field as follows:

> It is said that at three inches or thereabouts below the sea of breath is the Jade Pond or the lower cinnabar field, which shelters the vital essence and is the place where the medicine is gathered. It is flanked on the left and right by the Hall of Light (Mingtang) and the Cavern Chamber (Dongfang) and measures 1.2 inches for each side. At this point, there are two orifices communicating with the internal kidneys.

This cinnabar field is also called "Jade Furnace" on the *Chart*. On the Nanning version, a text explains that the Jade Furnace is the starting point for success and soaring to immortality:

> The divine immortals perfectly understood where the Jade Furnace was to be found. From this point, everyone has access to the Great Way. The Jade Furnace burns long and its smoke covers the three thousand worlds. The heated yang exchanges with [the yin] and spreads, completing the transformations. The hermit of the mountain shows you the way of life or death. By the movement of inversion and return, thanks to the true flower, we accomplish immortality. The sword of wisdom is actually the smoke of the Jade Furnace. Eventually the body stabilizes and the search within it continues. We fly to Perfection, transformed into a winged being, in resonance with the great awakening. We ascend to the Heaven of the Great Network in the Obscure Capital.

The lower cinnabar field is shown on the Chart, between the legs crossed in the lotus position, as a circle divided into five sections and is similar to the Yanluozi diagrams, to the drawing of the commentary on the *Classic of the Difficulties*, and to the *Great Rites of the Numinous Treasure and Upper Clarity* by Wang Qizhen 王契真 (fourteenth century), a text related to Divine Empyrean rites (Fig. 4.1).[53] This latter text includes a drawing titled "Diagram of Inner Contemplation" ("Neiguan tu" 內觀圖). The narrative accompanying this illustration states that the celebrant must first enter his meditation chamber and visualize the five viscera and then the lower cinnabar field. But the colours specified for each sector do not correspond to those given in the *Chart for the Cultivation of Perfection* and in the *Most High Lord Lao's Book on the Centre*

53 *Shangqing lingbao dafa* 上清靈寶大法 [Great rites of numinous treasure and upper clarity] (DZ 1221), 2.23b.

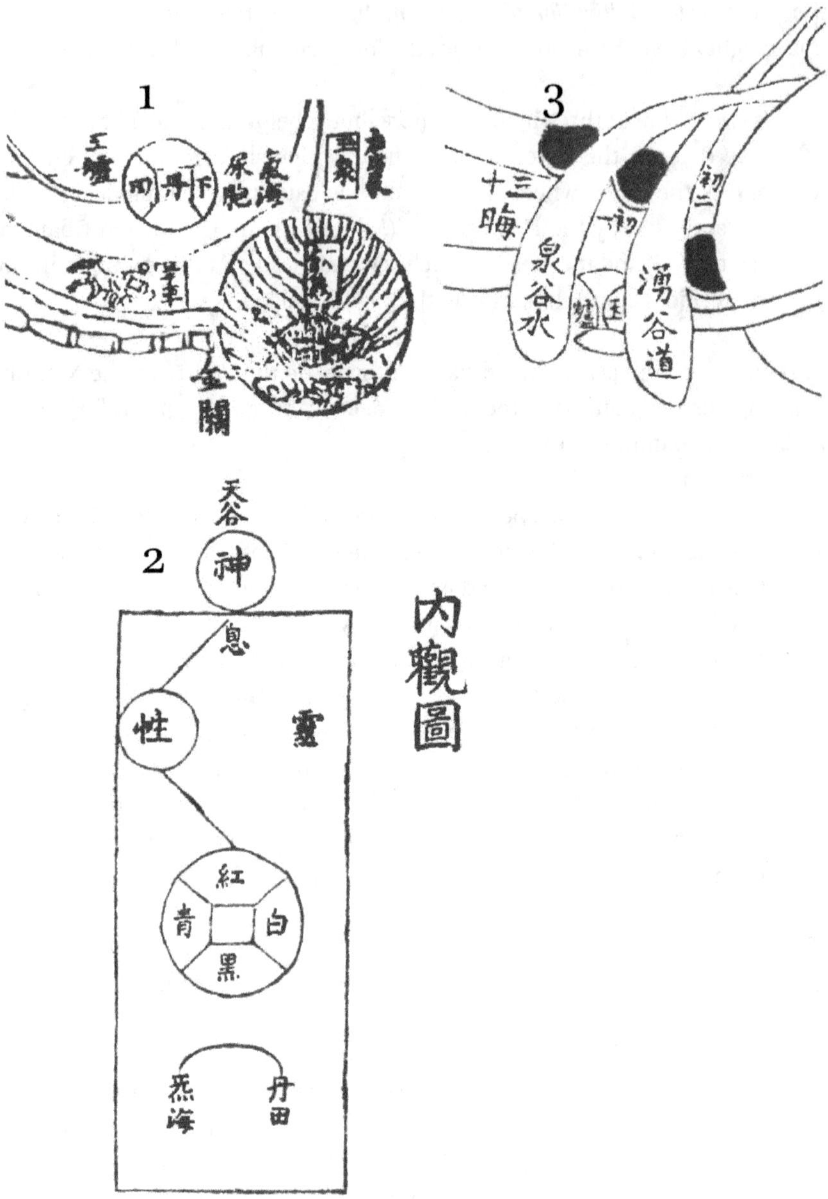


FIGURE 4.1 1. Tenth-century drawing of the lower cinnabar field on the Yanluozi diagram. 2. Fourteenth-century drawing of the "inner contemplation" (*neiguan* 內觀) with the five colours of the lower cinnabar field, *Shangqing lingbao dafa* (DZ 1221), 2.23b. 3. Drawing of the *Chart for the Cultivation of Perfection.*

which place the red in the centre and follows the classical correspondence between the cardinal points and the colours, that is to say green on the left (East), white on the right (West), red on the top (South), black on the bottom (North) and yellow in the centre.

On the *Chart*, the lower cinnabar field is also represented as an area and place of meditation by another drawing, evoking its function of moving the Primordial Breath compared to thunder. This is a spiral drawn below the kidneys with above and below the inscriptions Jasper Pond (*qiongchi*) and Lapis Lazuli Pond (*liuchi*). To the left of the spiral and below the trapezium, an inscription on the lower cinnabar field begins by giving the four colours that compose the breath, and then continues by enumerating the various symbols or functions of the cinnabar field. These terms refer to different stages of the transformation process, referring allegorically to different states of awareness or perceptions that an adept will experience. For example, the Palace of Fusang 扶桑, a mythical tree associated with the sun, indicates that internal brightness will shine at a stage of practice. The abode of the infant refers to the process of rebirth and a feeling of something moving in the lower abdomen. The text reads (fig. 3.6, text 18):

> In this field, the [Original] Breath is blue to the left, yellow to the right, black on the bottom, and white on the top. This is the lower cinnabar field, the perfected tiger, the land of Kan, the abode of the infant, the Palace of Fusang [Tree],[54] the Sea of Breath, the Crystal Palace,[55] the Female Gate. The cavity in the centre of the Obscure Female is the true essence. The Peduncle of the Vital Force (*mingdi* 命蒂) is three inches above.[56] [This cinnabar field] is actually the field of transformations, the root of heaven

---

54 The Fusang 扶桑 is a mythical tree mentioned in the *Classic of Mountains and Seas* (*Shanhai jing* 山海經), 9.3a (trans. Mathieu 1983: 45). Located at the top of the bubbling valley, ten suns are drying, nine on the lower branches and one on the upper branch. It is represented on the banner excavated from the tomb No.1 at Mawangdui 馬王堆 (see Loewe 1979: 50 sq.). In Inner Alchemy, the first occurrence of the term Fusang is found in the *Wuzhen pian*: "At the summit of the Huashan, the tiger roared. Near the Fusang tree at the bottom of the sea, the female dragon whistles." *Wuzhen pian zhushi* 悟真篇註釋 (DZ 145) 2.7a. According to Xue Daoguang 薛道光, the Fusang Tree is a metaphor for the rising sun, and the dragon is the animal corresponding to the East. The rising sun is the apparition of yang in the yin, which is represented by the central yang line in the trigram *kan* (water).

55 See the technique called *zhouhou jinjing* 肘後金晶 [The golden crystal behind the elbow], which consists of making the breath that gives birth to the seminal essence rise upwards, an energy compared to a drop of light or of crystal.

56 It means the umbilicus, where the breath is generated.

> and earth, where the old white-haired man can blacken his hair again. This is the place that makes it possible for me to establish my kingdom. The Real One, in other words, the metal that comes from water and that is called Metal Essence is my supreme essence prior to heaven. It is also said that this is the tiger born in water, the hexagram of "return" (*fu*), i.e., the birth of a yang, the *zi* period (11pm–1am),[57] the moon at the bottom of the sea, the birth gate, and my root. Those who cultivate perfection should know these few metaphors.[58]

The text that is closest to the above description is, as with the upper right text, the *Thus I Have Heard* (1834), one of the few sources we found, with the *Path of the Great Fulfilment* attributed to Liu Huayang 柳華陽, mentioning a Hall of Light and a Cavern Chamber at the lower cinnabar field.[59]

### 3.2 *The Median Cinnabar Field*

According to the *Master who Embraces Simplicity*, the median cinnabar field is "located below the heart ... some place it in the bronze watchtower and in the Scarlet Palace under the heart."[60] On the *Chart for the Cultivation of Perfection*, in the upper right text, the description of the median cinnabar field is similar to those of the *Path of Great Fulfilment* and The *Thus I Have Heard*: "At 3.6 inches below the Scarlet Palace is the Earth Furnace or the cavity of the Yellow Court, that is to say the median cinnabar field. It is flanked to the left by the Hall of Light and to the right by the Cavern-Chamber. On the left is the liver where abides the Non-pareil Lordling (Wuying), to the right, the lung is the residence of the White Prime. The centre is empty, it measures 1.2 inches and is the abode of the breath, the cauldron where it is refined."[61] According to this text, the median cinnabar field is 3.6 inches from the Scarlet Palace, itself situated below the heart. Therefore, the position of the median cinnabar field shifts. It is not located near the heart as in the Six Dynasties, but lower, at the level of spleen and stomach.

---

57 Among the twelve two hours periods in a day, the period *zi* corresponds to that of the reapparition of the yang after the apogee of yin between 23h and 1h, hence the use of the hexagram *fu* 復 [Return] formed by a yang line below and five yin lines above, as a symbol of the emergence of yang in the yin of the kidneys.

58 The version of the White Cloud Temple has *shuming* 數名. The Mount Wudang version has *jiaoming* 教名, "the teached names." The text of the Sichuan version by Duan Fu is shorter.

59 *Dacheng jiejing* 大乘捷徑, 4b.

60 *Baopu zi neipian jiaoshi*, 18.296.

61 *Rushi wowen*, 2b.

## 3.3 *The Upper Cinnabar Field*

The text describing the upper cinnabar field on the *Chart for the Cultivation of Perfection* is also similar to the *Thus I Have Heard*, and mentions only three of the nine cases of the classic upper cinnabar field, which is typical of the late Qing sources. Apart from this, the description is consistent with the classical descriptions according to the Upper Clarity tradition. In the right-hand text, an overview of the body (fig. 3.6, copy 2), it is described as follows:

> The Niwan is the upper cinnabar field. It measures 1.2 inches. This hole is an empty pass (*xuguan* 虛關) in which the spirit abides. It is a court located right in the centre when you enter in the head from the space between the two eyebrows. From the Heavenly Gate,[62] enter one inch inside the head and you will arrive at the Hall of Light. If you penetrate one inch more, you arrive at the Cavern Chamber and again one inch to the Muddy Pellet.

Recall the description in the left-hand text: "The Muddy Pellet has nine cavities; it corresponds to the nine heavenly palaces.[63] The brain bones form eight sectors that correspond to the eight directions. Like the heavens, they extend like a vast net, the Jade Emperor Palace, or the Heavenly Palace Pure Yang. The centre is a cavity called 'Palace of the Primordial Spirit' (*Yuanshen gong*) or the 'Heaven of the Obscure Immensity'." And further: "In reality my divine chamber and the nine orifices of the Muddy Pellet Palace are the Palace of the Heavenly Sovereign. In the centre is a cavity in the shape of a hen's egg, the Lotus Terrace and Mount Kunlun."

From the middle of the fourth century, there are at least nine instances in which the upper cinnabar field and its resident deities are described.[64] The visualisation of these nine palaces and their respective deities is re-used, often with simplifications, by the writings on Inner Alchemy "Formula to conserve and visualize the nine palaces," a text probably written by Yanluozi and situated after his drawings in the *Ten Books for the Cultivation of Perfection*, indicates:

> The head consists of nine palaces, which are like the nine heavens above, and nine lands below. The body has nine orifices and the

62 This means the space between the eyebrows.

63 See *Shangqing dadong zhenjing* (DZ 6), 2.18b.

64 See *Shangqing lingsu shangpian* 上清靈素上篇 [The upper chapters on the spirit immaculate of upper clarity] (DZ 1371), 7b–8a. A similar description is given in *Dongzhen Taishang suling dongyuan dayou miaojing* (DZ 1314), 13–19, and *Dengzhen yinjue* 登真隱訣 [Secret instructions for the ascent of perfected] (DZ 421), 1.3–4.

> twelve-storey pagoda (trachea). If, from the space between the eyebrows, one penetrates an inch into the head, one arrives at the Hall of Light where the Lord of the Great One (*Taiyi jun* 太一君) resides. On his left is the Purple Room, on the right the Vermilion Gate. He is dressed in brocade, has the appearance of an infant, and governs the self and the body. If you penetrate two inches further, you will arrive at the Cavern Chamber Palace (*Dongfang gong*) where the three Perfected reside: on the left, the Non-pareil Lordling, on the right, the White Prime (*Baiyuan*), in the centre, the Yellow Clouds (*Huangyun* 黄雲). If you penetrate three inches, you will arrive at the Cinnabar Field Palace (*Dantian gong* 丹田宫), after four inches, you will arrive at the Rolling Pearls Palace (*Liuzhu gong* 流珠宫), after five inches, at the Jade Emperor Palace (Yudi gong). One inch from the Hall of Light is the Palace of the Heavenly Court (*Tianting gong* 天庭宫), one inch from the Cavern-Chamber is the Palace of Extreme Perfection (*Jizhen gong* 極真宫), one inch from the cinnabar field is the Palace of the Obscure Cinnabar (*Xuandan gong* 玄丹宫), and one inch from the rolling pearls is the Palace of the Heavenly Sovereign (*Tianhuang gong* 天皇宫)."[65]

The *Chart for the Cultivation of Perfection* repeats more succinctly this description of the nine palaces also evoked by the inscriptions located on the front part of the head. In addition to these nine palaces, it refers to a cavity in the shape of a hen's egg, the Lotus Terrace and Mount Kunlun, which usually refer to the whole head. Also, note the correlation established between the upper cinnabar field and the Miluo Heaven Palace of the Jade Emperor, and the residence of the Primordial Spirit (*yuanshen*). This is a conception specific to Inner Alchemy.

## 4 The Three Passes on the Back

If, in the front of the body, or more precisely in the middle of the body, the most important places for the alchemical work of transmutations are the three cinnabar fields, in the back, following the spinal cord, there are three locations

65 *Xiuzhen shishu* (DZ 263), 18.6a; also in *Yuqing wuji zongzhen Wenchang dadong xianjing zhu* 玉清無極總真文長大洞仙經註 [Commentary on the great cavern scripture according to Wenchang], ed. Wei Qi 衛琪 (1309), DZ 103, 3.26b. Text similar in *Dongzhen Taishang daojun yuandan shangjing* 洞真太上道君元丹上經 [Superior scripture of the mysterious cinnabar], with the difference that the last palace is called Taihuang gong 太皇宫 (DZ 1345, 8a), as well as in *Dengzhen yinjue* (DZ 421), 1.3b–4b.

corresponding also to different levels of the alchemical process. The Three Passes are three places on the spine where the breath circulates with difficulty when rising in the Control Vessel (*dumai*). They are locations specific to Inner Alchemy and they correspond to three stages. Their name and location varied in the early days,[66] but were formalized by the Song dynasty. They are named the Caudal Pass, the Spinal Handle Pass, and the Jade Pillow Pass and are respectively located at the coccyx, the middle of the back and the neck (fig. 4.3).

### 4.1 *The Caudal Pass*

The "Caudal Pass" (*Weilü*), at the base of the backbone designates the coccyx region in Inner Alchemy. This term, also common in traditional medicine, is associated with an ancient myth. Zhuangzi, a fourth-century BCE Taoist philosopher writes that Weilü is the name of a hole in the bottom of the sea that allows their waters to flow away and not overflow. Beihairuo 北海若, addressing the Duke of the Yellow River, boasted of his grandeur and power, said: "To you who have left your banks, who have seen the immense sea and have thus grasped your mediocrity, we can speak of the universal order. Of all the waters of the world, the greatest is the sea. Countless rivers pour their water into it constantly, without being able to fill it. The Caudal Pass drains the water indefinitely without being able to empty itself. It remains the same in spring and autumn; it knows neither flood nor drought. It immeasurably surpasses the Blue River and the Yellow River."[67]

Taoists and doctors considered the Caudal Pass (i.e., the coccyx) as the place where the bone marrow flowed from the brain into the spine to diffuse sperm.[68] They thought this loss exhausted the brain and the marrow; the latter two were viewed as one and the same. In the West, the same belief circulated in the schools of Hippocrates and Galen of Pergamon (129–210 CE), a prominent Greek physician and philosopher in the Roman Empire.[69] It was thus important in the ancient Taoist techniques such as internal alchemy to preserve the substances of the body and block the dispersal of the spermatic essence so as to nourish the bone marrow and the brain. In the techniques for nourishing life this was formerly referred to as "returning the essence to repair the brain" and, in Inner Alchemy, it is referred to by the expression "The flying

66 See Baldrian-Hussein 1984: 111.

67 *Zhuangzi jijie* 莊子集解 [Commentaries on the Zhuangzi], 17.249.

68 See *Huangdi neijing suwen*, chap. 10, *juan* 3, p. 62.

69 See for example Hippocrate, "De Generatio", 1. I have consulted the French translation by Joly, 1970: 43.

golden crystal behind the elbow" (*zhouhou fei jinjing* 肘後飛金晶). This pass is the beginning of the reversal path, the Return to the Great Way that gives access to heaven. In the body presentation text at the upper right of the *Chart*, it is presented succinctly as the starting point of the spinal cord, the path of yang ascension, and the pass communicating with the orifice of the internal kidneys. In the drawing of the spinal column, the circle at the bottom of the backbone symbolizes this pass and includes the following inscription (fig. 3.6, text 11):

> The Caudal Pass also bears these names: the Nine Orifices, the lion with nine heads,[70] the prince who shoots the nine successive bronze drums, the Yin Pass, the pass that is securely closed. The constant inability to cross this pass is symbolized by the nine successive bronze drums while the prince is a metaphor for the breath of pure yang. If one can manage to produce the ambrosia that flows from the top of the head, we can unblock [all passes] and connect them. This is why it is said that the prince pierces the nine bronze drums with an arrow. This pass is the start of the path up to heaven, the divine door of the earthly axis, the summit reaching for the sky, the cavity of the tiger and the dragon, the triple fork. Within the kidneys is a metal cauldron that enables communication between interior and exterior. Three paths go along the spinal cord and lead directly to the Niwan and to the summit of the head.[71] From here it can pass the spinal cord and connect the entire body.[72]

A number of elements of this inscription are found in a Taoist text of the thirteenth century transmitted by Huang Gongwang 黄公望 (1269–1354) to his disciple Jin Yueyan 金月岩. It appears before a chart of the Caudal Pass and its accompanying sixteen poems, the following text: "This Caudal Pass cavity is also called the tiger and the dragon, path of Cao Stream, nine successive bronze drums,[73] three fork bone, water chariot bone,[74] the gate of the sea of

70 The "nine-headed lion" (*jiutou shizi cao* 九頭獅子草) is the name of a plant, *Peristrophe japonica*, that tolerates drought, and for this reason, has become synonymous with long life.

71 The mention of these three pathways may be an influence of esoteric Buddhism, according to which there exists along the backbone a central channel, flanked on the right and the left by two channels.

72 The text of the Sichuan version is shorter and slightly different.

73 Further, the text cites a poem attributed to Lü Dongbin, in which he discussed "the nine caudal orifices that are the bronze drums." See DZ 281, 16b.

74 Sometimes it is referred to by the metaphor Yellow River.

breath, the summit which leads to heaven, the ladder for heavenly ascension. This bone (tailbone) has the shape of a metal cauldron bearing nine orifices (fig. 4.2) and allows communication between the interior and exterior."[75] Most of these designations are also in the chapter "Drawing of the reversal of light to illuminate the interior" (*Fanzhao tu* 反照圖) of the *Principles of the Tablets on the Innate Nature and the Vital Force* (text of the sixteenth century) mentioning in particular the terms "nine bronze drums, path of ascension to heaven, summit aimed heavenward, triple fork, the way of the Cao Stream, the cavity of the tiger and the dragon."[76]

## 4.2 *The Spinal Handle Pass*

This pass is twofold: it contains two winches that allow the current of fluids to flow upwards. On the left is the Taiyang, on the right the Taiyin. During inhalation yang rises, during the exhalation yin descends. A circle located in the middle of the spinal column carries an inscription on this pass (fig. 3.6, text 10):

> The path where the divine immortals rise and descend is the vessel of my body, it is the Gaohuang point 膏肓.[77] It's called the Double Pass, inside are two winches: Taiyang on the left, Taiyin on the right. This is the path where the yang rises in [the inhalation] and the yin descends in the exhalation. This path of ascension communicates with the cavity of the pillar of heaven, which is also called the dual internal forest and communicates with the dual external forest. It is in communication outside with thunder and is the vessel and pass of ascending yang. When the cavity starts to

75 *Baoyi zi Sanfeng laoren danjue* (DZ 281), 15b. Sanfeng laoren is the surname of Liu (see text, 6b). He was probably one of the masters of Huang Gongwang.

76 *Xingming guizhi* (seventeenth century), 1.21a.

77 The point Gaohuang yu 膏肓俞 is, according to the current arrangement of the acupuncture points, the 43rd acupuncture point on the bladder channel and is located at the fourth vertebra near the scapula. In a passage of the *Zuozhuan* 左傳 (the 10th year of Chenggong 成公), the term is divided in two parts, which the author considers a critical area of the body and difficult to access. The author reports the following dream of the Marquis of Jin: "The Duke dreamed that his illness was due to two children standing and having a conversation: 'This excellent doctor will scar us and wound us, how should we escape?' The other child replied: 'Let us take refuge above *huang* and below *gao*, what can he do?' When the doctor arrived, he exclaimed: 'I can not do anything against this disease, because it is above *huang* and below *gao*, I can neither attack nor expulse it by moxa, needle, or remedies.'" See *Zuozhuan*, in *Shisan jing zhushu* (1980): 1906c. This area was consequently, from the first centuries BCE considered important and delicate. The *gaohuang* point is not mentioned in the *Inner Canon of the Yellow Emperor Canon* (*Huangdi neijing*), a text compiled around the first century BCE or CE.

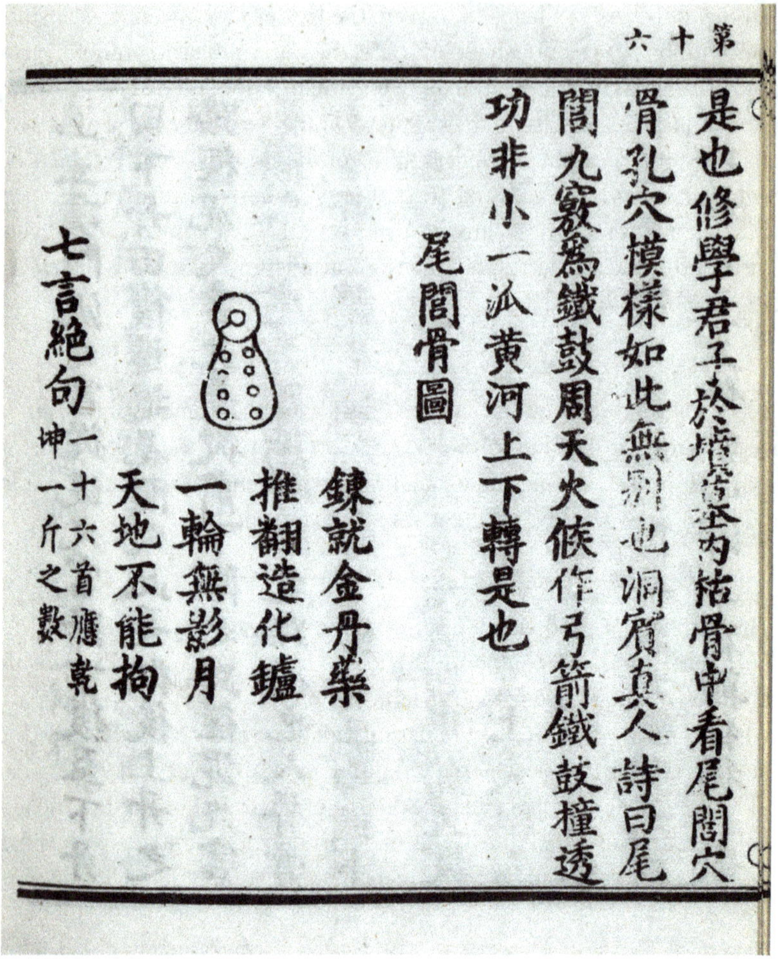


FIGURE 4.2 The nine holes of the Caudal Pass (Weilu 尾闾). *Baoyi zi Sanfeng laoren danjue* (DZ 281), 15b

bubble, yang rises from the rear, from the Bubbling Spring (*Yongquan*),[78] rises up to Muddy Pellet, then drops down through the Flowery Pond (i.e., the mouth) where it takes water, continues its descent through the Flowering Canopy [lungs], the seat of the five agents (i.e., viscera), the Cinnabar Field [lower], then inside the Peduncle of the Vital Force (*mingdi* 命蒂).

78 Point situated at the centre of the sole of the feet; it is the first point of the kidneys channel in acupuncture.

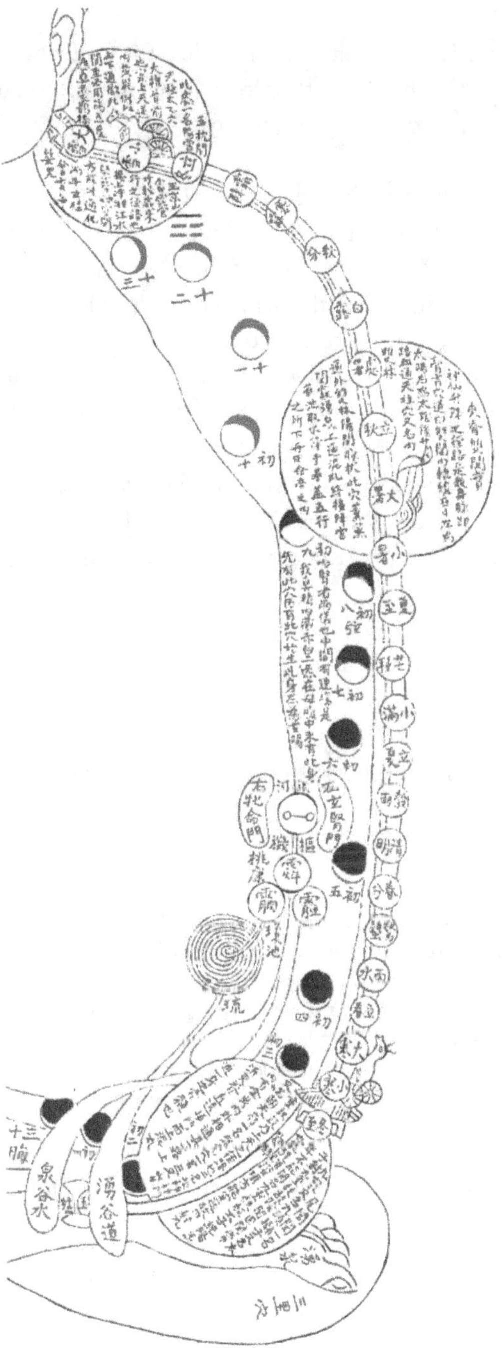

FIGURE 4.3
The three Passes on the back. Detail of the *Chart for the Cultivation of Perfection*

### 4.3 *The Jade Pillow Pass*

It is located at the occiput and is also called "iron enclosure" (*tiebi* 鐵壁) because it is difficult to breech.[79] On the *Chart*, the circle drawn at the level of the neck includes the following inscription (fig. 3.6, text 9):

> This place is called the Yang Palace, the Heavenly Pillar,[80] the Cavity of the Great one,[81] the Jade Capital Mountain.[82] In front of the sixth cervical lies the Palace of Thunder and Lightning (Leiting gong 雷霆宮); it is the strategic point for ascending to heaven and reaching the Yellow Dragon.[83] Through this inverted path, one can access to heaven and penetrate the dark and the subtle. Above and below are unblocked, the water of the Xiang flows in the opposite direction.[84] The yang breath is essential for crossing this very important pass, the door of which is guarded by a yin divinity. The true breath must reach the Bridge of the Magpies,[85] and suddenly burst through and unlock this pass. Then the cowherd and the weaver meet and beget the infant, nourished by the mother's milk.

## 5 Other Important Loci

### 5.1 *The Obscure Female*

The term "Obscure Female" comes from the sixth chapter of the *Book of the Way and its Virtue*:

---

79 The occiput was also called in the ancient times the "pillow bone" (*zhengu* 枕骨) (see *Suwen* 素問, 58.269; *Lingshu*, 13.1a). Yuzhen is currently the name of the ninth point of the bladder channel.

80 The heavenly pillar supports the sky. According to a legend, the demon Gonggong shook the heavenly pillar, so that the earth tilted towards the southeast (see Mathieu 1983: 38). In traditional Chinese medicine, the heavenly pillar is the 10th point of the bladder Meridian, it is also the place where the meridian goes deeper inside the body (*Lingshu*, 5.2a).

81 It is the name of the North Pole deity.

82 The capital of Jade Mountain is a city of heavenly paradise, home of the Celestial Emperor. It is said in the *Baopuzi*: "The Mountain of the Seven Gems of the Jade capital having a circumference of ninety thousand *li* is above the Daluo heaven." (Wang 1980: 295).

83 The yellow dragon is a term referring to the "Five Dragons upholding the Wise" (*wulong pengsheng* 五龍捧聖). It is thus a metaphor for the true deity (dragon) and the true intent (yellow).

84 Tributary of the Blue River often praised by poets.

85 Region in the mouth situated at the level of the nose. When the heat rises to the sinciput, fresh secretions descend from the brain and fill the mouth.

The spirit of the valley never dies,
This is called the obscure female.
The gateway of the obscure female
This is called the root of heaven and earth.
Existence and nonexistence, as a silk thread,
Its action is inexhaustible.

This obscure passage gave rise early on to diverse interpretations. One of the earliest commentators on this work, the Master of the River's Edge (Heshang gong 河上公) from the end of the second century, interprets this term of the obscure female in this way: "The obscure is the heaven in man; it is the nose. The female [refers to] the earth; in humans, it is the mouth. The sky feeds man with the five breaths that enter through the nose and hide in the heart."[86] Another comment, from the same period, attributed to Zhang Daoling 張道陵 (second century) or his grandson Zhang Lu 張魯 (ob. 216), gives the following interpretation: "The female is the earth in the image of the woman, the door of the yin orifice, organ of life and death, whose importance is primordial, which is why we say that it is the "root" [of heaven and earth]."[87]

In Inner Alchemy, this term is used in a sense close to that one just mentioned, but it takes a more specific sense, which also varies according to the sources. It most often refers to a place between the two kidneys. Zhang Boduan (ob. 1082) writes in his *Stanzas of Awakening to Perfection*: "We must rely the Obscure Female to establish the base and the root."[88] A text from the southern alchemical lineage, the "Chapter on the return to the Origin" (Huanyuan pian 還元篇) by Shi Tai 石泰 or Shi Xinglin 石杏林 (1022–1158), is more specific about the role of this Obscure Female: "An orifice has the name of the Obscure Female, it stores the breath and the spirit, but few know it, and should not search for it outside."[89]

On the *Chart for the Cultivation of Perfection*, the Obscure Female is divided in two, as it is on the "Drawing of the Obscure Female" reported by the *Collection on the Great Achievement of the Golden Elixir* by Xiao Tingzhi 蕭廷芝 (ca. 1260–1264) with the following commentary: "We take the centre from

86 Zheng Chenghai 1956: 9.

87 *Laozi Xiang'er zhu jiaozheng* 老子想爾註校證 [Xiang'er commentary to the Laozi, critical edition], ed. Rao Zhongyi 饒宗頤 (1991): 9. This is a document discovered in a grotto at Dunhuang in Central Asia. The meaning of the title Xiang'er is unknown; it is possibly the name of a person.

88 DZ 145, 2.21a. See also *Danfang baojian tu* 丹房寶鑑圖, in *Xiuzhen shishu* (DZ 263), 26.5; Needham, v.5 (1983): 97.

89 *Xiuzhen shishu* (DZ 263), 2.7a, poem 37.

*kan* ☵ which is full (yang) to transform the yin of the abdomen in the *li* ☲ palace. The valley of emptiness is the root of heaven and earth. The mystery in the obscure, it is the gate of marvels" (see fig. 4.4).[90]

In the explanation of the term given by the *Collection on the Zhong*[*li Quan*]'s *Transmission of the Way to Lü* [*Dongbin*]:

> At the moment of conception, the essence and the breath are still one. Once the breath and the essence separate, the kidneys are first to appear. One kidney is to the left, which corresponds to the obscure (*xuan*): it is the obscure that makes the breath rise and carries it up to the liver. One kidney is to the right, which corresponds to the female (*pin*). It collects secretions and carries them down to the bladder. The obscure female comes from what originally is not. Of which is not, we come to that which is. That is to say, the true breath of the father and mother is collected in the pure yin earth.[91]

Wang Wenqing 王文卿 (1093–1153) from the Divine Empyrean tradition gives in his *Song on the Mysterious Pearl* the following description: "The Obscure Female is the Ancestral [Original] Breath,[92] the root of Heaven and earth, the foundation of the vital force and of the innate nature. If the officiant knows that this orifice is the Way, when he will perform rituals, numinous spirits will all come, the breath and the spirit (*shen*) will transform into the essence of *kan* and *li*.[93] The *Thus I Have heard* writes:

> The yang is called obscure, the yin, the female, it is generally the obscure orifice. It is not in the body, or if it is considered to be in the body, it can be said that it is the root of what is and what is not, the ancestor of emptiness and fullness, the peduncle of yin and yang. Confucians call it the Great Ultimate, Taoists, the golden elixir, and Buddhists, the perfect

---

90 *Xiuzhen shishu* (DZ 263), 9.3a.

91 *Zhong Lü chuandao ji* 鍾呂傳道集 [Collection on the Zhong Liquan transmission to Lü Dongbin (DZ 263), 16.12a.

92 "Breath" translates the character *qi* 炁. The character was used in Taoism from the Song Dynasty on, to designate the "breath of the Anterior Heaven"; the graphy is written with the negation *wu* 无 and below the radical of the fire, because Taoists consider this breath as devoid of fire; by fire is meant in this context essentially the fire of the passions.

93 *Daofa huiyuan* (DZ 1220), 70.3b–4a.

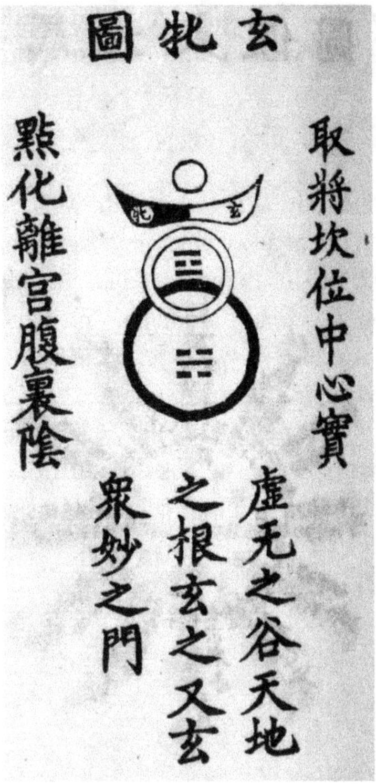


FIGURE 4.4
Drawing of the Obscure Female (*xuanpin* 玄牝). *Jindan dacheng ji*, in *Xiuzhen Shishu* 修真十書 (DZ 263), 9.3a

enlightenment. It appears only in the Great Voidness, and opens only when the calm is at its apogee.[94]

### 5.2 *The Life Gate* (*shengmen* 生門)

We can see in the middle of the Chart, a circle with the inscription "Life Gate." Above are inscribed the words "The navel is Life Gate."[95] The Great One remains there, he governs the innate nature and the vital force of the individual, he is the rector of the twelve thousand essences in the body."[96]

In the drawing on the "Washing of the Heart" in the *Principles of the Tablets on the Innate Nature and the Vital Force* attributed to Yin zhenren 尹真人 (17th cen.), we can see the expression "Life Gate," which corresponds to the

94 *Rushi wowen*, 2b.

95 Version of the stele of Canton. The version of the White Cloud Temple has "the navel is the life gate," while the version of the Mount Wudang writes, "The lungs are the life gate."

96 Thirteen thousand is the number found on the stele of Canton, on the Mount Wudang and the Sichuan versions, the later added the text "the root of the innate nature and of the vital force." The version of Guo of Black Sheep Palace and that of the White Cloud Temple have the number 12,000, the version of Moli has 22,000.

navel,[97] a significant place in alchemical practice.[98] It is already used in the *Precious Book of the Inner Landscape of the Yellow Court* (fifth century), but without precision of the significance.[99]

### 5.3 *The Throat*

The throat is a place of passage and communication with the outside. Most of the time, it is principally the trachea that is drawn as a twelve-storey pagoda or as twelve rings, as on our illustration (fig. 4.5).[100] This tiered pagoda is already mentioned in the *Precious Book of the Inner Landscape of the Yellow Court* and the *Book of the Great Clarity on Gymnastics and Nourishing Life* from the fourth or fifth century.[101] On the *Chart for the Cultivation of Perfection*, a text to the left of the twelve rings describes more precisely the region (see fig. 3.6, text 12): Under the tongue are two openings called Xuanying.[102] The posterior orifice is the pharynx; it permits the swallowing of solid food and liquids. The anterior orifice is the larynx, it consists of twelve rings that are called the twelve-storey pagoda, and is where the breath passes.

---

97 *Xingming guizhi*, 2.14b.

98 See *Xuanzhu ge* 玄珠歌 [Song on the obscure pearl] by Wang Wenqing, in *Daofa huiyuan* (DZ 1220), 70.7b: "The wheel of the navel is the Northern Dipper."

99 *Huangting neijing yujing zhu* (DZ 402), 1.22b: "The king of the waters of the two sectors faced at the life gate.

100 *Huangting neijing yujing zhu* is the earliest known text to mention a twelve-storey pagoda (DZ 402, 2.14b). The commentary by Liangqiu zi in the mid-Tang states, "There are twelve rings at the throat that stack above the heart." The heart is the Scarlet Palace, and the whole looks like a pavilion and its belvedere (*louge* 樓閣). The *Huangting waijing jing* (DZ 403) also mentions the Scarlet Palace and the twelve-storey pagoda. The *Taiqing daoyin yangsheng jing* 太清導引養生經 [Book of the great clarity on gymnastics and nourishing life] of the Six Dynasties writes, "The throat is like twelve silver rings stacked from uvula to the lungs." See DZ 818, 8.

101 See *Taishang huanting waijing yujing* (DZ 332), 1.1b and *Taiqing daoyin yangsheng jing* (DZ 818), 8a.

102 This term is found in the "Breath of the Lungs" chapter of the *Huangting neijing yujing zhu*: "Under the tongue, Xuanying is the shore of life and death." The commentary by Liangqiu zi says: "It is a metaphor. Xuanying is the bank that establishes communication with bodily fluids." (DZ 402, 1.11b). The term is also used in DZ 402, 3.14b: "Take the yang secretions at Xuanying and make enter them into the Hall of Light." The commentary by Liangqiu zi says: "The way to ingesting secretions necessarily goes through Xuanying to descend in the throat also called the tiered pagoda. The Hall of Light is located below the storey pagoda."

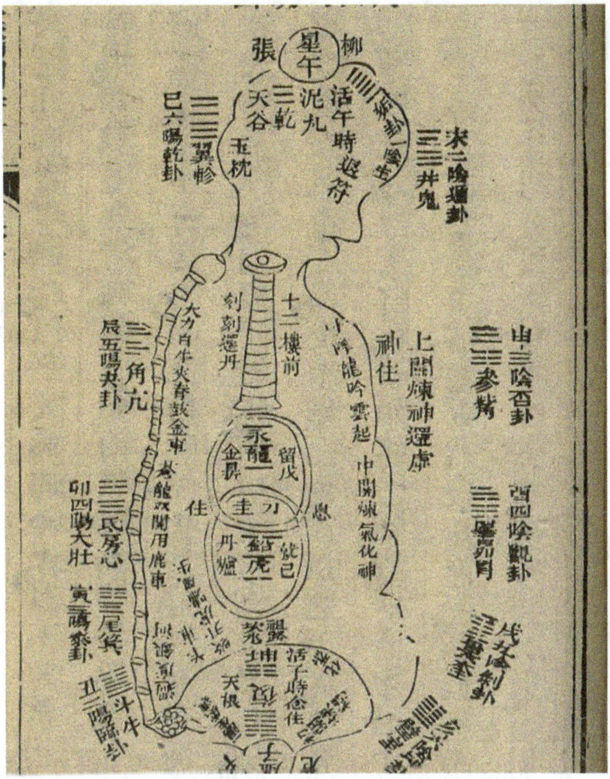


FIGURE 4.5 Representation of the body with the twelve-storey pagoda and the twenty-four spinal sections entitled "Drawing of the fire phasing and celestial revolution" (*Zhoutian huohou tu* 周天火候圖). *Qiaoqiao dongzhang*, 3.8a

## 6 The Eight Marvellous Vessels (*Qijing bamai* 奇經八脈)

Four encircled characters designate four of the eight marvellous vessels: Yangqiao 陽蹻, Yinqiao 陰蹻, Yangyu 陽俞 and Yinyu 陰俞. They probably designate places as in the *Book on the Eight Marvellous Vessels by Zhang Ziyang* (*Zhang Ziyang bamai jing* 張紫陽八脈經), an apocryphal text cited by Li Shizhen 李時珍 (1518–1593),[103] where it is written: "The Bursting Vessel (*chongmai* 冲脈) is at the rear of brain, the Function Vessel at the front, the

103 See Li Shizhen, *Qijing bamai kao* 奇經八脈考 [Research on the eight marvellous vessels], "Yangqiao mai" 陽蹺脈.

Control Vessel at the rear of the umbilicus, the Belt Vessel (*daimai* 带脈) at the abdomen, the Yinqiao 陰蹻 below the gonads, the Yangqiao 陽蹻 at the Caudal Pass (Weilü), the Yinyu 陰俞 at the front of the sinciput (at 1.3 inches), the Yangyu 陽俞 behind the sinciput (1.3 inches). Each individual has these eight vessels which all come under Yin Spirit (*yinshen* 陰神) and are closed. Only divine immortals can unlock them with the yang breath which can burst through and that is why they can obtain the Way. But the yang breath can only be gathered at Yinqiao. This point has many different names. It's called the Female Gate, the Gate of Death, the returning to the root orifice, the pass for recovering the vital force, the City of Darkness, and the root of life in the fields of death. A deity called Vigour of the Peach (Taokang) governs it. Towards the top, he communicates with the Muddy Pellet, and towards the bottom, he reaches the Bubbling Spring. It is from this Yinqiao that the true breath accumulates or disperses."[104] The names of the Control Vessel and Function Vessel are listed respectively on the *Chart for the Cultivation of Perfection* at the head (around the mouth), and down near the trapezium with the names of hells, they are not encircled as with the Yinqiao, the Yangqiao, the Yinyu and Yangyu, while the Bursting Vessel (*chongmai*) and the Belt Vessel (*daimai*) are not mentioned. Furthermore, for Yinyu and Yangyu, we find in medical texts the terms Yangwei and Yinwei. However, the term *yu* used herein refers in acupuncture to a specific kind of points situated on either side of the spinal column and associated with different organs. Its use here in reference to a meridian suggests an evolution of the conception of a channel to that of a place of passage, of connection. On the *Chart for the Cultivation of Perfection*, Yangyu is located near the lungs or heart, Yangqiao near the liver, and Yinyu Yinqiao at the lower corners of the trapezoidium. These sites do not correspond to those given in the text of Zhang Ziyang mentioned above. They would however be similar to those that we were given orally by a Taoist in Taiwan, Liu Peizhong 劉培中, who claimed to be an adept of the Wu-Liu School, who located Yinqiao at 1.3 inches from the perineum, Yangwei (Yangyu) at the heart, Yinwei (Yinyu) at 3 inches above the kidneys, and Yangqiao at the sacrum.

---

104 Translation from the version of the *Huiming jing* 慧命經 in *Wu Liu xianzong quanji* 伍柳仙宗全集 [Collection of the works of Wu Chongxu and Liu Huayang], 60a–b. There is a slightly different version in *Neiwaigong tushuo jiyao*), *xia* by Xi Yukang (1920), 331. This is translated in Despeux 1979: 44–45. The *Huiming jing* is a text written by the Chan Monk Liu Huayang (1735–1799) in 1794. It draws on the Inner Alchemy traditions of the Song and Yuan periods, joining them with Chan and Huayan Buddhism. See Esposito in Pregadio 2008: 520.

The Wu-Liu school has two patriarchs: Wu Chongxu 伍冲虛 (1574–1644), a man from Nanchang who would had among his teachers Wang Changyue and Liu Huayang 柳華陽 (1735–1799), also a native of Nanchang, which received the transmission of Wu Chongxu already dead. It is traditionally affiliated with the Dragon Gate movement. Both Wu and Liu advocate Buddhist Meditation to rediscover one's innate nature, and Taoist methods to replenish one's vital force.

CHAPTER 5

# The Body, World of Deities According to the *Chart for the Cultivation of Perfection*

In the aforementioned maps, the body is represented as a sacred place of paradises and hells, as well as divinities. When these supernatural elements are placed within the adept, his body becomes a divine realm that houses a pantheon of spirits. The idea that an individual has souls or spirits that enter (and exit) through the body is idea common in ancient time. Various sources confirm that when an individual is born, he carries with him two kinds of souls or spirits. The first is a celestial *hun* soul associated with the liver that ascends to heaven upon death. The second is a terrestrial *po* soul associated with either the lung or the rectum; after the death, the *po* soul remains on earth. For Taoists, this pair of souls is often referred to as the three *hun* and seven *po*. The latter have an ambiguous character and their possible maleficence brings them closer to another type of Taoist spirits, the three corpses or three kinds of vermin that corrode the vital principle. These spirits are mentioned on the Yanluozi chart but not on the *Chart for the Cultivation of Perfection*. With the desire of the mind and the pressure of life, these souls tend to escape and lose power. Here, the authors wish to prevent them from escaping or to be attacked and wounded.

By the Han dynasty, various models of the organised world were devised to explain the cosmos, the body and the society. All three domains were transposed onto the body, which integrated the natural and social environment of an individual. These early Taoists imagined the body as host to variety of anthropomorphic or animal deities. Each god was given a high rank in the administrative bureaucracy of the otherworld, and housed in a palace nestled among idyllic scenes of mountains and rivers. The number of these gods inhabiting the body varied according to Taoist schools, and changed over time. In Chinese medicine and Taoism, these spirits, which we would call in modern time psychic or emotional forces, have been associated with specific parts of the body and organs. Several Taoist writers of the late Han and Six Dynasties eras composed lists and detailed descriptions of these somatic gods, as well as methods of meditation and visualization to request their help in achieving longevity. The inner gods allow the human being to communicate with the corresponding gods of the celestial pantheon, serve as administrators of the human body, and preside over the balance of its functions. The main texts that

 | DOI:10.1163/9789004383456_007

document these early Taoist meditation practices are the *Most High Lord Lao's Book of the Centre*[1] and the *Book of the Yellow Court*.

The most known and most influential system in Taoism, including Internal Alchemy, is that of the Yellow Court tradition, which influenced the Upper Clarity Taoists, as well as other lineages from the Song such as the Correct Method of the Heart of Heaven, the Divine Empyrean and Pure Tenuity. In the *Chart for the Cultivation of Perfection*, the main gods are the six divinities of the six viscera and the nine divinities of the head. These former are the five viscera of the classical system of correspondence with the five agents (liver, heart, spleen, lungs, kidneys) along with the sixth viscera, the gallbladder. Meditating on these divinities enables the adept bring them into existence. As the *Book of the Yellow Court* attests, this kind of visualization practice guarantees an adept will reach longevity by protecting him or her from diseases and calamities. The transformation of one's body and the elaboration of his real self (*zhen* 真) exerts a powerful influence on one's own body, and will positively transform the surrounding community.

The transformation of bodily gods is especially significant for the currents growing out the Numinous Treasure tradition such as the Divine Empyrean (Shenxiao) Taoism, which arose in the Song. In these latter groups, it was prevalent that the inner cultivation of the self benefits both the individual and his or her ancestors. This form of bodily cultivation is also necessary to ensure the efficacy of the rites performed by an officiant. In Numinous Treasure rituals, the representation of heavens and hells in these texts ensures the salvation of ancestors, but also the therapeutic exorcism and salvation of souls more generally. By locating gods within his body, the ritualist becomes a kind of sacred area. The cosmic body and the body of the gods are imagined as a sacred interior site, and the adept would journey across the hells and the paradise. In the methods of culture of self as in rituals, the practitioner's body becomes a body full of divinities that are brought into existence by visualization, gestures of the hand, magic formulas, talismans, etc..

Few contemporary Taoists are able to explain how to use the *Chart* in a ritual setting. Most often, contemporary Taoists insert the body maps into manuscripts and use them as a guide for ritual activity. This is the case for the two charts drawn in a manuscript purchased in China over the past decade by Patrice Fava (fig. 5.1),[2] and the ten maps of a manuscript on a Lüshan therapeutic ritual claiming to be in the tradition of the Correct Method of the

1 *Taishang Laojun zhongjing* 太上老君中經 (DZ 1168).

2 See the introduction of *Lingbao Taiji lianfa* 靈寶太極煉法.

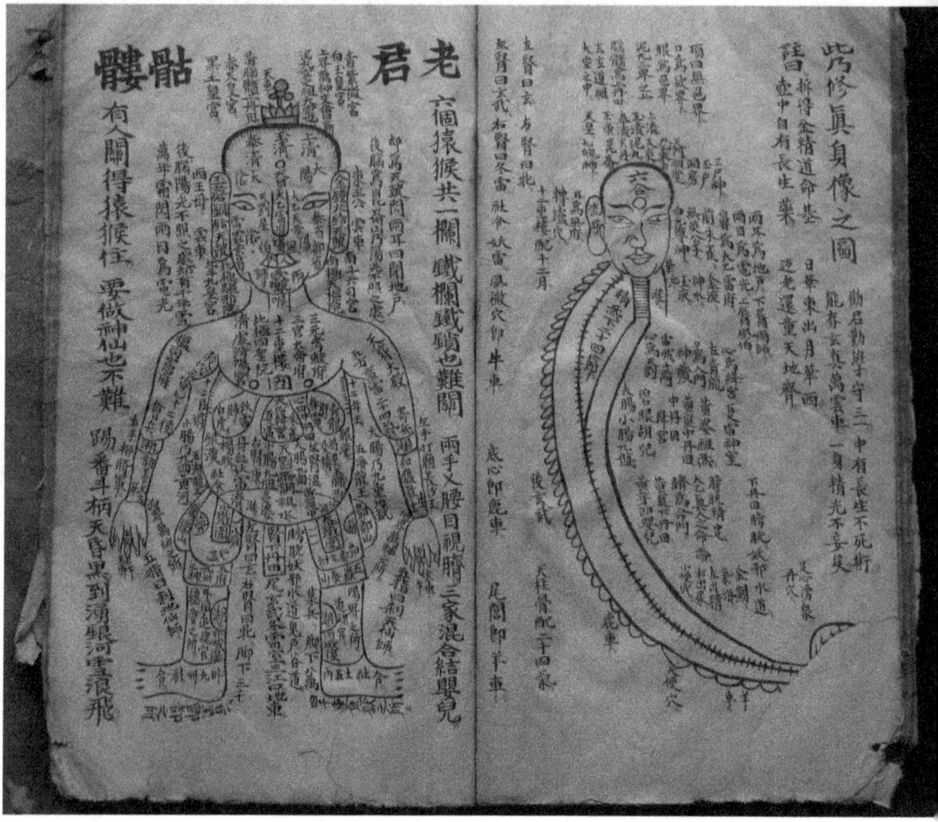


FIGURE 5.1 To the right: "Chart for the Cultivation of the True aspect of the body" (*Xiuzhen shenxiang zhi tu* 修真身像之圖). To the left: "Skeleton of the Lord Lao" (Laojun kulou 老君骷髏). From *Lingbao taiji lianbi* 靈寶太極煉秘 [Secret of the sublimation of the Great Pole according to the Numinous Treasure tradition], register belonging to *He Huaide* 何懷德, a manuscript which is the property of Patrice Fava

Heart of Heaven and the Divine Empyrean lineage.[3] Also, in a ritual observed by Brigitte Baptandier, the ten maps of the body serve as a support for the journey and ritual of the officiant. In the first course, the officiant invites the divinities (*qingshen* 請神) into his head. Here, according to the map, the hair is the seat of a thousand soldiers, the eyebrow that of the thunder and the mother of the lightning, and the forehead becomes a whole celestial pantheon. The officiant then continues to visualize his entire body, which is thereafter transformed into a talismanic map of the cosmos and its resident spirits.[4]

3 See Baptandier 2016.

4 See Baptandier 2016: 150–152.

The presentation of the ritual is two-fold. On the one hand, the officiant perceives the link between alchemical work and the unfolding of the ritual. On the other hand, he or she recognizes the gods throughout the body who can intervene through manipulation. As Baptandier explains, an adept visualizes his body as the microcosm of the universe in which the path of salvation could be traced. This is a mirror of the microcosm that the alchemist can recreate in his crucible: "By concentrating on the recreation of the cosmos in its own body, the master who performs this ritual is able to visualize the path to salvation to be travelled by souls lost in the abyss of purgatory."[5] Ultimately, the effectiveness of the ritual depends entirely on the realization and power of the master.

The sacred world that appears on the *Chart* is in line with the conceptions of the Numinous Treasure tradition founded on the *Book of Universal Salvation*. The latter text, which was greatly expanded in the early twelfth century, describes a journey in which an adept traverses the underworld. In the end, the adept completes his journey and is reborn by refining the self.[6] This text became the object of new interpretations starting in the Song dynasty when writers associated with Inner Alchemy, the Divine Empyrean School, and the Thunder Rites all studied this scripture.

## 1 The Hells

The body is the support of life, from which one can either sink to the underworld or access paradisiac realms. The hells are located in the lower part of the body, the paradises in the upper part. The reversal process, so important in alchemical methods, begins in the lower body, the realm of desire, and starts an ascent into the heavenly stratosphere of the upper body. The main process also consists of gradually eliminating the darkness and the opacity of the inner world that typically besets the ordinary man, and bring him to the light and lightness. The best way to destroy the inner hells is to increase spiritual clarity for the light of the spirit will dissolve the hells. The Taoist conceptions of hell were strongly influenced by the Buddhist representations of the world of darkness. In these two great traditions, their number and their characteristics vary according to the scriptures or the currents.

5 Baptandier 2016: 150.

6 See Schipper 2004: 1083.

### 1.1 *The City of Fengdu* 酆都

A city named Fengdu is mentioned on the Yanluozi diagrams (10th cen.), on the map of the commentary on the *Classic of the Difficulties* (*Nanjing* 難經) (late 13th cen.) and in the commentary by Xiao Yingsou on the *Book of Universal Salvation* (early 13th cen.). It is mentioned on all body maps known to date except on the *Chart on the Inner Landscape* kept in the White Cloud Temple. In the Song dynasty, Fengdu became the name of a small village not far from Chongqing in Sichuan, and was an important place of pilgrimage in subsequent centuries. With the construction of the Three Gorges dam, the town has been swallowed and its main monuments moved to a new place. From early on, Taoists located the underworld beneath a mountain called Mount Fengdu (Fengdu shan 酆都山) or Mount Luofeng (Luofeng shan 羅酆山), which occupied an inaccessible island far out in the South China Sea. On this mountain is a city where recently deceased people go, and is populated with ghosts and demons. The city also has an administrative bureaucracy similar to the human world, with an Emperor and judges overseeing the penal system. In short, Fengdu was imagined as a real society in the world of shadows (see fig. 5.2).

A passage from the *Master Who Embraces Simplicity* by Ge Hong is one of the oldest known sources about this hell city.[7] Some writings of the Upper Clarity tradition describe a hell city called Mount Luofeng (Luofeng shan or Fengdu shan) in similar terms to those used by Ge Hong.[8] However, hells play a minor role in the Upper Clarity tradition, while they are essential elements of the Numinous Treasure tradition and are subject to a very detailed set of descriptions.[9] A Six Dynasties text attributed to Ge Xuan 葛玄 (ca. 164–244), alleged founder of the Numinous Treasure tradition and great-uncle of Ge Hong, describes the underworld and Luofeng: "In the lower world of darkness is the black ocean of infinite evils, at the centre of which stands a mountain the top of which attains the Biluo 碧落 heaven, at the foot of which, the roots reach to

7 *Baopu zi neipian jiaoshi*, 3.118.

8 For the texts of the Upper Clarity describing Fengdu, cf. Robinet 1984: 137, she cites the *Zhen'gao* 真誥 [Declarations of the perfected] (DZ 1016), 13.1b–4a, 15.1a–3b and 15.11a; *Daoji lingxian ji* 道迹靈仙記 [Annals of transcendents, abstracted from the traces of the Tao] (DZ 597), 1a–2a; *Dengzhen yinjue* 登真隱訣 [Secret instructions for the ascent as a perfected] (DZ 421), 2.12a, *Shangqing tianguan santu jing* 上清天關三圖經 [Three limits scripture on the passes of heaven] (DZ 1366), lob–11b.

9 See Lagerwey 1987: 35 and 232–233; Chenivesse 1996: 61–86 and 1998: 287–339; Mollier 1997: 329–385.

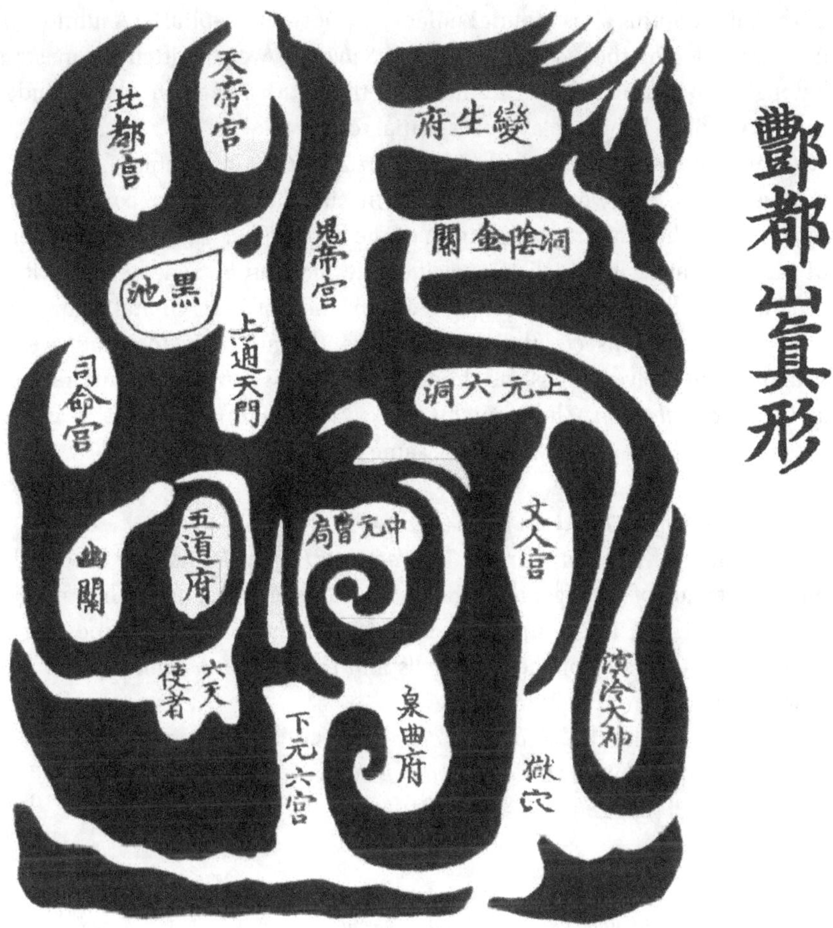


FIGURE 5.2 Drawing of the City of Fengdu. *Wushang huanglu dazhai licheng yi* (DZ 508), 40.5b

the source of the winds. It is called Mount Luo or the City of Fengdu. It reaches a height of one million one hundred and six thousand *li*."[10]

The location of this city in the human body appears in a commentary of the *Book of Universal Salvation*[11] from the thirteenth century: "The labyrinth, court

10 *Taishang cibei daochang xiaozai jiuyou chan* 太上慈悲道場消災九幽懺 [Water litany for the remission of sins, a ritual for the mercy of the most high] (DZ 543), 8.39.

11 This scripture, which dates from the fourth century, has already been thoroughly studied by Japanese and Western scholars. Mention may be made amongst other of: Gauchet 1941: 511 *sq*. Kaltenmark 1960–1961: 81–82, 1961–1962: 53–54, 1962–63: 50, 1963–64: 54. Strickmann 1975: 331–351. The first known commentary is that of Yan Dong 嚴東 (ca. middle of the fifth century).

of the Yellow Springs,[12] is Mount Luofeng, the northern capital."[13] A number of commentaries of the *Book of Universal Salvation* were written by masters belonging to the alchemical tradition of the South related to the Thunder Rites,[14] in which Fengdu plays an essential role.[15]

Commentaries of the *Book of Universal Salvation* establish analogies between the sacred world and the body. In Xiao Yingsou's 1226 commentary, for instance, there is a representation of the body called "Ascent and Descent of Yin and Yang," in which he specifies the location of Fengdu. He writes, "Below the kidneys are the City of Fengdu, the northern capital, the three corpses, the nine insects, the three officials, the nine directors, the twelve channels, the twelve springs and the streams."[16] In his commentary of the *Book of Universal Salvation*, Zhang Yuchu 張宇初 (1359–1410), a famous heavenly master of the Ming dynasty, gives the same location.[17]

### 1.2 *The Nine or Eighteen Hells* (*Fig. 5.3*)

Most versions of the *Chart for the Cultivation of Perfection* indicate nine hells; only the version of the Tiger and Dragon Altar lists eighteen hells. Their names are inscribed in a trapezium at the bottom of the body with nine points symbolizing the gates of the nine hells and the names inscribed below the points. They are, from right to left:

1. Bronze Column Hell (*Tongzhu diyu* 銅柱地獄)
2. Fiery Chariots Hell (*Huoche diyu* 火車地獄)
3. Vajra Hell (*Jingang diyu* 金剛地獄)

12 On this theme of the labyrinth, see Kaltenmark 1981: 48–49.

13 See *Yuanshi wuliang duren shangpin miaojing sizhu* 元始無量度人上品妙經四註 [Four commentaries on the *Book of Salvation*] (DZ 87), 2.29b. This text, like most others of the Numinous Treasure tradition, is imbued with Buddhist influences, and we can note in regard to the hells and Fengdu city, an influence of the *Sukhavatīvyuhasûtra* (T. 360 *Wuliang shou jing*), translated by Samghavarnam who arrived at Luoyang in 252, in which he refers to the "area of darkness" (*youming* 幽冥).

14 *Yuanshi wuliang duren shangpin miaojing tongyi* 元始無量度人上品妙經通義 [Comprehensive interpretation on the *Book of Salvation*] (DZ 89), a commentary by Zhang Yuchu (1359–1410), the fortieth heavenly master, who practiced Thunder Rites according to the Divine Empyrean tradition. *Yuanshi wuliang duren shangpin miaojing neiyi* (DZ 90), preface of 1226, a commentary by Xiao Yingsou (thirteenth century) of the tradition of the cultivation of perfection. *Yuanshi wuliang duren shangpin miaojing zhujie* 元始無量度人上品妙經註解 [Commentary on the *Book of Salvation*] (DZ 91) by Chen Zhixu (d. 1331), who made a synthesis between the southern and northern schools of Inner Alchemy.

15 See the ritual related to Fengdu analyzed by Chenivesse 1996.

16 *Yuanshi wuliang duren shangpin miaojing neiyi* (DZ 90), 3.25a.

17 *Yuanshi wuliang duren shangpin miaojing tongyi* (DZ 89), 2.14b.

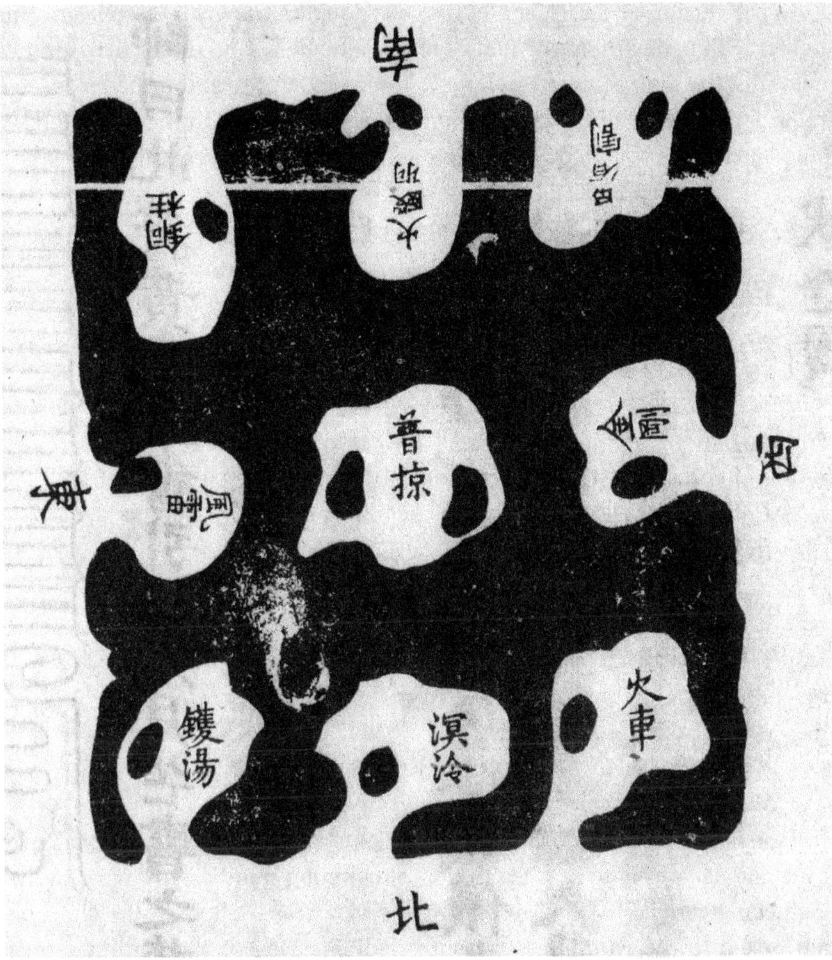


FIGURE 5.3 Chart of the nine hells lamps. *Wushang xuanyuan santian yutang dafa* (DZ 220), 14.15b

4. Mass Torture Hell (*Pulüe diyu* 普掠地獄)
5. Dark Ice Hell (*Mingleng diyu* 冥冷地獄)
6. Butchers Hell (*Tuge diyu* 屠割地獄)
7. Wind and Thunder Hell (*Fenglei diyu* 風雷地獄)
8. Boiling Cauldrons Hell (*Huotang diyu* 鑊湯地獄)
9. Unabated Hell (*Wujian diyu* 無間地獄)[18]

18 The names of the nine hells are the same on all versions.

In the version of the Tiger and Dragon Altar, the trapezium also bears nine points with below them the names of the nine hells, and under these, in two columns, the names of eighteen hells. It seems that the author had respected the original layout of the trapezium with nine points and nine names and in smaller characters added the names of eighteen hells as a commentary:

1. Hanging Tendons Hell (*Diaojin diyu* 吊筋地獄)
2. Crooked Columns Hell (*Youwang diyu* 幽枉地獄)
3. Flaming Pits Hell (*Huokang diyu* 火坑地獄)
4. City of Fengdu Hell (*Fengdu diyu* 酆都地獄)
5. Pulling Tongues Hell (*Bashe diyu* 拔舌地獄)
6. Peeling Skin Hell (*Bopi diyu* 剥皮地獄)
7. Wheel Crushing Hell (*Moya diyu* 磨挨地獄)
8. Pulverizing Pestles Hell (*Duidao diyu* 碓擣地獄)
9. Collapsing Chariot Hell (*Chebeng diyu* 車崩地獄)
10. Cold and Icy Hell (*Hanbing diyu* 寒冰地獄)
11. Removing the Shell Hell (*Tuoku diyu* 脱壳地獄)
12. Pulling Intestines Hell (*Chouchang diyu* 抽腸地獄)
13. Cauldrons of Boiling Oil Hell (*Youguo diyu* 油锅地獄)
14. Pitch Black Hell (*Hei'an diyu* 黑暗地獄)
15. Knife Mountain Hell (*Daoshan diyu* 刀山地獄)
16. Blood Lake Hell (*Xuechi diyu* 血池地獄)
17. Restless Hell (*Abi diyu* 阿鼻地獄)
18. Weighing the Scales Hell (*Pingheng diyu* 秤杆地獄)

In Taoism, the number of the hells, their name and their description vary over time and according to sources. The most common numbers are nine, twelve, eighteen, twenty-four, thirty-six or thirty-seven hells.[19] Those of the nine hells are linked to the Numinous Treasure tradition. One of the earliest sources mentioning them is a text attributed to Ge Xuan, but bears a preface of Li Hanguang (eighth century). The nine hells are distributed to eight cardinal points plus the centre as follows:

1. East: Wind and Thunder Hell
2. South: Flames Hell
3. West: Vajra Hell
4. North: Icy Hell
5. Centre: Devastating General Hell
6. Southeast: Bronze Columns Hell
7. Southwest: Butchers Hell

---

19 See Xiao 1989.

8. Northwest: Boiling Cauldrons Hell
9. Northeast: Fiery Chariot Hell[20]

This list differs from the *Chart for the Cultivation of Perfection*. The first eight hells are part of the list of the nine hells mentioned in Numinous Treasure scriptures and also used by the writings on the Thunder Rites. The last hell, however, the Unabated Hell, replaces the Flames Hell of the traditional list. Restless Hell is the central hell in the lists of thirty-seven hells.[21] It is well known in Buddhism and popular religion. Its name, Avici Hell, is the last of the eight hot hells, reserved for those who have committed the five fundamental transgressions of Buddhism. Its name is explained in different ways: the damned is subjected tirelessly to various tortures, or the damned shall fall forever or has the impression that the elapsed time is endless. As for the eighteen hells on the version of the Tiger and Dragon Altar, they correspond to the list given in chapter 11 of the well-known novel called *Journey to the West*. In this chapter, the spirit of Emperor Taizong is found in a place behind Mount Yin, where these eighteen hells are located. But there are many different lists of the eighteen hells.

## 2 The Paradises

### 2.1 *The Nine Empyreans (Jiuxiao 九霄) (See Fig. 5.4)*

The conceptions of paradises in the *Chart for the Cultivation of Perfection* adapts again from the Numinous Treasure tradition. The forehead is inscribed with the term "Nine Empyreans," each one governed by a celestial emperor.[22] The author of the *Book of Universal Salvation* describes these realms as follows: "From the yellow in the centre of the armillary sphere of the Three and the Five of the Jade Palace of the Divine Empyrean, the breaths are divided into Nine Empyreans. The breath emanating from the yang of chaos and from the original cosmic breath spreads everywhere; it is generated by transformation the nine heavens. As the models on which they operate are all recorded in the secret registers of the heavenly immortals of the Grotto-yang of the armillary

20 *Taishang cibei daochang xiaozai jiuyou chan* [Water litany for the remission of sins, a ritual for mercy most high] (DZ 543), 8.11a–12b.

21 See *Taishang cibei daochang xiaozai jiuyou chan* (DZ 543), 8.6a: "Mount Luo of the Feng capital has thirty-six hells distributed to the four directions, in the centre is the hell called Headquarters of Mount Luofeng of the North, the Avici hell without respite.

22 This entry is repeated on the nose in the version of the White Cloud Temple, while that of Mount Wudang has "nine palace" (*jiugong* 九宮) on the nose.

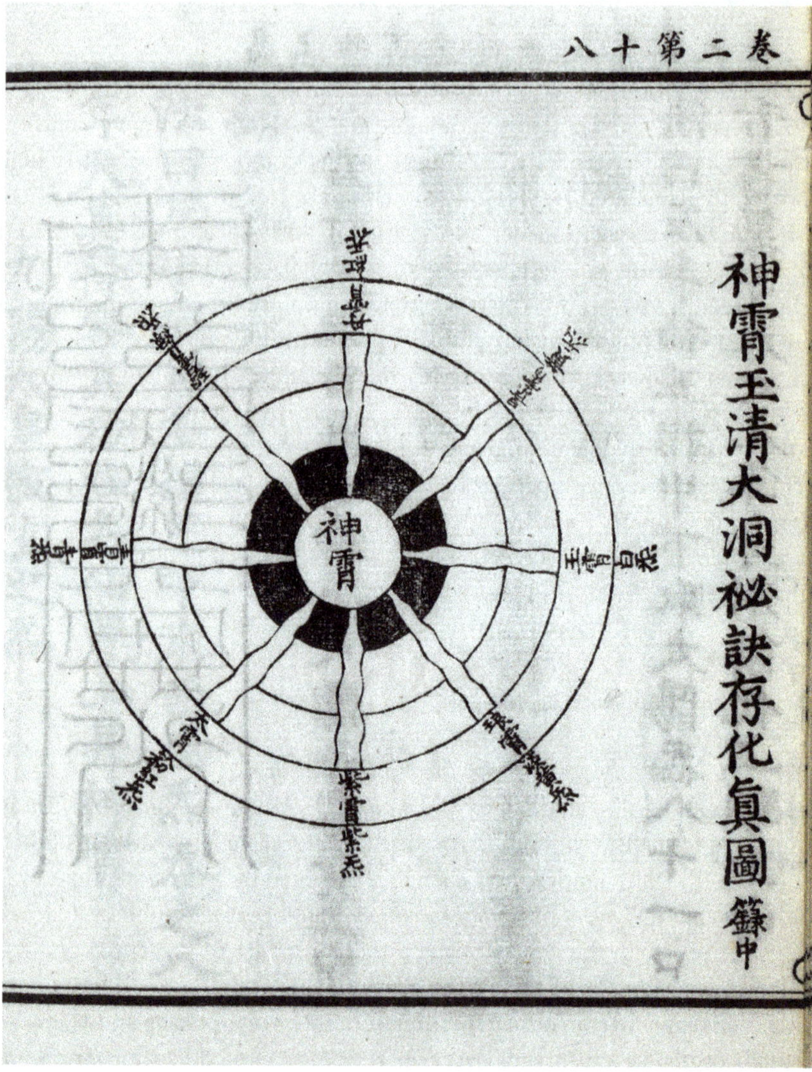


FIGURE 5.4 Diagram of the Nine Empyreans. *Gaoshang shenxiao yuqing zhenwang zishu dafa* (DZ 1219), 2.18b

sphere of the Three and the Five, it is unnecessary to describe them in detail here."[23]

23 *Lingbao wuliang duren shangpin miaojing futu* 靈寶無量度人上品妙經符圖 [Talismans and charts of the *Book of Universal Salvation*] (DZ 147), 2.5a. This text includes a foreword by Emperor Huizong of Song.

These Nine Empyreans are:[24]

1. Divine Empyrean (Shenxiao 神霄)
2. Lang-gem Empyrean (Langxiao 琅霄)
3. Purple Empyrean (Zixiao 紫霄)
4. Supreme Empyrean (Taixiao 太霄)
5. Blue Empyrean (Qingxiao 青霄)
6. Cyan Empyrean (Bixiao 碧霄)
7. Cinnabar Empyrean (Danxiao 丹霄)
8. Phosphor Empyrean (Jingxiao 景霄)
9. Jade Empyrean (Yuxiao 玉霄)

On the *Chart for the Cultivation of Perfection*, the text at the upper right of the chart alludes to these eight empyreans situated at the eight points of the compass card: "The bones of the brain include eight chambers in correspondence with the eight points of the compass."

### 2.2 *The Heaven of the Pervasive Net* (*Miluo* 彌羅) *or the Heaven of the Obscure Firmament* (*Xuanqiong* 玄瓊) *and Mount Yujing* 玉京山

On the upper left of the body map is the following inscription: "The bones of the brain are the Cosmic Heaven, the Jade Emperor Palace, the Heavenly Palace of Pure Yang. The centre is a cavity called the Palace of the Spirit, i.e., the ruler of the Obscure Firmament." The preceding body maps, such as the Yanluozi diagrams, the map in the commentary on the *Book of the Difficulties*, the one in Xiao Yingsou's commentary and the *Chart of the Inner Landscape* of the White Cloud Temple all write the Jade Net Heaven (*Yuluo tian* 玉羅天), which was mentioned in the *Book of Universal Salvation*. But all the versions of the *Chart for the Cultivation of Perfection* use the term Pervasive Net Heaven (*Miluo tian* 彌羅天), which has its *locus classicus* in the *Combined Scriptures on the Founding Acts of the Jade Sovereign on High* (13th cen.). The latter text also mentions the Heaven of the Obscure Firmament where the Jade Sovereign (Yuhuang) reigns; this heaven is mentioned in the upper-left portion of the text. This text enjoyed unprecedented popularity in the Qing dynasty, including under Emperor Kangxi (r. 1661–1722), that is at the period in which the *Chart for the Cultivation of Perfection* probably appeared. It became one of the texts read during the liturgy of the Complete Perfection School or the Dragon Gate tradition, and played a fundamental role in exorcisms.

24 See the "Diagram of the Nine Empyreans Generated by Transformation of the Breaths of Nine Radiances of the Red Writings in the Grotto-chaos," in *Lingbao wuliang duren shangpin miaojing futu* (DZ 147), 2.5b. A similar diagram is in *Gaoshang shenxiao yuqing zhenwang zishu dafa* 高上神霄玉清真王紫書大法 [Grand ritual from the purple book of the true king of the highest divine empyrean jade purity] (DZ 1219), 2.18b. See fig. 5.4.

The Jade Capital (Yujing 玉京) is mentioned on the *Chart for the Cultivation of Perfection* in the text inscribed near the third pass on the neck. It reads, "This place is called the Yang Palace. It is the Jade Mountain Capital, the heaven to which belong the Palace of the Great One and the Palace of Thunder and Lightning." The Jade Mountain Capital is quoted in the *Scripture of Universal Salvation* for this scripture is depicted as "a venerable and wonderful text, the only one giving access to the Jade Capital."[25] That text also mentions "the upper capital of Jade Mountain and of the Sagebrush Terrace" (*Xiaotai yushan shangjing* 蕭臺玉山上京).[26] According to the commentary by Xiao Yingsou, in "the Great Net Heaven is Mount Jade on which is built the Mysterious Terrace of seven jewels. In the city of seven jewels, there is the Great Hall of the Jade Clarity where the Jade Sovereign resides."

## 3 The Celestial Palaces[27]

The *Chart for the Cultivation of Perfection* comprises the name of four palaces. They are related to palaces mentioned in at least two scriptures of the Taoist Canon. First, the *Book of Universal Salvation*, a text that several Song commentators interpret with vocabulary of Inner Alchemy and thunder rites. The palaces also appear in the aforementioned *Essentials of the Combined Scriptures of the Founding Acts of the Jade Emperor on High*, a text that is often linked to the Heaven of the Pervasive Net and an important text in the Dragon Gate tradition.

### 3.1 *The Fire Palace of the Vermilion Mound (Zhuling huofu* 朱陵火府*)*

The Fire Palace of the Vermilion Mound is the place of salvation that follows the refinement of the body. It often is used to describe the destination of the deceased, but can also be applied to the adept refining his self through Inner Alchemy. This palace is located on the *Chart for the Cultivation of Perfection* in the heart. In addition, one can read in this area the inscriptions "Upper Palace of the South Brightness" (*Nanchang shanggong*) and "Scarlet Palace" (*Jianggong*).[28]

---

25 *Yuanshi wuliang duren shangpin miaojing sizhu* (DZ 87), 1.22a.

26 *Ibid.*, 2.10a.

27 *Yuanshi wuliang duren shangpin miaojing neiyi* (DZ 90), 2.9b.

28 A description and a list of the various heavenly palaces according to the tradition of the Numinous Treasure are given in *Lingbao wuliang duren shangpin dafa* 靈寶無量度人上品大法 [Great rites of the *Book of Universal Salvation*] (DZ 219), 29.2a–3b.

Vermilion Mound (*Zhuling* 朱陵) is already a well-known place in the ancient Chinese mythology and Taoism. There is a passage in the *Collection on the Ten Continents* attributed to Dongfang Shuo 東方朔 (ca. 154–93 BCE) that reads, "Following the master, I reached the porch giving access to the Vermilion Mound (Zhuling) and Fusang Tree."[29] This is also cited in the *Inner Biography of Emperor Wu of the Han*: "The Queen Mother told the Lady of the Upper Origin, 'Install the vermilion fire, the cinnabar mound, eat the magic gourd, enjoy its sweetness, and you will live seven thousand years.'"[30]

The idea that the soul of the deceased through refinement can be reborn as human is already present in the *Book of Universal Salvation* which mentions this place without specifying that it is a palace: "The spirits pass the Vermilion Mound where they are refined and reborn." According to Xue Youqi's 薛幽契 (ca. 754) commentary, Vermilion Mound designates a palace located to the South.[31] The role of the Vermilion Mound Palace is described in greater detail in a passage of a later text (1406) by Zheng Sixiao 鄭思肖, who links it to the thunder rites and describes a ritual by explaining the interior character of this rite:

> Enter in the chamber and sit-up straight. Purify the heart, calm the mind, regulate the breath, and after a while, concentrate on the true breath of the lower cinnabar field which becomes a fire like a red jade pearl. Afterwards, turn nine times to the left and right. Practice until it becomes very clear. After a while, you feel that the Jade Pond is filled with secretions; it is the moment that the water will rise from the kidneys. This true fire pill starts to rise into the heart palace or the Scarlet Palace called The Upper Palace of South Brightness or the Fire Palace of the Vermilion Mound. From the court where the fire burns, ascend the fumes that melt the metal. Imagine that this fire consumes completely your own body. After a while the body will be transformed into an infant that is sitting upright in the Scarlet Palace. Gradually, the infant goes up the twelve-storey pagoda, passes the Jade Chamber, the Bronze Tower, and attains the Muddy Pellet Palace at the top of the head. He will transform into the body of a celestial worthy, and sit at the centre of the palace.[32]

---

29 *Shizhou ji* 十洲記 [Records on the ten continents], in *Yunji qiqian* (DZ 1032), 26.1b.

30 Schipper 1996: 105.

31 *Yuanshi wuliang duren shangpin miaojing sizhu* (DZ 87), 2. 27b.

32 Zheng Sixiao (1241–1318), *Taiji jilian neifa* 太極祭鍊內法 [Inner method of Taiji for sacrificing to and sublimating the deceased] (DZ 548), 1.1b–2a. This palace is also mentioned in Lu Shizhong's 路時中 *Wushang xuanyuan santian yutang dafa* 無上玄

### 3.2 *The Upper Palace of the South Brightness* (*Nanchang shanggong* 南昌上宫)

This palace is mentioned in the *Book of Universal Salvation* alongside ministers and assistants of various heavens.[33] According to the commentary by Xiao Yingsou, "the minister and the assistant breaths can establish the evolutions and transformations. They are the lords and gods of the Great Net Heaven, and the upper palace of the South Brightness is the Palace of the Vermilion Mound, which is inside the Yang Heaven and the red light of the infant."[34]

This palace is often considered as the same as the Vermilion Mound Palace, as asserted by the text by Zheng Suonan of the Divine Empyrean tradition already quoted in relation with the Vermilion Mound Palace: "The South Palace is high up in heaven the place where the principal fire refines the souls of the dead to transform them into immortals. The South Dipper is a configuration of the stars high up in heaven, where are kept the long-life registers of *hun* souls belonging to the World of darkness. The various sovereigns of the South Pole are the deities of the various palaces below the Muddy Pellet. The Upper Palace of the South Brightness is the Fire Palace of the Vermilion Mound, i.e., the Scarlet Palace within the human body."[35]

The Scarlet Palace is an important place in the alchemical process. It seems in any case distinct from the heart. Zhang Jixian 張繼先 (1092–1127), the thirtieth Heavenly Master of the Orthodox Unity tradition, a Taoist adored by the Song Emperor Huizong, composed a poem called "Nanchang is not the Heart," in which he writes:

> This orifice of the Obscure Pass stores yin and yang,
> In the beginning the heart and the kidneys are not places of water and fire.
> The master of sublimation with penetrative insight told me this,
> "Do not take the palace of the heart for the South Brightness."[36]

元三天玉堂大法 [Great ritual of the Jade Hall of the three heavens of the supreme mysterious origin] (DZ 220), 15.10ab.

33 *Yuanshi wuliang duren shangpin miaojing sizhu* (DZ 87), 3.20b.

34 *Yuanshi wuliang duren shangpin miaojing neiyi* (DZ 90), 3.20b.

35 *Taiji jilian neifa* (DZ 548), 3.6b.

36 Zhang Jixian 張繼先 (1092–1127), *Mingzhen powang zhangsong* 明真破望章頌 [Stanzas of understanding truth and refuting error] (DZ 979), 3b.

### 3.3 *The Cinnabar Hall of the Spirits of the Cold (Hanling dandian* 寒靈丹殿)

The inscription "Cinnabar Hall of the Spirits of the Cold" is engraved at the centre of the representation, to the right of the standing infant symbolizing the breath. This palace belongs to the Upper Palace of the Purple Tenuity (*Ziwei shanggong* 紫微上宫), which according to the *Essentials of the Combined Scriptures of the Founding Acts of the Jade Emperor on High* is one of the palaces where the Jade Emperor installed the perfected scripts.[37] It is clear that the *Jade Emperor Scripture* is an essential scriptural source for the *Chart for the Cultivation of Perfection.*

### 3.4 *The Palace of Thunder and Lightning (Leiting fu* 雷霆府)

On the *Chart for the Cultivation of Perfection*, the upper part of the nose bears the inscription Leifu, probably a shortened version for *Leiting dufu* 雷霆都府 [Palace of thunder and lightning], the name of a heavenly palace linked to the methods of the thunder rites. The Celestial Worthy of the Universal Transformations of the Nine Heavens (*Jiutian puhua tianzun* 九天普化天尊) governs the five thunders and magically transforms the nine heavens. He is the governor general of the Palace of Thunder and Lightning, which is associated with two courts: the Court of The Five Thunders (*Wulei yuan* 五雷院) and the Court for Exorcising Evils (*Quxie yuan* 去邪院).[38] It is therefore normal that the name of the Palace of Thunder and Lightning is inscribed on the Chart at the head since the head is metaphorically the heaven. In addition, according to the *Taoist Methods, United in Principle*, "the spirit corresponds in the heaven to thunder and in the earth to fire, or in the human body to the heart."[39] Another text on the Thunder Rites describes this palace as follows:

> What are the thunder and the lightning? The yang, or the One, is the thunder; the yin, or the two, is the lightning. The yin and yang [Original] Breaths increase and decrease. When the yin is buried in the yang and when yang reaches the peak, you should let it shoot up and stimulate it: a roll of thunder occurs in the sky, while the earth quakes.[40]

---

37 See *Gaoshang yuhuang benxing jijing* 高上玉皇本行集經 [Combined scriptures of the founding acts of the Jade Emperor on high] (DZ 10), 2.3b.

38 See *Lingbao lingjiao jidu jinshu* 靈寶靈教濟度金書 [Golden book of salvation according to the numinous treasure tradition] (DZ 466).

39 *Daofa huiyuan* (DZ 1220), 67.9.

40 See Wang Weiyi 王惟一 (ob. 1294), *Daofa xinchuan* 道法心傳 [Spiritual tradition of Taoist rites] (DZ 1253), 11a. The author, Wang Weiyi, belonged to the Divine Empyrean

## 4 The *Hun* 魂 Souls and the *Po* 魄 Souls in Inner Alchemy

The term *hun* designating the celestial souls and that of *po* the terrestrial souls are ancient. *Po* is already used in Chapter Ten of Laozi: "When carrying on your head the *po*, can you embrace the One and not let go?" According to the early commentary by the Master of the River Bank (Heshang gong 河上公), one must understand: "Carrying the *hun* and the *po*." His commentary says:

> *Yingpo* [Carrying the *po*] must be understood as *hun po*, 'the *hun* soul and the *po* soul.' Man needs the *hun* souls and the *po* souls to be alive, he must cherish and nurture them. Joy or anger makes the *hun* soul disappear; sudden anguish hurts the *po* soul. The *hun* soul abides in the liver, the *po* soul in the lungs. Tasty dishes and delicious alcohol deteriorate the lungs. If the *hun* soul is in peace, if while aspiring to the Way we keep the mind untroubled, the *po* soul is in peace and we can live a long time.[41]

According to the writings of the Master of Huainan 淮南子, a collection of essays that resulted from a series of scholarly debates held at the court of the Master sometime before 139 BC, the *hun* soul is the celestial breath while the *po* soul is the terrestrial breath."[42] In his article on the term "numinous treasure," Max Kaltenmark highlights the link between the *po* soul whose character includes the "white" 白 element, and the skeleton, where abide the vital principles represented by marrow and seminal essence.[43] He adds that "Just as the witch Bao 保 sexually united with spirits (*ling* 靈 or *shen* 神),[44] we can imagine between the *hun* and the *po* souls a kind of hierogamic link that certain practices should help to establish or maintain. Internal Alchemy in particular is built on this theme, where alloys and transmutations of vital elements are described in terms of marriage and birth."[45]

The numbers of three *hun* and seven *po* souls are attested only from the time of the *Master Who Embraces Simplicity*. Techniques to monitor and control the vital spirits are developed from Jin onwards and are particularly prevalent in the Tang Dynasty. In the Song texts on Internal Alchemy, they are also commonly mentioned. In the text on the deity of the liver in the *Chart*

---

tradition. He exposes alchemical processes related to those of the Southern tradition and often cites Zhang Boduan and Bai Yuchan.

41 *Laozi Heshang gong zhu jiaoli* 1971: 55–56.

42 *Huainan zi*, 9.127.

43 See also Ikeda 1953.

44 Mentioned in the poem "Shao siming" of the *Chuci*. *Chuci zhangju* 楚辭章句 (SKQS), 2.12.

45 Kaltenmark 1960: 580.

*for the Cultivation of Perfection*, it is said: "Harmonize and master the *hun* souls, the *po* souls and the bodily fluids," which is a citation of the *Book of the Yellow Court*. It is also said: "In the liver abide the three *hun* souls respectively named Serene Numinous Spirit (*Shuangling* 爽靈), White Light (*Baiguang* 白光) and Obscure Essence (*Youjing* 幽精)." The seven *po* souls are also mentioned in the text on the lungs, with their respective names. The earliest known text which describes the *hun* and *po* souls, giving a representation of them and their names, dates from the middle of the ninth century: the *Scripture of the Most High for the Protection of Life through the Elimination of the Three Corpses and the Nine worms*. The three *hun* souls have a human form, but the seven *po* have a demonic one, because they are "heaps of yin." Each of the three *hun* souls has an essential function. The Serene Numinous Spirit has a protective function, the White Light nourishes and the Obscure Essence preserves life.[46] On the 3rd, 13th and 23rd of each month, these spirits leave the body to make a report on the conduct of the individual to the heavenly emperor; it is therefore necessary to retain them within the body by methods such as calling them three times. The seven *po* souls, attracted by dirt, activate the three corpses. During the nights of the new and the full moon, dirt, demons, blood, bodies, and sex attract them, and they must be particularly controlled. The representations of the three corpses are included in the Yanluozi diagrams (fig. 5.5), in the commentary of the *Classic of the Difficulties*,[47] in some ritual texts (fig. 5.6) or in scholarly works (see fig. 5.7), but they disappeared from the *Chart for the Cultivation of Perfection*.

In Inner Alchemy, the three *hun* souls and the seven *po* souls are seldom mentioned; more often there is only the mention of one *hun* and one *po*, and they have lost their anthropomorphic and divine characters. Instead, they become vital forces integrated with various other major forces associated with each of the five viscera. Here, for example, is how the *Principles of the Tablets on the Innate Nature and the Vital Force* describes them:

> The "cloud" (*yun* 云) and "demon" (*gui* 鬼) characters together form the character *hun* 魂. The "white" (*bai* 白) and the "demon" characters put

46 A fragment of a Zhengyi text is conserved in the *Yunji qiqian* (1024); in these teachings of the Zhengyi Taoist Zhao Sheng (趙昇) of Mount Heming (Sichuan), the text is far from presenting the three *hun* as beneficial to man. *Yunji qiqian* (DZ 1032), 54.1–2.

47 Yanluozi's *Chaozhen tu*, in *Xiuzhen shishu* (DZ 263), 18.2b. See *Huangdi bashiyi nanjing zhuyi tuxu lun* (DZ 1024) by Li Jiong (1269). These representations are also given in *Wushang sanyuan santian yutang dafa*, DZ 220, 3.5b–6a (fig. 5.6). They are also found in the *Yuhan bizhi* 玉函秘指 of the *Yimen guangdu* (late 16th cen.) (fig. 5.7) and in *Xingming guizhi*, 1.32b.

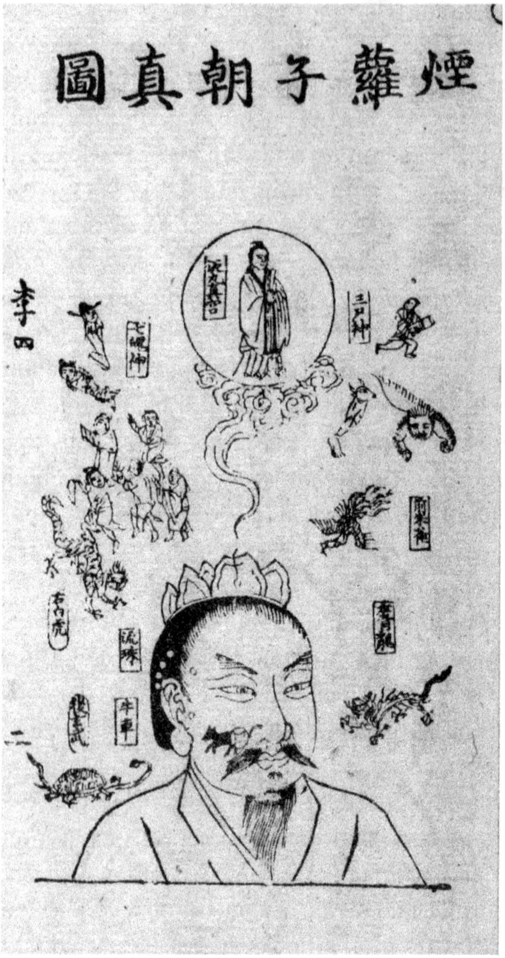


FIGURE 5.5 The three corpses and seven *po* souls. Yanluozi's drawings, in *Xiuzhen shishu* (DZ 263), 18.2a

together form the character *po* 魄. The cloud corresponds to the wind, and the wind, to wood. White corresponds to the breath and the breath corresponds to metal. The wind disperses and gives lightness and purity. This causes the *po* to rise, and this is followed by the *hun*. The breath is metal, corresponding to the heavy and impurity. When it is heavy and unclean, the *hun* descends, and is followed by the *po*. It is the reason why the sage moves the *hun* and *po* souls together, while the ordinary man only preserves the *hun* and *po* souls. During the day, the *hun* resides in the eyes, during the night, in the liver, and this is what allows you to see

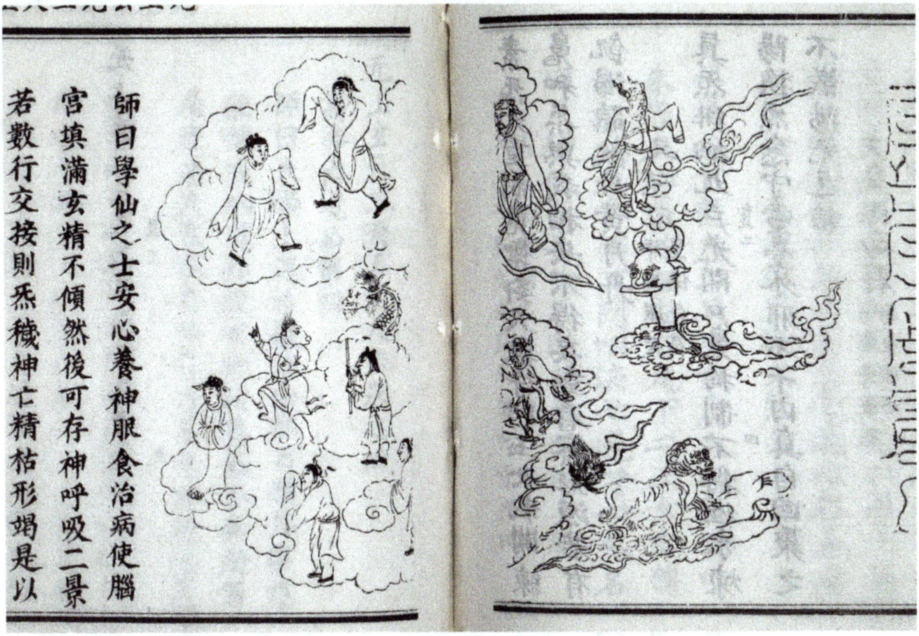
師曰學仙之士安心養神服食治病使腦
宮填滿玄精不傾然後可存神呼吸二景
若數行交接則炁穢神亡精枯形竭是以

FIGURE 5.6 The three corpses, the three *hun* and the seven *po*. *Wushang xuanyuan santian yutang dafa* (DZ 220), 3.5b–6a

> and dream. If you have many dreams, it is that the *po* controls the *hun*. If instead the mind is lucid, the *hun* masters the *po*. But the essence exists because of the *po*, and due to the essence, there is the *hun*, and due to the *hun*, there is the spirit (*shen*), and due to the spirit, there is creative thinking (*yi*) and because of creative thinking, there is the *po*. The *hun* and the *po* souls move into an uninterrupted cycle.[48]

Two texts on the Chart present these two souls:
(fig. 3.6, text 15)

> It is called the Azure Dragon of the East Sea. It corresponds to the celestial stem *jia*, to the wood liquor, the trigram Zhen, the East. Of the five agents, it corresponds to wood. In the Way it remains the residence of the *hun* souls, that is to say innate nature. It is the mother of the fire god and among the five viscera, it corresponds to the liver. In the sky, it corresponds to the sun. It is really where my hun souls abide.

48 *Xingming guizhi*, 1.32b.

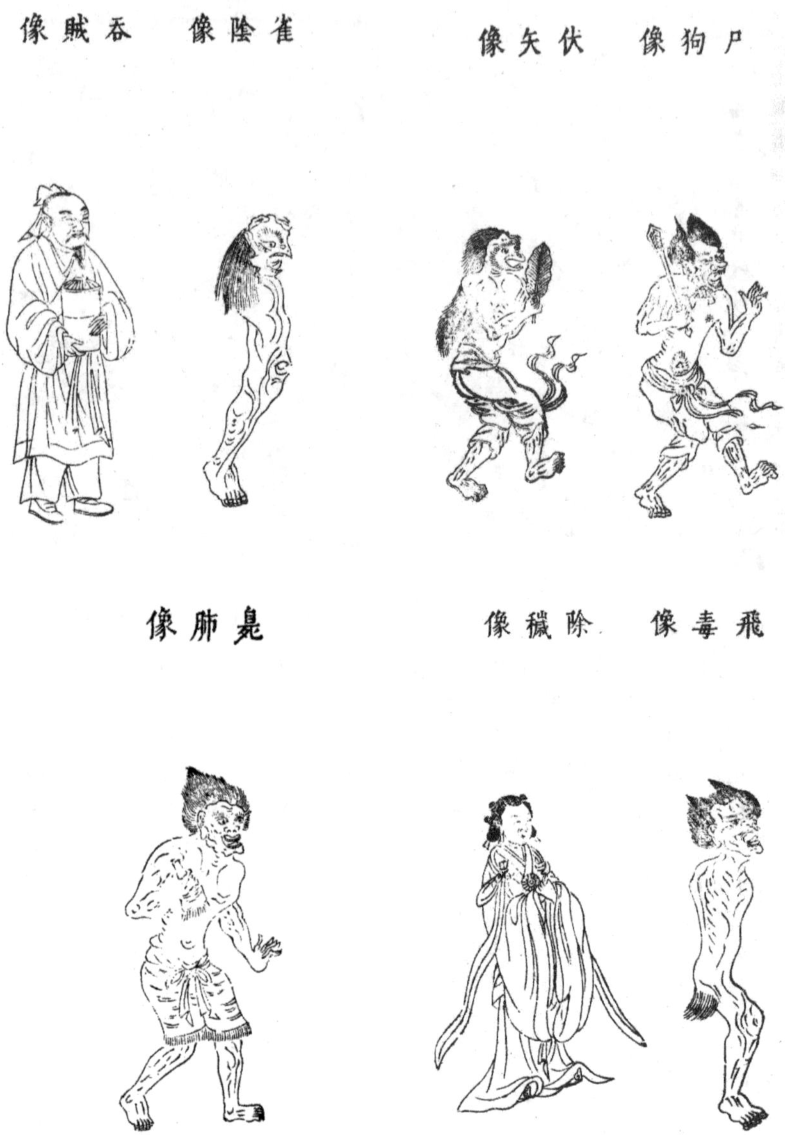


FIGURE 5.7 Drawing of the seven *po* souls. *Yuhan bidian* 玉函秘典, in *Yimen guangdu* 夷門廣牘 by Zhou Lüjing 周履靖

(fig. 3.6, text 14)

It is called the White Tiger of the Mountain of the West. It corresponds to the celestial stem *geng*, to the essence of the metal, the trigram Dui, the West. Of the five agents, it corresponds to metal. In the Way, it is the *po* souls, that is to say the passions. It is the mother of the water essence, and corresponds to the lungs. In the sky, it corresponds to the moon. It is really where my *po* souls abide.

## 5 The Inner Gods in the Yellow Court Tradition

### 5.1 *The Yellow Court (huangting* 黄庭*)*

There are two similar scriptures describing deities inside the body: the *Book of the Inner Landscape of the Yellow Court* and the *Book of the Outer Landscape of the Yellow Court*. They were written between the Later Han (late second century) and the fourth century respectively.[49] Various specialists have divergent positions on the precedence of one over the other, some considering the *Book of the Inner Landscape* as the earlier, other supporting the inverse position.[50] The study of these texts became widespread in the Tang Dynasty (618–907)[51] and continued to be part of the most common practices of meditation on the body. During the Song dynasty (960–1271) they were integrated to the southern alchemical practices, notably by the currents practicing the thunder rites.[52]

49 *Huangting neijing jing* and *Huangting waijing jing*. There is a stele from 337 of the *Huangting waijing jing* calligraphied by Wang Xizhi 王羲之 (303–379).

50 See Wang 1984: 324–371, considering the *Neijing* as being older, such as I. Robinet (1979, p. 86). K. Schipper takes the opposite position in the introduction to his *Concordance du Houang-t'ing king*. The title *Huangting jing* is cited in *Liexian zhuan* 列仙傳, a work dating of the Late Han (cf. p. 179 of the translation by Mr. Kaltenmark), and in "Xialan" 暇覽, the eighteenth chapter of the *Master Who Embraces Simplicity*.

51 There remains two commentaries from this time: one by Liangqiu zi (or Bai Lüzhong 白履忠) written in 722 during the reign of Emperor Xuanzong, and one by Wucheng zi 務成子, which from the third paragraph on, is in fact the commentary of Liangqiu zi. See the introduction of Schipper 1975.

52 Some writings of the Yellow Court tradition are included for example in *Xiuzhen shishu* (DZ 263). These include the *Huangting neijing wuzang liufu buxie tu* 黄庭內景五藏六府補瀉圖 [Chart on the procedures of tonification and purgation of the six receptacles and five viscera according to the inner landscape of the Yellow Court], by Hu Yin 胡愔 (DZ 263), 54.1–24; *Huangting neijing yujing zhu* (DZ 263), *j.* 55–57; and *Huangting waijing yujing zhu* (DZ 263), *j.* 58–60. On the relationship between the tradition of the Yellow Court and the Xiuzhen, see Needham 1983: 67 *sq*.

Both of the aforementioned texts on the Yellow Court present the inner landscape of the body, i.e., the major organs and the hundred and eight deities abiding therein, the orifices, the locations of passage and transmutation. The adept who visualizes the deities of these viscera is safe from all diseases and evil influences, as stated in one of the two texts: "This scripture must be carefully studied; whoever recites it ten thousand times can access the three heavens, destroy the thousand calamities, cure diseases; he will no longer fear the ferocity of tigers and wolves, and he may counteract aging and live a long time."[53]

The term Yellow Court is attested from the second century onwards, since it is used in an "Inscription on Laozi" by Bian Shao 邊韶 dating from 165.[54] This term is also used in the *Most High Lord Lao's Book on the Centre* dating from the late second century, which reads: "Imagine that, under the breasts, the yellow essence and the red breath emanate from the sun and the moon, enter the Scarlet Palace, then penetrate again into the Yellow Court and the Purple chamber."[55] The Yellow Court is a central element of the inner vision of the body. The term "court" suggests that it is a place where abides a deity and the colour yellow indicates that this place is central. Yellow, after all, is associated with the centre and with the earth according to the correlation system of the five agents. Nevertheless, in both scriptures, no precise information is given about this Yellow Court and its location is not specified. Only a late commentary by Liangqiu zi 梁丘子 (ca. 722) provides us with clarification. He writes, "The spleen is the central position of the earth, which is why (its deity) is called Permanent Residence (*Changzai* 常在). This is the Palace of the Yellow Court."[56] This later localisation, equating the Yellow Court to the spleen, is not the only one. In Internal Alchemy, it is located either at the spleen or below the navel, and can sometimes be confused with the Lower Cinnabar Field. A twelfth century writer poses the question, "Where is the Yellow Court?" and answers "The Yellow Court having the shape of a hen's egg is located above the bladder, to the front of the kidneys and the spleen, behind the navel, to the right of the liver and to the left of the lungs."[57] In the different versions of

53 *Huangting neijing yujing zhu* (DZ 402), 1.3ab.

54 "Laozi ming" 老子銘. This inscription includes the following sentence: "He enters and exits by the cinnabar cottage, he rises and falls from the Yellow Court." See Seidel 1969: 47–48.

55 *Taishang Laojun zhongjing* (DZ 1168), 1.6b–7a. Prior to this, the writer claims that "the Perfected of the Yellow Court is the father and mother of the Dao, the place where the child is conceived."

56 DZ 402, 1.15b. Cf. *ibid.*, 2.4a: "The spleen is the Palace of the Yellow Court."

57 Chapter "Hundred Questions" in *Daoshu* (DZ 1017), 5.17a.

the *Chart for the Cultivation of Perfection*, the inscription "Yellow Court" is located at the Median Cinnabar Field in the central circle. To the side we can see the character *zhong* 中 [centre]. Therefore, on this body map, the Yellow Court is probably identified with the spleen.

### 5.2 *Importance of the Gallbladder in the Yellow Court Tradition*

The bodily functions described in this text include six viscera (*zang* 藏), not five as was common in medical texts in the Han dynasty and thereafter. To the usual correlation system with the five agents and the five viscera (liver, heart, spleen, lungs, kidneys), is added the gallbladder, classified in the medical system as one of the six receptacles (*fu* 府), and coupled with the liver.[58] The presentation of the five viscera, with the gallbladder added is a relic of an ancient tradition of which there are traces in the *Inner Canon of the Yellow Emperor*, which was competing with the tradition of the five viscera and six receptacles, and attributed a prominent place to the gallbladder. Thus, in the chapter "Treaty on the Viscera" in the *Inner Canon of the Yellow Emperor*, we found a passage that claims that the arbiter of the eleven organs is the gallbladder.[59] In chapter eight of this same text, the writer further clarifies: "The gallbladder is the official of the centre and of righteousness, decisions and verdicts emanate from it."[60] This tradition probably comes from the masters of esoterica (*fangshi* 方士), as suggested by another passage:

> The Yellow Emperor said: "I learned that some masters of techniques consider the brain and the spinal cord, the intestines and the stomach as viscera (*zang*), while others consider them as receptacles (*fu*), what about these contradictions?" Qibo replied, "The marrow, the brain, the bones, the vessels, the gallbladder, the womb, the six are generated by the breath of the earth. Their storage is associated with yin; they are in the image of the earth. Hence, they store and don't drain. They are called 'independent and marvellous receptacles' (*qiheng zhi fu* 奇橫之府)."[61]

---

58 The six receptacles (*liufu*) are, in the system of traditional Chinese medicine, the stomach, the gallbladder, both intestines, the bladder and the triple heater (*sanjiao* 三焦), an organ which, in traditional Chinese medicine is considered as having a function but no form.

59 *Huangdi neijing*. This book consists of two parts: *Questions about the Emergence of Life* (*Suwen*) and *Pivot of Numinous Spirits* (*Lingshu*). It was probably written around the first century BCE, and uses documents belonging to different schools and from various periods; for this point it may be compared to the Hippocratic corpus. See chapter 9 of *Suwen* ("Liujie zangxiang lun" 六節藏象論), 2.60.

60 *Ibid.*, ch. 8 "Linglan midian lun" 靈蘭秘典論, 3.49.

61 *Ibid.*, ch. 11 "Wuzang bielun" 五藏別論, 3.67.

In the correspondence between the grades of officials and the body elements, a Taoist text generally dated from the Later Han or from the Three Kingdoms, gives the gallbladder the highest rank, i.e., the Son of Heaven (Emperor).[62] As for the *Book of the Inner Landscape of the Yellow Court*, it considers that "the palace of the gallbladder is the quintessence of the six receptacles", and the commentary by Liangqiu zi adds that "according to the *Book of the Great Peace*, the accumulation of essence becomes azure (*qing* 青), which is why the gallbladder is the quintessence of the six receptacles."[63] In the *Book of the Inner Landscape of the Yellow Court*, the gallbladder is presented as follows:

> The palace of the gallbladder area,
> Is the quintessence of the six receptacles.
> Within it remains a young boy,
> Called Vapours of the Dragon with Majestic Brightness.
> To the eight directions arise thunder and lightning,
> The jade banners are deployed.
> The dragon flag covers the sky,
> And the fire bell tinkles continuously.
> This young boy governs all breath, controls the armies of tigers,
> And corresponds outwardly with the pupil and the edge of the nose.
> His boldness makes the hair stand on your head.
> He wears a brocade garment of nine colours and a flowered green skirt,
> He wears a gold belt with the insignia of the tiger.
> Anyone able to visualize Majestic Brightness,
> Will straddle the splendorous clouds.
> He will further be served by all the gods,
> And will have an audience with the Three Origins.[64]

## 5.3 *Animal Images of the Deities of the Six Viscera*

In the Tang period, several texts related to the *Book of the Yellow Court* appeared. They give much more detailed descriptions of the viscera than before, and were often accompanied by illustrations of gymnastic and breathing techniques, as well as visualizations. Two of these texts had a relatively important diffusion.[65]

---

62 *Taishang lingbao wufu xu* 太上靈寶五符序 [The five talismans, powerful treasure of the most high] (DZ 388), 1.20a.

63 *Huangting neijing yujing zhu* (DZ 402), 2.2b.

64 *Huangting neijing yujing zhu* (DZ 402), 2.2b–3b.

65 *Shangqing huangting wuzang liufu zhenren yuzhou jing* 上清黃庭五藏六府真人玉軸經 [Precious scroll of the perfected being on the six receptacles and five viscera of the Yellow Court of upper clarity] (DZ 1402), a version of which is in the *Yunji qiqian, juan* 14, bears the title of *Huangting dunjia yuanshen jing* 黃庭盾甲緣身經 [Book of the

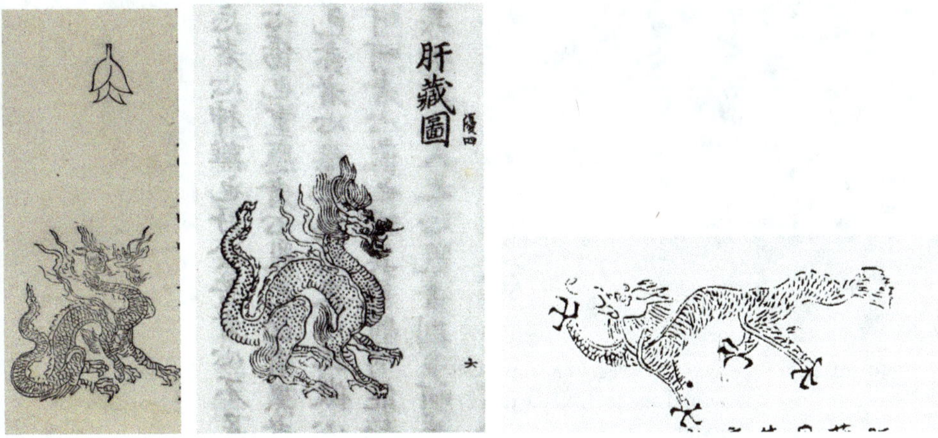


FIGURE 5.8 Deity of the liver (dragon). Left, *Shangqing huangting wuzang liufu zhenren yuzhou jing* (DZ 1402), 5a. In the middle, *Yunji qiqian* (DZ 1032), 14.7b, and on the right, *Chart for the Cultivation of Perfection*

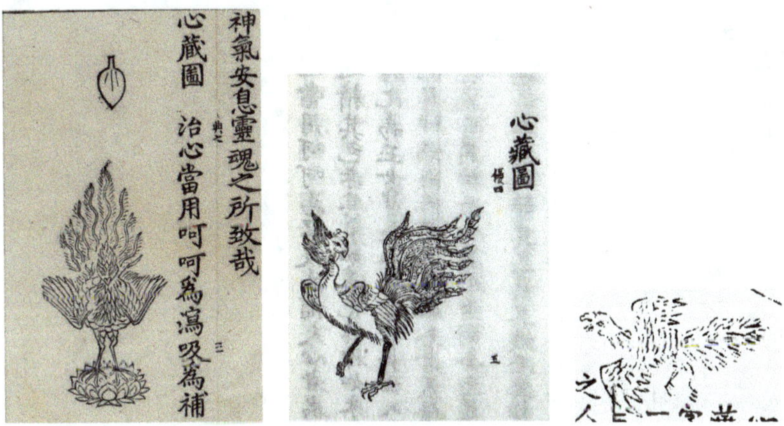


FIGURE 5.9 Deity of the heart (vermilion sparrow). Left, *Shangqing huangting wuzang liufu zhenren yuzhou jing* (DZ 1402), 3b. In the middle, *Yunji qiqian* (DZ 1032), 14.6a, and on the right, the *Chart for the Cultivation of Perfection*

hidden period and the causal karma body of the Yellow Court] and is anterior to 1024, the date of compilation of *Yunji qiqian*. The animal forms are represented in a different manner from those of DZ 432 and we can see above them the shape of the organs (see fig. 38–43). *Huangting wuzang liufu buxie tu* (DZ 432) with a foreword of 848, written under Emperor Xuanzong and attributed to Hu Yin 胡愔 or Jiansu zi 見素子, a Taoist woman of the Upper Clarity tradition who lived at Mount Taibai. A version of this text is included in the *Xiuzhen shishu, juan* 54. The five viscera are qualified as "viscera" (*zang*) and the gallbladder as a "receptacle" (*fu*), in accordance with the orthodox system. The name of the organ deities is not given in the text. In her preface, Hu Yin said she consulted representations of organs of different shapes; she adds that these visualizations help strengthen the viscera, to communicate with the great harmony, and to be protected on the left by the deities of the six *yang* signs *jia* and on the right by the deities of the six yin *ding*.

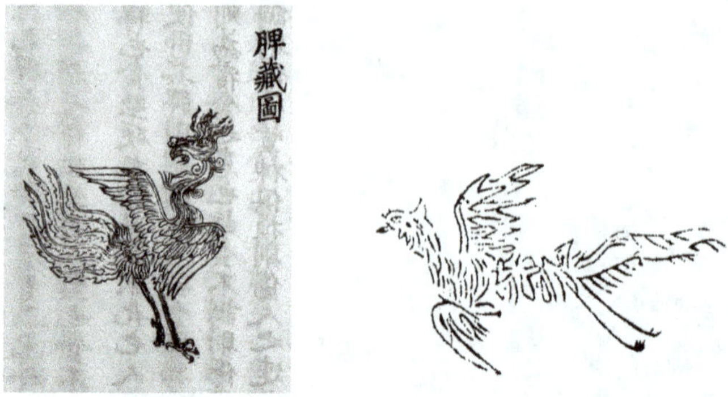


FIGURE 5.10 Deity of the spleen (phoenix). Left, *Yunji qiqian*, DZ 1032, 14.9a, and on the right, the *Chart for the Cultivation of Perfection*

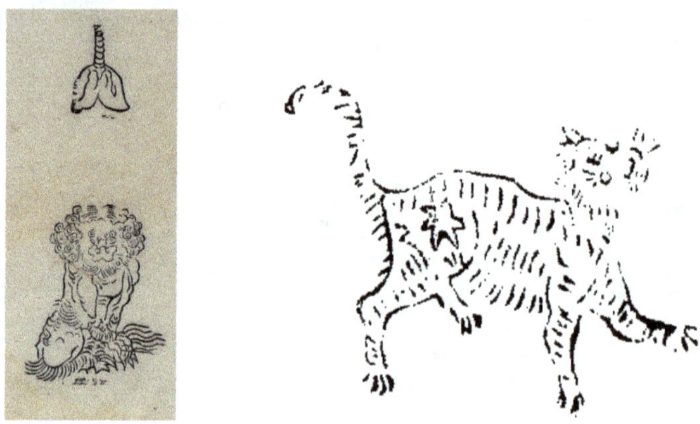

FIGURE 5.11 Deity of the lungs (Tiger). Left, *Yunji qiqian* (DZ 1032), 14.4b, and on the right, the *Chart for the Cultivation of Perfection*

According to them, the deities of the viscera correspond to the image of an animal: a dragon for the liver, a turtle entwingled by a snake for the gallbladder, a deer with two heads for the kidneys, a vermilion sparrow for the heart, a white tiger for the lungs and a phoenix for the spleen (see fig. 5.8–5.13).[66] This list includes the four numinous animals (*siling* 四靈) corresponding to the four directions: the dragon in the East, the vermilion sparrow in the south, the tiger in the west and the turtle and the Snake in the North, to which were added the phoenix and the two-headed deer. The four numinous animals correlated with the four directions are attested from the Han dynasty onwards.[67] Taoist adepts

66 On the viscera in the tradition of the Yellow Court, see Robinet 1979: 103–120.

67 See the work of Rudolph Richard (1951), who studies representations of these four animals found in Han tombs. These are similar under the Six Dynasties. Thus, Lin Shuzhong

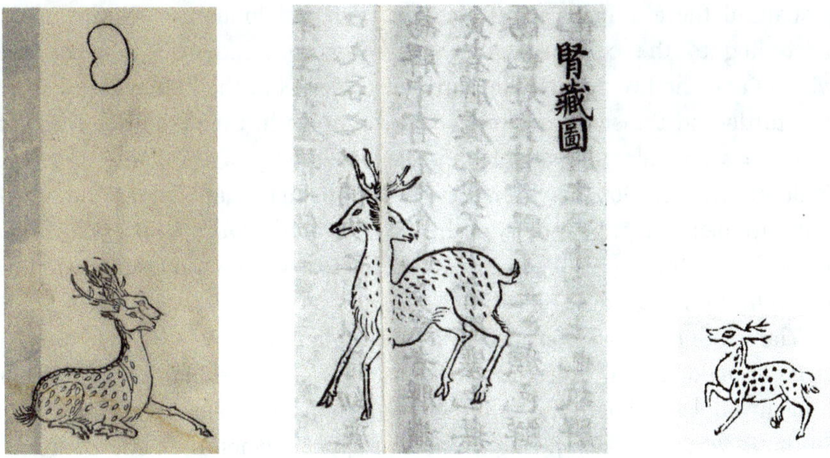


FIGURE 5.12 Deity of the kidneys (deer with two heads). Left, *Shangqing huangting wuzang liufu zhenren yuzhou jing*, DZ 1402, 8a. In the middle, *Yunji qiqian* (DZ 1032), 14.10b–11a, and on the right, the *Chart for the Cultivation of Perfection*

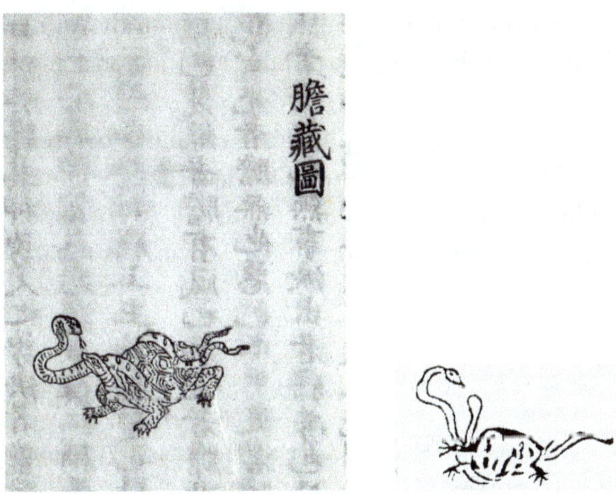


FIGURE 5.13 Deity of the gallbladder (turtle and snake). Left, *Yunji Qiqian* (DZ 1032), 14.12a, and on the right, the *Chart for the Cultivation of Perfection*

visualized these animals for protection from evil influences. Nevertheless, according to the conventional system of correspondences between the viscera and the five agents, the north corresponds to the kidneys, and since the turtle and the snake are related to the north in the system of the four numinous animals, they should represent the deity of the kidneys. In the Yellow Court tradition, however, they correspond to the gallbladder, and a deer with two heads is given as deity of the kidneys. On the *Chart for the Cultivation of Perfection*, the deer is black, but according to several writings of the Yellow Court tradition, it should be white.[68]

The white deer was considered in Chinese antiquity as a happy omen. It is mentioned several times in the *Classic on Mountains and Seas* and other ancient books.[69] According to a chapter on talismans and auspicious signs in the *History of Liu-Song*, "the white deer appears when the benevolence of the sovereign reaches the inferiors."[70] In the *Magnificent Ceremonial Rites of the Northern Dipper*, which quotes a Tang source, the writer claims, "When the sovereign rules under the sign of the water and when his government is peaceful, the Northern Sea brings white deer."[71] In the latter text, the deer is matched with water, which could explain the choice of deer for the kidneys in the Yellow Court tradition since the water corresponds to the north and to the colour black.[72]

The correspondence of the spleen with the phoenix is unknown before the Yellow Court tradition. This choice is possibly due to the fact that the phoenix was supposed to have feathers of five colours and therefore could correspond to the centre.[73] It is also possible that it was a relic of a previous correlation system because, according to the *Ceremonial Rites of the Northern Dipper*, the

---

(*Wenwu* 1977.1: 15) presents these animals found drawn on clay from tomb # 3 in Danyang (Jiangsu province). This article also gives on p. 15 the drawing on clay of Xuanwu, i.e., the turtle and snake, from the district Deng 登 (Henan) (fig. 5.14 and 5.15). The earliest known representations of the tiger and the dragon are made with shells and were found in a tomb. See *La Chine* 3 (1988): 36–37.

68 *Huangting dunjia yuanshen jing*, as quoted in the *Yunji qiqian* (DZ 1032), 14.11a.

69 *Shanhai jing* 山海經 [Book on mountains and seas], 2.30b; translated by Mathieu 1983, note 4.

70 "Furui zhi" 符瑞志 in the *Songshu* 宋書.

71 *Lidou weiyi* 禮斗威儀 [Magnificent ceremonial rites of Northern Dipper]. In *Huangshi yishu kao* 黃氏遺書考, 1.14a; citation in the *Yiwen leiju* 藝文類聚, 99.1714.

72 See *Zhenzhong jing* (DZ 1422), 2a–b.

73 See Diény 1989–1990: 1–14.

phoenix corresponds to the earth.[74] The only known animal related to the centre in Taoist writings is that given by the *Five Talismans, Numinous Treasure of the Most High*,[75] which is the yellow unicorn.[76] The unicorn and the phoenix are two of the four numinous animals, the two others being the dragon and the turtle.[77]

Nevertheless, the phoenix appears in Taoism in the Tang dynasty, but in a different context: the rituals of the Orthodox Unity related to the practice of "walking on the star network" (*bugang* 步罡), in which the officiant meets a nine-headed phoenix responsible for summoning the strength of the North Star to destroy impurities.[78] In this text, however, the animal is not associated with the centre.

In the *Chart*, the turtle and the snake are here associated with the gallbladder, which immediately suggests a relationship between this organ of the body and the North, as both animals are from the Han onwards related to the North and also to the Dark Warrior (Xuanwu),[79] who subjugates all demons, and whose exorcist and protective function already has a strong foothold under the Tang.

In the *Precious Scroll of the Perfected Being on the Five Viscera and the Six Receptacles of the Yellow Court of the Upper Clarity*, the gallbladder is considered as a viscera (*zang*) and not a receptacle (*fu*), unlike the traditional system developed in the medical context and repeated by many Taoist texts, according to the classical system, the gallbladder is coupled with the liver. In the *Precious Scroll on the Five Viscera*, it is coupled to the bladder, the two organs being related to water. This text asserts that the energy of the gallbladder is "the essence of metal and the water breath,"[80] and is associated with the trigram *kan* and is related to water. Therefore, there is a correlation between the gallbladder and the turtle, entwined with a snake corresponding to the north and to water. It is said in the same text that the gallbladder comes from

---

74 It is said in the *Lidou weiyi*: "If the sovereign rules under the sign of earth and if the government knows the great peace, the phoenix will gather in the forests and parks." *Huangshi yishu kao*, 13a; citation in *Yiwen leiju*, 99.1707.

75 *Taishang lingbao wufu xu* (DZ 388). See Yamada 1989: 99–124.

76 *Taishang Lingbao wufu xu* (DZ 388), 1.22b: "First visualize the five animals, the blue dragon, the white tiger, the vermilion sparrow, the Dark Warrior and in the centre, the yellow unicorn."

77 See *Liyun*, transl. Couvreur 1950, I.2, 524.

78 See Andersen 1989–1990: 43–44.

79 Recall that on the version of the White Cloud Temple the drawing of the turtle and the snake is juxtaposed with the inscription, "Dark Warrior" (Xuanwu).

80 *Shangqing huangting wuzang liufu zhenren yuzhou jing* (DZ 1402), 9.

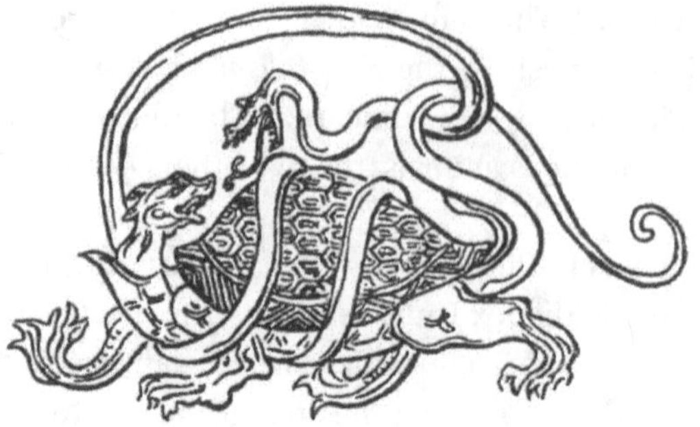

FIGURE 5.14
Terracotta drawing of Xuanwu from Deng district. "Danyang Qi Nan linmu zuanyin Bihua tantao," p. 65

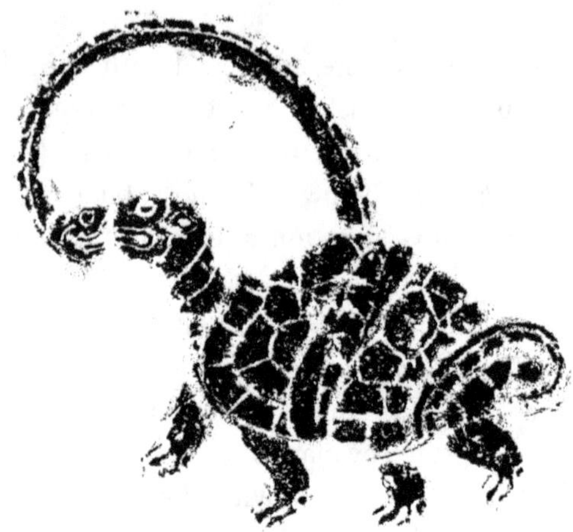

FIGURE 5.15
Turtle and snake represented in the engraving n.3 in Danyang (Jiangsu). "Danyang Nan Qi linmu zuanyin bihua tantao," p. 65

metal, and metal is born of martial virtue.[81] This also justifies the association of the gallbladder with the warrior element and its mastery of demons.

In the *Book of the Yellow Court*, the gallbladder controls the armies of tigers, exorcist animals par excellence. Moreover, the text of Hu Yin on these animal deities bears in the title of the *Cloudy Bookcase with Seven Labels* version the term *dunjia* 盾甲 "hide the (six) cyclical signs *jia*," which refers to exorcist techniques for the protection against evil.[82] Elsewhere in the paragraph on the gallbladder, this text describes the following exercise in conjunction with the North: "Regularly on the Meng 孟 months,[83] in the correct position, visualize

81 *Ibid.*, DZ 1402, lob.

82 Hu Yin writes in her preface to *Huangting neijing wuzang liufu buxie tu* (DZ 432, lb), that in heaven, we can call at the left six yang deities of the six *jia* and at the right the six yin deities of the six *ding*.

83 Each of the four seasons includes one month Meng. In the traditional lunar calendar, it corresponds to the first, fourth, seventh and tenth months.

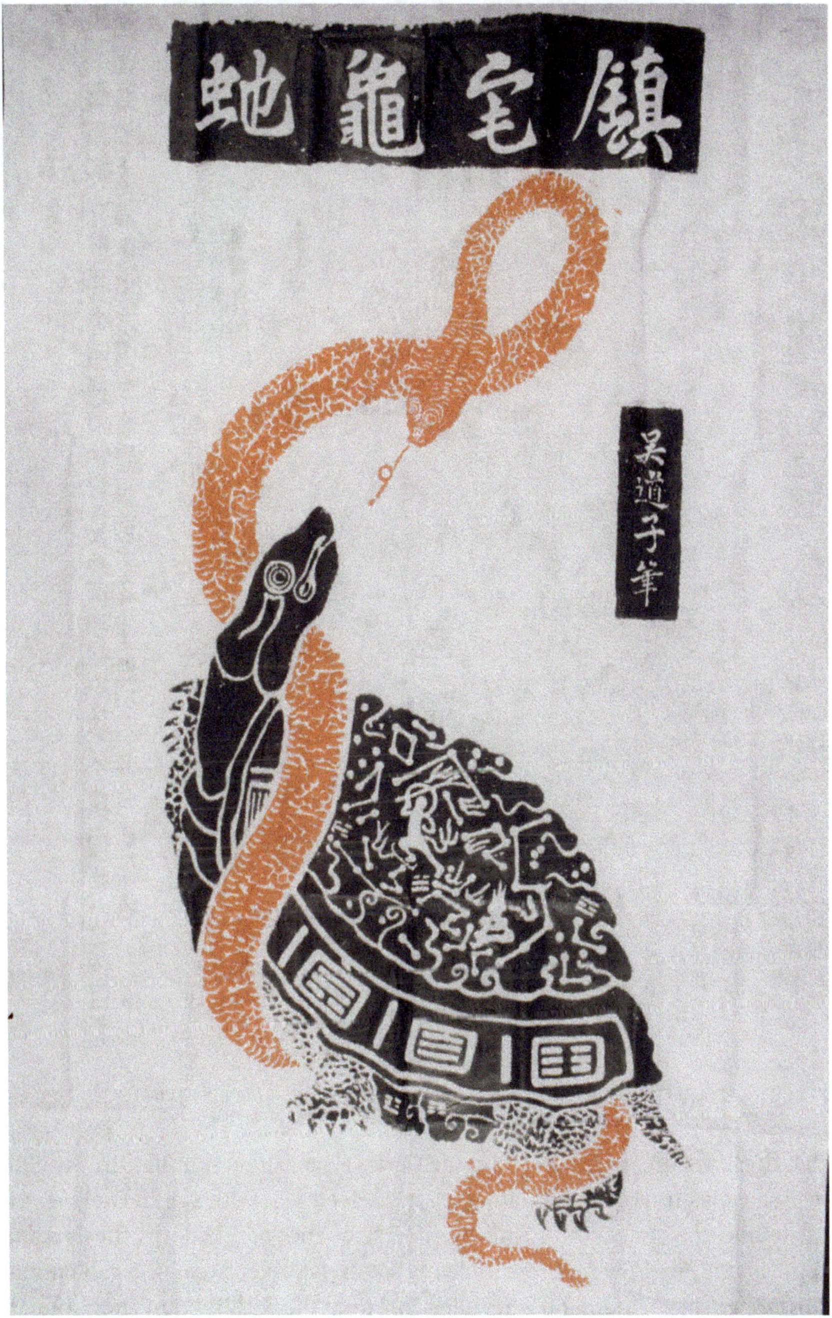


FIGURE 5.16 Representation of the turtle entwined by a snake from Wudao zi 吳道子, a famous Tang painter. A stamp from the White Cloud Temple in Beijing

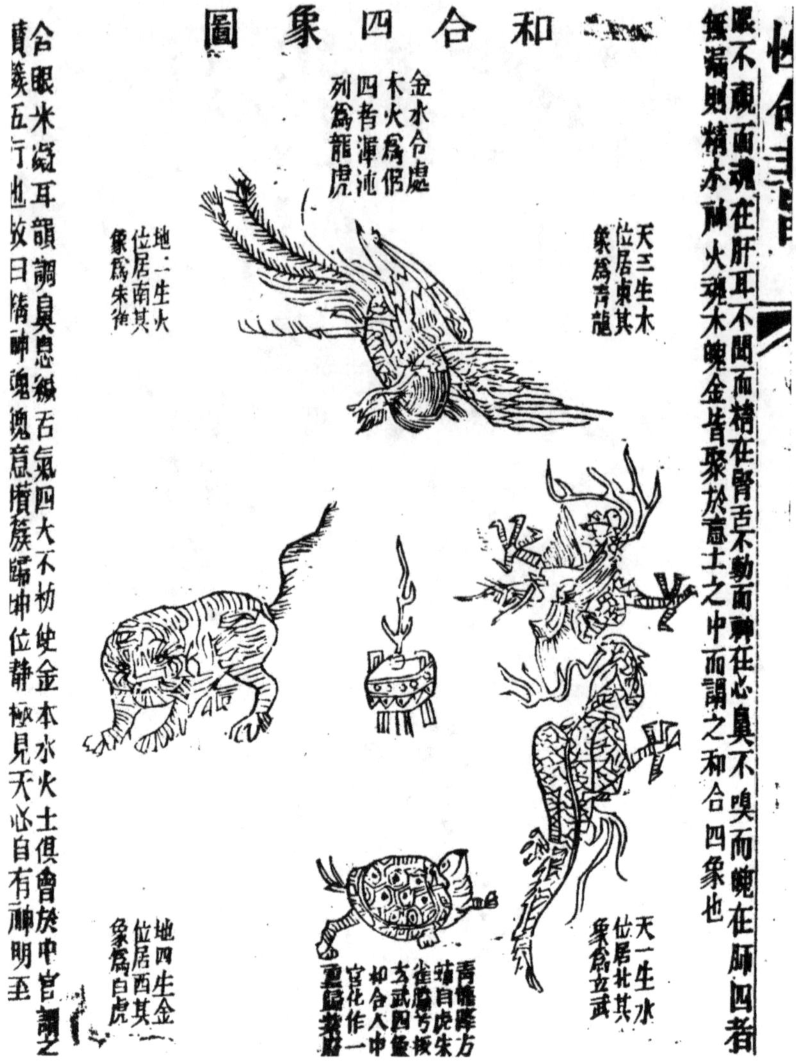


FIGURE 5.17 Representation of the four numinous animals. *Xingming guizhi*, 1.37b

that the black breath sucked from the Dark Palace enters your mouth. Swallow it nine times to repair the damage, and to feed you with the flavours of the turtle and the snake and drink the nectar of the Jade Lad." In the *Precious Scroll on the Five Viscera*, there is clearly a correlation between the gallbladder, the north, the water and the dark Warrior, the latter being not directly designated. The turtle and the snake, its two emblematic animals, suggest this association.

## 6 The Inner Gods of the Yellow Court Tradition Integrated to the *Chart for the Cultivation of Perfection*

The *Chart for the Cultivation of Perfection* contains the divinities of the six viscera according to the tradition of the Yellow Court, both in the pictographic representation and in the description of the viscera and the gods. Let us recall that the Yellow Court tradition was integrated during the Song dynasty by the three main currents related to the thunder rites: the Correct Method of the Heart of Heaven (*Tianxin zhengfa*), the Divine Empyrean (*Shenxiao*) and the Pure Tenuity (*Qingwei*) traditions, which can therefore be at the origin of this *Chart for the Cultivation of Perfection*, especially since the other gods on this Chart belong to these currents, as we will see.

### 6.1 *The Image of the Six Viscera on the Chart*

The *Chart for the Cultivation of Perfection* surrounds the body map with the six animals corresponding to the deities of the six viscera according to the Yellow Court tradition. These drawings vary from one version to another, and are in colour in modern versions. They are also somewhat different from the representation of these six animals that came to us in the Taoist Canon edited during the Ming dynasty (1445), by an illustrated text of the eighth century belonging to the Yellow Court tradition: the *Chart on the Procedures for Filling and Emptying the Five Viscera and the Six Receptacles according to the Inner Landscape of the Yellow Court* by Hu Yin. The drawing of the snake and the turtle is similar to that of the tomb of Danyang 丹陽 (figs. 5.14 and 5.15) dating from the Southern Qi (479–502) and the representation of Wudao zi 吳道子 (680–740) kept in the White Cloud Temple in Beijing (see fig. 5.16). In contrast, the representation of the tiger and the dragon is closer to the drawings found in the *Charts of the Precious Alchemical Mirror*[84] and the *Principles of the Tablets on the Innate Nature and the Vital Force* (fig. 5.17).[85] As for the representations of the Vermilion Sparrow and of the phoenix, they are quite different from those accompanying the text of Hu Yin.

### 6.2 *The Texts on the Six Viscera on the Chart*

Besides the drawings of the six animals, the *Chart for the Cultivation of Perfection* has six texts on the six viscera, which are an adaptation of the descriptions

84 *Danfang baojianzhi tu* in *Xiuzhen shishu* (DZ 263), 26.5. Texts and drawings included in *Shangyangzi jindan dayao tu* (DZ 1068), 8a.

85 *Xingming guizhi*, fasc. 2, p. 166.

given in the two main Tang texts of the Yellow Court tradition cited above.[86] For a better understanding of these texts, we will give a summary of the correlations used in Chinese medicine and in Taoism between the organs which are divided in two types, the "viscera" (*zang* 藏) and the "receptacles" (*fu* 府), and the other elements of the body and the universe. Here is a table of these correspondences:

Correspondences between the constitutive elements of a person

| | | | | | |
|---|---|---|---|---|---|
| FIVE AGENTS (*Wuxing* 五行) | wood (*mu* 木) | fire (*huo* 火) | earth (*tu* 土) | metal (*jin* 金) | water (*shui* 水) |
| VISCERA | liver (*gan* 肝) | heart (*xin* 心) | spleen (*pi* 脾) | lungs (*fei* 肺) | kidneys (*shen* 腎) |
| FUNCTION | general (*jiangjun* 將軍) | sovereign (*junzi* 君子) | granary (*cangku* 倉庫) | minister (*shangshu* 尚書) | women of the harem (*hougong* 後宮) |
| RECEPTACLE | gallbladder (*dan* 膽) | small intestine (*xiaochang* 小腸) | stomach (*wei* 胃) | large intestine (*dachang* 大腸) | bladder (*pangguang* 膀胱) |
| BODY PART | tendons (*jin* 筋) | vessels (*mai* 脉 [脈]) | flesh (*rou* 肉) | skin and hair (*pimao* 皮毛) | bones and marrow (*gusui* 骨髓) |
| LIQUID | tears (*lei* 淚) | sweat (*han* 汗) | saliva (*xian* 涎) | mucous (*ti* 涕) | sputum (*tuo* 唾) |
| BODILY APERTURE | eyes (*mu* 目) | tongue (*she* 舌) | lips (*chun* 唇) | nose (*bi* 鼻) | ears (*er* 耳) |
| FLAVOR | acid (*suan* 酸) | bitter (*ku* 苦) | sweet (*gan* 甘) | spicy (*xin* 辛) | salty (*xian* 鹹) |
| FEELING | anger (*nu* 怒) | joy (*xi* 喜) | thinking (*si* 思) | sadness (*bei* 悲) | fear (*kong* 恐) |
| SPIRIT | hun 魂 | spirit (*shen* 神) | imaginative spirit (*si* 思) | po 魄 | aspiration (*zhi* 志) |
| NUMINOUS ANIMAL | Azure Dragon (*qinglong* 青龍) | Vermilion Sparrow (*zhuque* 朱雀) | Yellow Dragon (*huanglong* 黃龍) | White Tiger (*baihu* 白虎) | Dark Warrior (*xuanwu* 玄武) |

86 DZ 432 and DZ 1402.

Here is the translation of the six texts on the six viscera on the *Chart for the Cultivation of Perfection.*

A) The deity of the liver (text at the upper right) (fig. 4.2, text 3)

> The deity of the liver has the form of a blue-green dragon. His name is Dragon Vapour (Longyan 龍煙)[87] and his byname is Containing illumination (Hanming 含明).[88] The liver, near the heart, appears like a suspended gourd.[89] It has three petals to the left and four to the right; the one next to the gallbladder is shorter. It weighs four pounds and four ounces. It is the mother of the heart and the son of the kidneys.[90] The three *hun* souls, called Shining Numinous (Shuangling 爽靈), White Light (Baiguang 白光) and Obscure Essence (Youjing 幽精), abide in the liver. The eyes are the palace of the liver. The left eye corresponds to the cyclical sign *jia*, the right eye to the sign *yi*.[91] When a man reaches sixty, his liver breath weakens, the petals of his liver become thinner, his gallbladder gradually decreases, and his eyesight diminishes.[92] The liver correlates to the tendons, and its vessels are linked with the element of wood; it is the organ of the *hun*. Its secretions are tears. When a pathogen enters the liver, tears abound. The gallbladder is the receptacle corresponding to the liver and coupled with it. It is stated in the *Book of the Yellow Court*: "Harmonize and master the *hun* souls, the *po* souls and the bodily secretions. On the outside, the liver is in resonance with the eyes and with the quintessence of sun and moon. If you are suffering from any disease, visualize assiduously for seven days the Non-pareil Lordling, and you will fully recover your health.[93]

B) The gallbladder (text at the middle right) (fig. 3.6, text 4)

---

87 The name is absent from the version of the White Cloud Temple.

88 There are the names given to this deity in the *Book of the Yellow Court.*

89 The text is the same as in DZ 1402.

90 The description of the liver "it weighs four pounds four ounces, has three petals to the left and four to the right" is already in chapter 42 of the *Classic of the Difficulties*, a medical apocryphal of the Late Han.

91 Both *jia* and *yi* signs are related to the east and to wood.

92 See DZ 432, 1.lob.

93 This last passage is taken from the second chapter on the liver in *Huangting neijing yujing zhu* (DZ 402), 1.20a.

The gallbladder is the essence of metal and the breath of water. Its colour is dark blue.[94] It lies beneath the liver's shorter petal. Gallbladder (*dan* 膽) is homophonous with "boldness" (*gan* 敢). When the gallbladder is big, man is free from fears. Its deity is called Dragon Sparkle (Longyao 龍耀) and its byname is Majestic Brightness (Weiming 威明).[95] It has the shape of a turtle wrapped by a snake. It has the shape of a suspended sack and weighs three ounces and one sixteenth of an ounce. In traditional Chinese medicine, the gallbladder is coupled with the liver and called a receptacle (*fu*) rather than a viscera (*zang*). In this formulation, however, the gallbladder receives the breath of water and has the same path as the trigram of water, *kan*.[96] Consequently, it cannot be integrated into the receptacles, and is considered as one of the viscera. It is coupled with the bladder and in the upper body, governs body and head hairs.[97] It is said in the *Book of the Yellow Court*: "The gallbladder governs the strength of the different breaths and controls the armies of tigers. On the outer part of the body, it corresponds to the pupil of the eye and to the space between the eyebrows. It is coupled with the brain and the hair. Its deity wears a brocade garment of nine colours and a skirt of blue-green flowers.[98]

C) The kidneys (text at the lower right) (fig. 3.6, text 5)

The kidneys correspond to the north and to the trigram *kan*.[99] Their deity has the shape of a two-headed dark deer. It is called Obscure Darkness (Xuanming 玄冥) and its byname is Numinous infant (Ling'er 靈兒). The kidneys have the shape of pebbles and are located at the level of the navel and suspended each side of the backbone. They weigh one pound two and three tenths ounces. Their principal function consists of separating water and breath and then distributing them throughout the body. The kidneys are like the roots of a tree. The left kidney is called

---

94 See *Huangting dunjia yuanshen jing*, in *Yunji qiqian* (DZ 1032), 14.12a.

95 See *Huangting neijing jing*, version of the *Yunji qiqian* (DZ 1032), 11.23b.

96 "Transform" on the Mount Wudang version.

97 It is written in the *Huangting dunjia yuanzhen jing* (*Yunji qiqian*, DZ 1032, 14.12ab): "The gallbladder is coupled with the bladder, above, it regulates hair and the hair."

98 *Huangting neijing jing*, ch.14 on gallbladder as recorded in *Yunji qiqian* (DZ 1032), 11.33b–34a. According to the commentary of Liangqiu zi, the green flower skirt is an image for the membrane of the gallbladder, and the colour of the brocade is that of the nine breaths of the East. See DZ 402, 2.3a–b.

99 The version of the White Cloud Temple has more "correspond to water."

the gate of the kidneys (*shenmen* 腎門), the right, the Gate of the Vital Force (*mingmen* 命門). They reside in the Palace of the Original Breath, the gate of death.[100] If you preserve them, you will have a long life; if you overuse them, you will be exhausted. They are the mother of the liver and the son of the lungs. The ears are their palace. When heaven gave birth to me, the circulating breath turned into a vital breath, of which coming and going creates the spirit (*shen*). The holy man stores emotions and knowledge in his kidneys.[101]

The left kidney corresponds to the cyclical sign *ren*, and the right kidney to *gui* (two cyclical signs related to the north and to water).[102] Among the twelve-day periods, they correspond to *zi* (11 pm–1 am) and *yin* (3 am–5 am). For the six breaths, they correspond to *chui*. Among the secretions, they correspond to saliva, and for the body parts, they correspond to the bones. The kidneys channel is related to the upper heater, the nourishing breath is related to the median heater and the protective breath, to the lower heater. In the chapter on the area of the kidneys in the *Book of the Yellow Court*, it is said: "Within the Obscure Pass, resides an infant called Upper Obscurity, who governs the six receptacles,[103] and is the source of the nine secretions. On the outer part of the body, the kidneys correspond to the two ears and govern the bodily secretions."[104]

D) The deity of the heart (text at the upper left) (fig. 3.6, text 6)

The deity of the heart has the form of a vermilion sparrow. The heart is like an inverted hanging lotus flower. It can transform water into blood. Its divinity is called Origin of Cinnabar (Danyuan 丹元) and its byname is Guardian of Numina (Shouling 守靈). It weighs twelve ounces, and is located one inch below the turtledove's tail. It has the colour of a ripe orange. It has seven cavities and three hairs. A man of superior wisdom has all the cavities unlocked and pervaded with brightness; a man of medium wisdom has only five cavities through which the breath enters; a man of inferior wisdom has none of the orifices unlocked, so that

100 The Mount Wudang version lacks the term "gate."

101 The term "knowledge" (*zhi* 智) is absent from the version of the White Cloud Temple.

102 Both *ren* and *gui* cyclical signs are associated with the north and water.

103 Version of the *Huangting jing*. The Mount Wudang representation has *xuefu* "palace of cavities"; the White Cloud Temple's version has *zhu xueqi* 諸穴氣 "the various breaths of the cavities."

104 DZ 402, 1.21b–22a.

light and breaths do not flow through the heart.[105] The heart is the son of the liver and the mother of the spleen. The tongue is its palace. The *jue*[106] orifices communicate with the ears. The left ear corresponds to the cyclical sign *bing* and the right ear to the sign *ding*. Its secretion is sweat. If an evil element of the kidneys enters the heart, the sweat overflows. The heart's associated flavour is sweet, and its corresponding receptacle is the small intestine. The *Book of the Yellow Court* says: "The palace of the heart is like a lotus flower in bud with closed petals, under which lies an adolescent named the Origin of Cinnabar.[107] He is the divinity of the heart. Below the heart there is the Scarlet Palace.

E) The deity of the lungs (text at the middle left) (fig. 3.6, text 7)

The deity of the lungs has the shape of a white tiger. The lungs have the shape of a hanging musical stone. They dwell above the five viscera and envelop them like a cover. Facing each other with the womb, they form a flowered canopy. Their deity is named Hoary Flower (Haohua 皓華), its byname is Vacuous Attainment (Xucheng 虛成). They weigh three pounds and three ounces. They are composed from eight parts: six petals and two ears. The lungs are the son of the spleen and the mother of the kidneys. They contain the seven *po* souls,[108] similar to children. They are called Corpse Dog (Shigou 尸狗), Buried Cadaver (Fushi 伏尸) Sparrow Demon (Queyin 雀陰), Devouring Robber (Tunzei 吞賊) Flying Poison (Feidu 飛

105 DZ 1402, 4a: "Amongst people of superior intelligence, the heart has seven orifices, for those of medium intelligence, five, for those of lower intelligence, three, those of reduced intelligence, two, for ordinary men, one, and for stupid men, none."

106 Perhaps this is an allusion to the *jueyin* meridian of the heart envelopment (*baoluo* 包絡), which was later identified as the pericardium, particularly in Chinese medical sources of the nineteenth century.

107 DZ 402, 1.18a.

108 As for the three visionary souls, seven vegetative souls were represented on the Yanluozi drawings and in the *Taishang chu sanshi jiuchong baosheng jing* 太上出三尸九蟲保生經 [Scripture of the most high for the protection of life through the elimination of the three corpses and the nine worms] (DZ 871), in which we find the same names as here. These drawings have been included in the *Yimen guangdu* 夷門廣牘, a Ming text written by Zhou Lüjing.

毒),[109] Expulsor of Dirt (Chuhui 除穢) and Stink Hunter (Bichou 辟臭).[110] The nose is its palace. The left part is the cyclical sign *geng*, the right part is the cyclical sign *xin*.[111] The corresponding breath is coughing; among the fluids they correspond to nasal mucus. As for the physical parts of the body, they correspond to the skin and the hair. Flowing upwards, the breaths attain the brain and flowing downwards, they enter the spleen; all breaths are a matter for the lungs. The lungs are the origin of breathing. It is said in the *Book of the Yellow Court*: "We must rapidly focus on White Prime when suffering a body discomfort due to breathing difficulties.[112]

F) The deity of the spleen (text at the lower left) (fig. 3.6, text 8)

The spleen corresponds to the centre and the earth and reigns throughout the four seasons. It is the Yellow Emperor. Its deity has the shape of a phoenix with spread wings. This deity is named Eternal Residence (Changzhu 常住) and its byname is *Hun*-soul Court (Hunting 魂庭). It is located just above the navel and is covered by the stomach. It is the breath of the trigram *kun* and the quintessence of earth. Located three inches below the heart, it weighs one pound and two ounces. It is three inches wide and one foot long. It is the son of the heart and the mother of the lungs. On the outer part of the body, it communicates with the eyebrows. The mouth is its palace. Its deity is very jealous. The spleen has no fixed structure, it governs earth and yin, and therefore it is the pivot of the five viscera. The orifice with which it is correlated is the mouth. As for the physical elements of the body, it corresponds to the muscles. The spleen channel originates in Hidden White (Yinbai 隐 白),[113] which is the basis of the flesh. It is [the source of] creative

109 The Mount Wudang version. The Moli, White Cloud Temple and Tiger and Dragon Altar versions have *fei shengmu* 非生母. *Shengmu* is a decomposition and a misreading of the character 毒 [Poison]. For *fei*, instead of the character *fei* meaning flying, it is the character *fei* for the negation, as on the Mount Wudang version.

110 According to the Mount Wudang version. Those of Moli, of the White Cloud Temple and of the Dragon and tiger Altar have *qunchou* 群臭 "various smells." The list of the seven names given by the Mount Wudang version is the classic list as it can be found for example in *Taishang chu sanshi jiuchong baosheng jing* (DZ 871), 3a–b, with the exception of the second Buried Dung (Fushi 伏矢) and of the last Stinky Lungs (Choufei 臭肺).

111 The cyclical signs *geng* and *xin* correspond to the metal and to West.

112 DZ 402, 1.17b.

113 In acupuncture, it is the name of the first point of the spleen meridian located 0.1 inches (*cun*) back from the internal angle of the nail of the big toe.

thinking (*yi* 意) and thoughts. It is said in the *Book of the Yellow Court*: "It cures all the diseases of mankind and digests food; its deity wears a yellow garment with a purple belt bearing the insignia of the tiger and the dragon.[114]

### 6.3 *The Deities of the Head on the Chart*

Two circles that form a halo surround the head. In the ring formed by the inner circle and the outer circle are inscriptions coming from Chapter Seven of the *Book of the Inner Landscape of the Yellow Court*, and from passages of the commentary to this chapter by Liangqiu zi. This seventh chapter, titled the "Supreme Way" ("Zhidao zhang" 至道章), describes the head palaces and their gods:

> No effort is required in the supreme path,
> Simply visualize with determination the Perfected.
> Each articulation of the Muddy Pellet has its deity.
> The hair deity is called Jet-black Flower,
> Its byname is Supreme Origin.
> The brain deity is called Upper Light,
> Its byname is Mystery of the Efflorescence.
> The nose deity is called Jade Mound,
> Its byname is Numinous Strength.
> The ears deity is called Serene Emptiness,
> Its byname is Peaceful Field.
> The tongue deity is called Life Force Communicator,
> Its byname is Ethic and Righteousness.
> The teeth deity is called Sharp Blade,
> Its byname is Merciless Crusher.
> All the gods of the face revere the Muddy Pellet.
> Each of the Nine Perfected of the Muddy Pellet has his cave.
> Abiding at the centre of the nine chambers measuring one square inch,
> They wear a purple garment and a suit of fine gauze.
> Just maintain your intent on this area to acquire an infinite life,
> Don't visualize each of them separately in the brain.
> They are sitting, facing outward,
> Towards those visualized in the heart.

114 DZ 402, 2a–b.

The names of the Nine Perfected of the Muddy Pellet in the ring on the *Chart* are the same as in the aforementioned chapter seven of the *Book of the Yellow Court*:[115] the High Perfected (Gaozhen 高真), the Realized Perfected (Zhizhen 至真), the Supreme Perfected (Taizhen 太真), the Void Perfected (Xuzhen 虛真), the Immortal Perfected (Xianzhen 仙真), the Mysterious Perfected (Xuanzhen 玄真), the Superior Perfected (Shangzhen 上真), the Divine Perfected (Shenzhen 神真) and the Heavenly Perfected (Tianzhen 天真). This list corresponds to the classical list of the Nine Perfected given in the texts of the Upper Clarity tradition, except the fourth (Xuzhen) which is replaced with the name Numinous Perfected (Lingzhen 靈真).[116]

The other inscriptions arranged in the disc around these nine names are:

On the upper part: The chamber measures one square inch. The brain has nine petals." The first four characters are an abbreviated form of the twelfth verse of Chapter Seven of the *Book of the Yellow Court*: "The Nine Perfected abide in the centre of this chamber which measures one square inch." The second inscription of four characters is an abbreviation of the commentary by Liangqiu zi on the twelfth verse of chapter seven: "The chamber measures one square inch. The brain has nine petals."

To the right in the disc an inscription of ten characters is arranged on two lines:

> "The path of the non-extinction consists of visualizing the Nine Perfected of the Muddy Pellet." This sentence is similar to the one in the commentary by Liangqiu zi.
>
> On the left in the disk we can see two lines of ten characters: "The garments of the Nine Perfected have for each of them the colour of their corresponding breaths, they are light and floating", which is also a sentence of the commentary by Liangqiu zi on the thirteenth verse of the seventh chapter: "Each of the Nine Perfected wears a purple garment and a suit of fine gauze."

115 In the representation of Chengdu similar to ours published by Needham, the pairs are contained in the same circle.

116 The commentary to the seventh chapter of the *Book of the Yellow Court* by Liangqiu zi cites the Nine Perfected and their orientation according to the *Basu jing* 八素經: the Superior Perfected face upwards, the Higher Perfected face south, the Supreme Perfected face southeast, the Divine Perfected face southwest, the Mysterious Perfected face north, the Immortal Perfected face northeast, the Heavenly Perfected face southeast, the Numinous Perfected face southwest, the Jade Perfected (Yuzhen 玉真) face northwest.

> At the bottom of the disc is the character *shen* [Spirit], of the triad "essence, breath and spirit," referring to the three basic ingredients in Inner Alchemy that correspond to the three levels of the three cinnabar fields.

In the drawings affiliated to the Yanluozi diagrams, there is only mention of the Lord of Muddy Pellet, whereas here there are numerous details about the deities of the head, on the six animal deities of the six viscera; this reflects the importance of the Yellow Court tradition in this body map. But the mention in the centre of the ring evokes divinities that do not belong to the tradition of the Yellow Court, but rather to the Numinous Treasure School of the Song dynasty. A standing man is drawn in the centre of the ring, with a shaved hair in the White Cloud Temple version, but his hair is tied up and he is dressed in a Taoist robe on the other versions, as on the Yanluozi diagrams despite minor pictographic differences. He is flanked to the right by a seven-character inscription: "The Perfected of the Primordial Destiny of the Muddy Pellet Palace." To his left is the inscription: "The Sovereign of the Obscure Firmament or the Jade Emperor Palace." The Perfected of the Primordial Destiny is central in the texts like the *Taoist Methods, United in Principle*[117] or the *Pearls Retrieved from the Sea of Rites*. The adept visualizes an infant who becomes identical to the adept: that is the Perfected of the Primordial Destiny.[118] The Sovereign of the Obscure Firmament is another name for the Jade Emperor, a high god in the Thunder Rites. In the Numinous Treasure system, the Nine Perfected are subordinated to the Celestial Worthy of Original Commencement:

> The Celestial Worthy of the Numinous Treasure is the ancestor of the Nine Perfected, the eminent holy man of the Upper Clarity, the Original Breath of the Way. According to the Taoist teachings, the Original Commencement belongs to the Dongzhen, but in this context it is differentiated as Dongxuan, it means that he, the Jade Aurora, received the Way of the Universal Salvation of the Numinous Treasure and is a disciple of the Original Commencement, the patriarch of the Upper Clarity.[119]

---

117 See *Daofa huiyuan* (DZ 1220).

118 See for example an exorcistic and therapeutic ritual in *Fahai yizhu* (DZ 1166), 2.16a or a visualisation for purifying the heaven and the earth during a *zhai* 齋 in *Shangqing lingbao dafa* (DZ 1221), 24.4b.

119 *Shangqing lingbao dafa* (DZ 1221), 10.1b.

## 7 The Deities Related to the Numinous Treasure and the Thunder Rites

The other names of deities mentioned on the Chart, either on the head or on the abdomen, correspond to the pantheon of the Numinous Treasure and the Thunder Rites traditions.

### 7.1 *Deities Related to the Tradition of the Numinous Treasure*

In the Numinous Treasure tradition, the supreme god is the Celestial Worthy of Primordial Commencement (Yuanshi tianzun 元始天尊). He transmitted the *Book of Universal Salvation* to the Most High Lord Lao (Taishang Laojun 太上老君), and claimed that reciting this holy scripture would ensure salvation for oneself and for his ancestors. The Celestial Worthy is the source of all the transformations, the mysterious breath of the Way. The salvific power of the *Book of Universal Salvation* resides in the fact that it contains the names of the celestial emperors, the secret name of demons and spirits and the sounds of the heavens.

In the *Book of Universal Salvation*, the divine cosmology is presented as follows: "The [Celestial Worthy of] Original Commencement fixes and stabilises the jade characters of the five red writings, the eight majestic ornaments in the form of a dragon, he controls the revolution of the cosmic cycles (kalpa), in order that heaven will exist for a long time. The cosmic breath encompasses all; the ten thousand models emanate from it and open out. They revolve without specific colour, then spread in the ten directions."[120]

In this formulation, the body is transformed by the establishment of a cosmic network linking it to the underworld and paradises, and also gods. There are five main deities that correlate with the five directions and the five agents, and in the alchemical commentaries of the *Book of Universal Salvation*, they also correlate with the five viscera. The latter commentaries define these five deities as follows:

> Within the Perfection, there are the Great Lord of Long Life (Changsheng dajun 長生大君), the Non-pareil Lordling (Wuying gongzi 無英公子), the True Worthy of the White Prime (Baiyuan zhenzun 白元真尊), the Rector of Fate, Great One (Taiyi Siming 太乙司命, and Vigour of Peach, Union to Longevity (Taokang heyan 桃康合延). The latter holds a talisman and the registers for preserving the destiny and the root of life. Above, they saunter in the Upper Clarity, they come and go in the flowery chamber,

120 *Yuanshi wuliang duren shangpin miaojing neiyi* (DZ 90), 1.7b–9b.

> enjoy the eight darknesses and penetrate into the infinitely subtle. Down here, in the human body, they calm and stabilize the Muddy Pellet and the Scarlet Palace. They regulate the five breaths, mingle and unite the hundred deities. They make numinous spirits and the ten thousand breaths turn ten times, and make you reach the rank of transcendent.[121]

These five deities were integrated in the pantheon related to the thunder rites, mixing elements of the Upper Clarity tradition and of the Numinous Treasure tradition, as in the text entitled the *Great Rites of the Numinous Treasure and the Upper Clarity* placing on top the Great One, on the left Non-pareil Lordling, on the right Worthy of the White Prime, at the centre Rector of Fate and in the south Vigour of Peach of the gate of the vital force.[122]

The *Chart for the Cultivation of Perfection* includes the names of four of these deities: the Non-pareil Lordling, the Worthy of the White Prime, the Lord of the Great One, and Vigour of Peach. It lacks the Great Lord of Long Life if we refer to the *Book of Universal Salvation* and the Rector of Fate if we refer to the *Great Rites of the Numinous Treasure*. The Great One is mentioned in connection with the navel: "The navel is the Life Gate. The divinity of the Great One resides there. He regulates the innate nature and the vital force of the individual. He is the rector of the thirteen thousand essences in the body." Three of these deities, the Non-pareil Lordling related to the liver, the Worthy of the White Prime related to the lungs, Vigour of Peach related to the kidneys are also deities of the Yellow Court tradition. On the *Chart for the Cultivation of Perfection*, their names are inscribed in the drawings of the liver and the lungs and beside the kidneys, where a short text describe Vigour of Peach (fig. 4.2, text 17):

> The Lord Vigour of Peach wears a lotus flower hat, a red garment and looks like a Perfected. He resides in the palace of the kidneys. There are cyan, purple, yellow, white, green, azure, red, and blue-green breaths that are a transformation of the eight heavens of the North.

Vigour of Peach is thus described in the *Book of the Inner Landscape of the Yellow Court*: "The infant Peach leading to longevity generates rays of flowery

121 *Ibid.*, 4.13b–14.

122 Wang Qizhen 王契真 (fourteenth century), *Shangqing lingbao dafa* 上清靈寶大法 [Great rites of the Numinous Treasure and the Upper Clarity] (DZ 1221), 4.16b. On the drawings of the five deities, see Wei Qi's 衛琪 (1309) commentary in *Yuqing wuji zongzhen Wenchang dadong xianjing zhu* 玉清無極總真文長大洞仙經註 [Commentary on the *Great Cavern Scripture* according to Wenchang] (DZ 103), 1.23b.

light; after man and woman unite nine times, Vigour of Peach will be found."[123] According to the commentary by Liangqiu zi, "the Infant Peach is the deity of yin and yang that is also called Earl Peach (Botao 伯桃). According to the *Classic on Immortality*, in the navel palace or the Gate of the Vital Force (*mingmen* 命門), there is "a great lord, the Infant Peach, whose nickname is Union to Longevity. He wears a red garment and a purple hat shaped like a hibiscus.' Before you sleep at night, visualize him so that the six *ding* and six *jia* deities come to serve you. He sheds light, prevents the yin and yang breaths from withering. When man and woman unite, they must visualize the three Cinnabar Fields. Vigour of Peach is the deity abiding under the Cinnabar Field and governing yin and yang, who unites the three with the nine."[124] The *Perfected Scripture of the Great Cavern of the Upper Clarity*, a fundamental document of the Upper Clarity tradition, gives a slightly different description of this divinity: "I reverently pray to the Lord of the Gate of the Vital Force or Vigour of Peach, whose nickname is 'Union of the Essence' (Hejing 合精), to constantly keep the Pass at the centre of the navel, the gate of the morbid breaths inside the palace of the Gate of the Vital Force, in order to keep the good omens in the navel, the floating yellow clouds coating the three vital forces, the life root which untie the knots of the embryo."[125]

In the Numinous Treasure School and the commentaries of the *Book for Universal Salvation*, from the Song, Yuan and Ming dynasties, Vigour of Peach is not one deity, but two. According to the commentary of the *Book of Universal Salvation* by Xiao Yingsou, the "Non-pareil Lordling is the deity of the liver, White Prime the deity of the lungs, Great One is the chief of the hundred deities, Rector of fate is the perfection above the South, Vigour of Peach and Union to Longevity are the deities of the left and right kidneys."[126] According to the commentary by Xue Jizhao 薛季昭 of the Yuan dynasty, "the deities Non-pareil Lordling, White Prime, Great One, Rector of Fate, Vigour of Peach and Union of longevity are Perfected of the Northern Dipper. Great One is in the brain, Rector of fate in the heart, Vigour of Peach in the umbilicus to the left, and Union of Longevity in the right kidney."[127] According to the commentary by Zhang Yuchu, "the Non-pareil Lordling is the deity of the liver, White Prime that of the lungs, Great One the leader of the hundred deities, the Rector of

123 *Huangting neijing yujing zhu* (DZ 402), 2.5b.

124 According to *Taishang huangting neijing yujing* (DZ 331), 5b, this should be read as Taohai 桃海.

125 *Shangqing dadong zhenjing* 上清大洞真經 [Perfected scripture of the great cavern of upper clarity] (DZ 6), 2.16a.

126 *Yuanshi wuliang duren shangpin miaojing neiyi* (DZ 90), 4.13b.

127 *Yuanshi wuliang duren shangpin miaojing zhujie* (DZ 92), 2.31a.

the fate, the deity of the heart. Vigour of Peach and Union of longevity are the deities of the two kidneys."[128]

But the commentary of the *Book for Universal Salvation* that is closest to the text of the Chart belongs to Chen Chunrong 陳椿榮 of the Southern Song who describes Vigour of Peach with a lotus flower hat:

> Great One is in the brain and governs all the deities, the Rector of Fate is the governor of the heart, and Vigour of Peach and Union to Longevity are the deities of the two kidneys. Vigour of Peach remains in the navel and guards the root of the essence. He is called the deity of the meeting and the union. His family name is Peach, his given name Vigour. He wears a purple garment and a lotus hat; he holds in his hand the jade registers of long life and is standing at the lower left part. Union of Longevity resides in the kidneys and guards the Gate of the Vital Force. His nickname is the Lord of the Gate of the Vital Force. He is also called Peach; his byname is Huihai and his nickname "Union of the Essence." He wears a red garment, a hat with the form of a hibiscus; he holds the talisman in the image of the heavenly Sovereign and stands at the lower right part.[129]

## 7.2 *Deities Related to the Thunder Rites*

### 7.2.1 The Dark Warrior (Xuanwu) (fig. 5.18)

The representation bears in the lower petal of the cruciform drawing the inscription "the killing breath of the Dark Warrior" (*Xuanwu shaqi* 玄武煞氣). The Dark Warrior was, from the Han onwards, the emblem of the seven constellations of the North, the essence of water and supreme yin, symbolized by a turtle and a snake. By the Tang dynasty, the Dark Warrior was identified with a legendary immortal of the Han dynasty, an exorcist and alchemist who won immortality at Mount Wudang and to whom the heavenly Emperor conferred the North.[130] Because of a taboo on the character *xuan* under the emperor Zhenzong (998–1023) of the Song, his name was changed to Zhenwu, the "Perfected Warrior." In 1118, Emperor Huizong was evoking this deity with the Taoist Lin Lingsu 林靈素, a specialist of the methods of the Divine Empyrean tradition, and the Dark Warrior appeared to him. He first saw

---

128 *Yuanshi wuliang duren shangpin miaojing tongyi* (DZ 89), 3.8b.

129 Chen Chunrong 陳春榮, *Taishang dongxuan lingbao wuliang duren shangpin jingfa* 太上洞玄靈寶無量度人上品經法 [Scriptures and rituals for the *Book of Universal Salvation*] (DZ 93), 3.11b–12.

130 See Grootaers 1952:139–181.

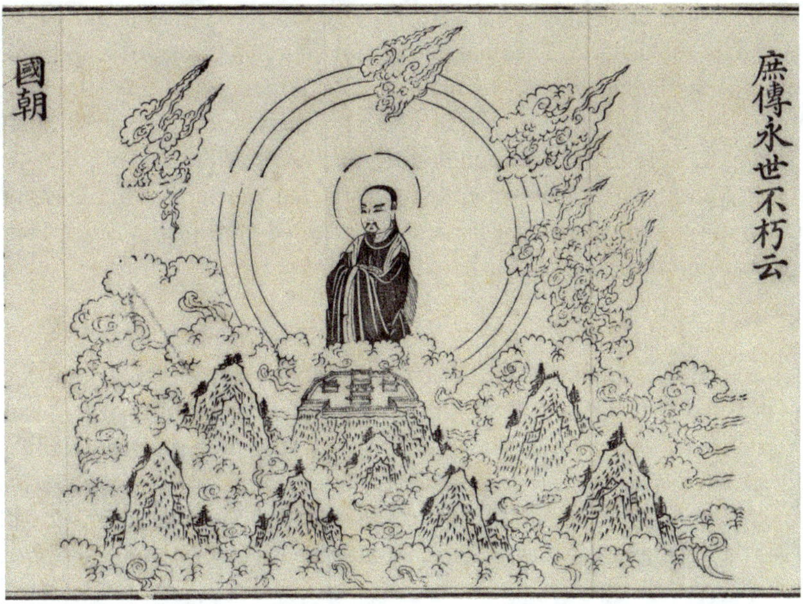


FIGURE 5.18 Manifestation of the "Supreme Emperor of the Dark Heaven" (Xuantian Shangdi 玄天上帝), that is to say Zhenwu 真武, above the Mount Wudang in 1413. *Da Ming Xuantian shangdi ruiying tulu* 大明玄天上帝瑞應圖錄 (DZ 959)

amongst the thunder and lightning a turtle and a snake, as well as a ten-foot man covered in a golden breastplate who was carrying a sword.

A later hagiography of Zhenwu, probably dating from the Yuan Dynasty,[131] tells us that the Perfected Warrior cultivated the Way for forty-two years according to the instructions of the Primordial Princess of the Purple Emptiness (Zixu yuanjun 紫虛元君), Wei Huacun 魏華存 (252–334), the matriarch of the Upper Clarity tradition. The celestial thearch ordered him to pacify the demons.[132]

131 See *Xuantian shangdi qishenglu* 玄天上帝啟聖錄 [Records of the epiphany of the supreme ancestor of the dark heaven] (DZ 958), 1.2b, which tells the story of the transmission to Xuandi by Zixu yuanjun.

132 The Heavenly Sovereign and Great Emperor (*Tianhuang dadi*) is mentioned in the general text on the body, in the upper left corner of the Chart.

With his hair untied, he led the army of the six cyclic signs *jia* and the six *ding* to fight the demons. The demon king turned into a black turtle and a big snake, but the Perfected Warrior trampled them underfoot. Under the Ming dynasty, his cult gained in importance. During the *yongle* reign (1369–1424), Emperor Chengzu ordered the building of a road and the undertaking of major works at Mount Wudang, to venerate the Perfected Warrior. During the Qing dynasty, the title of "Holy and Protecting Perfected Lord of the North Pole" (*Beiji yousheng zhenjun*) was conferred upon him.

### 7.2.2 The Black Killer (Heisha 黑煞)

The *shaqi* 煞氣 [Killing breath], designates this black killer associated with the Perfected Warrior and the North. This is a fundamental divinity in all exorcist rituals using the Thunder Rites (fig. 5.19). The *Secret Essentials of the Most High Principal Perfected Assisting the Country and Saving the People* mentions a magic talisman of the "black Killer" or "Formula of the Emperor of the North."[133] The *Great Rites of Upper Level of the Book of Universal Salvation* mentions the "killer breath of the Northern Thearch of the Supreme Mystery" (Taixuan Beidi shaqi 太玄北帝煞氣) corresponding on the inside of the body to the kidneys.[134]

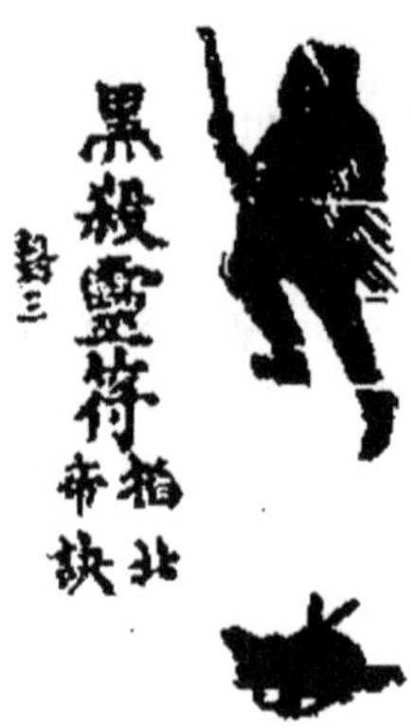

FIGURE 5.19
"Magic talisman of the Black Killer" (Heisha lingfu 黑煞靈符). *Taishang zhuguo jiumin zongzhen biyao* 太上助國救民總真秘要 (DZ 1227), 3.12b

133 See Yuan Miaozong's 元妙宗 preface to *Taishang zhuguo jiumin zongzhen biyao* 太上助國救民總真秘要 [Secret essentials of the most high principal perfected that assists the country and saves the people] (DZ 1227), 3.12b. The scripture also contains the following passage: "It is the great general Black killer. Visualize the true breath of the seventh star of the Northern Dipper concentrated at the point of the brush." (DZ 1227, 3.23a).

134 *Lingbao wuliang duren shangpin dafa* (DZ 219), 14.9b.

### 7.2.3 The Great Emperor of Purple Tenuity (Ziwei dadi 紫微大帝)

The inscription "Purple Tenuity" (*Ziwei* 紫微) is written on the forehead below the left hand point. It is difficult to determine if this designates the Palace of Purple Tenuity or the deity. The Great Emperor of Purple Tenuity is the deity of the North Pole. "Deity of the North Pole" is inscribed at the bottom of the illustration near the legs. This emperor was a primordial deity of the Correct Method of the Heart of Heaven. He chairs to the "Court of the North Pole which chases evil influences" (*Beiji quxie yuan*). In the *Correct Method of the Heart of Heaven, of the Upper Clarity Tradition*, there is a passage concerning this deity: "The Great Emperor of the Purple Tenuity of the North Pole straddles the purple clouds and leads the thirty-six generals under the command of Marshal Tianpeng 天蓬 who, with courage and ferocity, performs the rituals, straddle the purple clouds and completely cover the Dharma body."[135]

### 7.2.4 The Jade Emperor (Yudi 玉帝)

Yudi, "Jade Emperor" or Yuhuang dadi 玉皇大帝 "Great Sovereign Jade Emperor," is one of the most popular deities of the Taoist pantheon, particularly from the Song onwards.[136] Emperor Zhenzong (r. 997–1022) conferred to him a title in 1012, and almost all temples then included his statue. His elevated status in the Taoist pantheon was conferred in the Song dynasty with the text *Combined Scriptures of the Founding Acts of the Jade Emperor on High*.[137] He is related to the heaven of the Pure Tenuity and for this reason is also important in the Pure Tenuity tradition. According to this text, the Celestial Worthy of Original Commencement is located in the palace of the Jade Sovereign, in the mysterious garden with seven jewels, at the golden porte of the Jade Capital, in the Heaven of the Pure Tenuity, exposing the non-duality. The Jade Sovereign stands to his right, manifesting the six supernatural powers. The Sovereign of the Heaven of pure light and wide emptiness pronounced this stanza in praise of the Jade Emperor:

---

135 *Shangqing tianxin zhengfa* 上清天心正法 [Correct method of the heart of heaven] (DZ 566), 2.3b. See also *Wushang xuanyuan santian yutang dafa* on the commandment of Ziwei dadi (DZ 220, 27.7a). The Dharma body is a Buddhist expression, designating the Absolute, the nature of Buddha.

136 See Ma 1990: 28–37.

137 *Gaoshang yuhuang benxing jijing* (DZ 10); Liu Chuyuan 劉處元, *Gaoshang yuhuang benxing jingsui* (DZ 12).

In homage to the Sovereign of the Obscure Firmament of the golden
portico,[138]
Worthy Superior and Jade Emperor,
Whose marvellous signs cover Heaven,
Whose lamp of love illuminates the three worlds.[139]

The Jade Emperor is asked to transmit the teachings of the jade chapters of the Numinous Treasure to those who were unaware of their existence. Then the five emperors ascend to the Cinnabar Hall of the Spirits of the Cold and could then show the perfected writings.

138 Term engraved on the *Chart for the Cultivation of Perfection* in the central circle above the head.

139 The Buddhist model of this character is Amitāyus or Amitābha.

CHAPTER 6

# Alchemical Methods According to the *Chart for the Cultivation of Perfection*

The methods of Inner Alchemy are meditative rituals that an adept uses alone in his chamber or in a quiet place of the natural world. The process culminates in the realization of the Way, what Taoists often call "obtaining of the Way." In writings on Inner Alchemy, these practices are described with a vocabulary that draws on many sources beyond operative alchemy, such as terms adapted from Chinese cosmology, myths and the plant world.

Many of these terms are related to agricultural work; they often detail ways that an adept produces a plant of immortality. If the metaphorical melting of metals within the body corresponds to the production of spiritual light shining like gold, the production of the plant of immortality corresponds to the transformation of the life force into an inexhaustible source of energy that constantly renews itself. A seed is planted in the carefully ploughed "perfected earth" (*zhentu* 真土), and is cared for by carefully cultivating its "jade peduncle" (*yudi* 玉蒂) or its "golden flower" (*jinhua* 金花), after which it is harvested. In this way, the "medicine of longevity" (*changsheng yao* 長生樂), also simply called "medicine" (*yaowu* 藥物), is cultivated as follows:

> Each person has the medicine of long life,
> But foolishly casts it aside.
> When the ambrosia descends, heaven and earth unite.
> Where the yellow sprout grows, *kan* [water] and *li* [fire] unite.[1]

The life in the body functions like the cosmos. The cosmos is conceived of a series of transformations that start with chaos and result in unity. From the Song dynasty onwards, this unity is called the Taiji [Great ultimate]. This initial unity, the One, is divided into yin and yang breaths, as well as the five agents and the eight trigrams. The evolution and transformation of these entities create the multiplicity of phenomena in a well-ordered space-time. In this vein, the *Classic of Changes* (*Yijing* 易經) and the symbolism of the trigrams (figures of three lines, in group of three, broken lines symbolizing yin and continuous lines symbolizing yang) are a constant reference in writings

1 Zhang Boduan, *Wuzhen pian zhushu* (DZ 141), 2.13a–b.

 DOI:10.1163/9789004383456_008

on Internal Alchemy. The evolutions of the yin and yang breaths in the body following a specific rhythm of time are usually expressed by using the eight trigrams or the sixty-four hexagrams (figures of six yin or yang lines) from the *Classic of Changes*. For example, the appearance of inner heat arising from the lower abdomen during meditation is designated by the hexagram *fu* 復 ䷗ [Return], which contains one yang line (heat) on the bottom and five yin lines (quiet mind) on top. This signifies that in the lower part of a person's yin body appears a heat, a yang element. Using a hexagram to represent heat frees the process from physiology, as it frees it from specific space of the body to integrate it into a general process, that of the yin and yang transformations in the world.

All of this symbolism creates a complex system, and the alchemical charts of the body integrate the different metaphors and constitute a synthesis in images of the alchemical process. The elements represented in these charts are rooted in the system of Internal Alchemy that the Taoist writers of a given era wished to transmit. Similarities can be found in the terminology and in descriptions contained in the *Chart* with texts such as the *Stanzas of Awakening to Perfection* of Zhang Boduan or the writings included in the great compilation of the late 13th or early 14th centuries, the *Ten Books on the Cultivation of Perfection*. But the similarities also concern writings of later Taoists, such as Chen Zhixu 陳致虛 (ca. 1331), Li Daochun 李道純 (ob. 1306), Chen Xubai 陳虛白 (fl. thirteenth century) and Li Jianyi 李簡易 (ca. 1264). These authors have already made a synthesis between certain elements of the traditions of the Northern and the Southern alchemical traditions. In fact, each of these two main branches displays a remarkable variety of doctrinal statements and forms of practice.

One of the most noticeable features of the *Chart* is that Internal Alchemy was intimately related to ritual activity. The latter is an external use of the forces developed by an adept, who becomes an officiant, notably in thunder ritual, which will be described in more detail in the next chapter.[2] At present, it is not possible to reconstruct in detail all the alchemical processes evoked by this map, but I shall address the principal ones. The most common and key idea in Inner Alchemy concerns the three stages of the sublimation around the "three jewels" (the essence, the breath and the spirit), which take place in the three cinnabar fields. During these three stages, the main processes are an inversion of the typical operation of all things. The Dao

2 For an example of the links between Inner Alchemy and thunder rites, see Chao 2009: 104–120.

is imagined to act in this inversion, for it is a return from multiplicity to unity, and a reversion, with the rise of the breath along the vertebral column and the crossing of the three passes along the spine.

During this journey backwards, there is an exchange and a union between opposing elements that bring about the transformations of the breaths of the five viscera. These opposites are expressed in terms of natural elements such as the water and fire trigrams (*kan* and *li*) and other alchemical symbols. These symbols, though not numerous on the *Chart*, are sometimes difficult to decipher because they can take on different meanings according to the tradition that employs them and according to the stages of the process.

Finally, in the elaboration of self in comparison with the melting of metal in order to extract a luminous and brilliant gold, one of the essential links is the work of the blacksmith, who, with his bellows, properly stirs fire. The mastery of the fire regiment is a sine qua non for the success of these exercises. In Internal Alchemy, the regime of fire consists in knowing how to distinguish psychophysiological changes that occur in themselves with the aid of "martial fire" (i.e., respiration) and then of "civil fire" (i.e., creative thought) that accompany transformations of the self.[3] These are modelled on the course of macrocosmic time and install an internal time in harmony with the external weather, according to the cycle of days, months and years.

## 1 The Three Stages of the Process

### 1.1 *The Vital Essence, the Breath and the Spirit*

The main Inner Alchemy traditions from Song onwards consider three basic ingredients of the alchemical process: the vital essence (*jing* 精), the breath (*qi* 氣) and the spirit (*shen* 神).[4] These three elements are located within the three Cinnabar Fields and correspond to three basic steps: refining the vital essence and transform it into breath, refining the breath and transform

3 It is the interpretation given in *Tianxian zhengli zhilun* 大仙止理直論 by Wu Chongxu, fourth chapter "Classic on the Fire Phasing" (*Huohou jing* 火候經) and in most of the Qing texts.

4 Zhang Jixian's (1092–1127) *Mingzhen powang zhangsong* (DZ 979, 1b) mentions the three jewels of the body as the primordial essence, the primordial breath and the primordial spirit. Lu Shizhong 路時中 (twelfth century), in his *Wushang sanyuan santian yutang dafa* 無上玄元三天玉堂大法 [Great method of the jade hall of the three heavens, the supreme mysterious origin] (DZ 220, 18.9a), writes, "Heaven has three powers (*sancai* 三才): the sun, the moon and the stars. Earth has three powers: the three time markers *yi*, *bing*, and *ding*. Man has three powers: the vital essence, the [original] breath, and the spirit. When the vital essence is strengthened, the breath is complete, and the primordial spirit appears."

it into spirit, refining the spirit and return it to emptiness.[5] On the *Chart for the Cultivation of Perfection*, there are three characters for the "vital essence," the "breath" and the "spirit" listed from the bottom to the top in the middle of the body. The character "essence" is written near the Lower Cinnabar Field surmounted by a standing child, "breath" is written in the Median Cinnabar Field surmounted by a sitting child and "spirit" is inscribed at the bottom of the circle above the head and surmounted by a standing Taoist. A text in the middle of the body map describes this three-stage process: "When the body is still, the essence is established; when thought is motionless, the spirit becomes agile and efficient; when the heart is quiet, the breath becomes stronger." A quite similar formulation is also used in the *Collection on the Centre and the Harmony* by Li Daochun in reference to the exchange between *kan* and *li*.[6] The "Centre and the Harmony" (*zhonghe* 中和) was the name of the meditation room of Li Daochun in Nanking. He was a major author of the Yuan dynasty. His principal affiliation was with the Southern School as he was a disciple of one of Bai Yuchan's pupils, but he later became acquainted with masters of the Complete Perfection School and his own disciples were considered a part of this lineage.[7] This book is probably one of the sources of the *Chart for the Cultivation of Perfection*.

### 1.2 *The Reversal Path*

The fortieth chapter of the *Book of the Way and its Virtue* includes the verse:

> Reversal is the motion of the Way,
> Weakening is its modus operandi.

In alchemy, this reversal (*fan* 反) or "inversal" (*ni* 逆) is a cornerstone of the process. While the normal course of things leads to death, its reversal by an inverse movement leads to immortality. In the body, the inner breath normally circulates from top to bottom or more precisely from the brain to the coccyx and genitalia. The inversion of the direction of this movement and the arising of the breath along the backbone is the beginning of the alchemical work. This primordial breath is conveyed by the seminal essence. If the essence follows its

---

5 These three steps and three ingredients are presented in several Taoist texts such as the *Qingwei danjue* 清微丹訣 (DZ 278), 1.

6 Li Daochun's (ob. 1306) *Zhonghe ji* 中和集 (DZ 249), 2.2a. The inscription of the *Zhonghe ji* differs for one character with most of the versions of the *Chart for the Cultivation of Perfection*, but is identical with that of the Sichuan version by Duan Fu.

7 On Li Daochun, see Schipper and Verellen 2004: 1264.

normal course, it gives birth to an external being. After returning, it gives birth in the self to the embryo of immortality.

Evolution in the normal course leads from unity to multiplicity; by reversing the course, it goes from multiplicity to unity. Chaos is divided into two (yin / yang), three (heaven, earth, man), five (wood, fire, earth, metal, water), eight (eight trigrams), and so on. As it gradually unfolds, its will expand and manifest the ten thousand beings. In Inner Alchemy, the reversal of the process consists of gradually uniting in the body the multiple breaths, including those of the five viscera corresponding to the five agents, those of the three cinnabar fields, and of yin and yang, to achieve the return to the One within a great void. This unit is sometimes called the "[Original] Breath of the One" (*yiqi* 一炁) as in the Tiger and Dragon Altar's version of the *Chart for the Cultivation of Perfection*, or "Great Ultimate" (Taiji 太極). It is located at different places in the human body according to the sources: sometimes it is three inches below the navel,[8] but most often between the two kidneys.[9] It can have no particular place and is often equated to the light principle from which the self returns to the Origin.[10]

This reversal is indicated on the *Chart for the Cultivation of Perfection* by an inscription of twelve characters written on either side of the centre of the body: "The normal direction leads to the secular world; the reversal leads to holiness." Li Daochun also uses this phrase in the aforementioned *Collection on the Centre and the Harmony* when relating the three stages of the process.[11]

Chen Zhixu (ca. 1289–1331), a contemporary of Li Daochun, composed or perhaps revised an alchemical chart named The *Chart of the Normal or Reversal Reading of the Great Ultimate* (*Taiji shunni tu* 太極順逆圖) representing the reversal movement for achieving the cinnabar. Two identical drawings are side by side. The first is the "Chart of the Great Ultimate" (*Taiji tu* 太極圖) by Zhou Dunyi 周敦頤 (1017–1073), which itself represents the normal direction and the second is the alchemical map, whose drawings are identical but bear different legends (see fig. 6.1). During the Song dynasty, the cosmological pattern of the Great Ultimate developed and led to several representations using the circle as model.[12] In the context of Inner Alchemy, a number of representations similar to that of Zhou Dunyi appeared, sometimes with a different title. Inserted in Song and Ming documents, they schematize the main transformation processes at

8 *Daofa huiyuan* (DZ 1220), 69.3b.

9 *Daoshu* (DZ 1017), 7.11a–13a.

10 *Shangyangzi jindan dayao* (DZ 1067), 6.2a–18a.

11 *Zhonghe ji* (DZ 249), 2.2a.

12 On the concept of Taiji in Inner Alchemy, see Robinet 1990: 373–411.

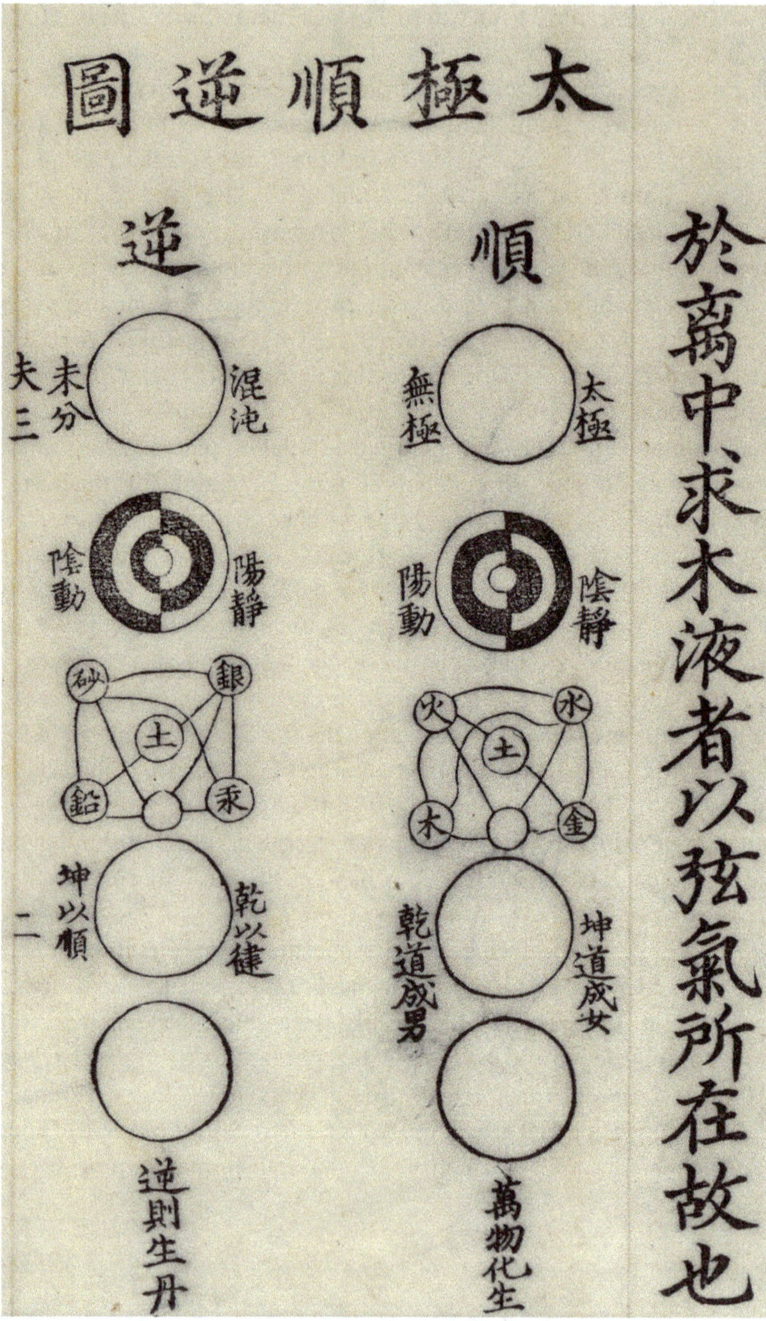


FIGURE 6.1 "Chart of the normal or reversal reading of the Great Ultimate" (*Taiji shunni tu* 太極順逆圖). *Shangyangzi jindan dayao tu* (DZ 1068), 3a

work in the human body.[13] This is the case of the *Chart of the Normal or Reversal Reading of the Great Ultimate* where the terms of "Great Ultimate" (*taiji* 太極) and "Non-Ultimate" (*wuji* 無極), which are inscribed on the top of the Zhou Dunyi diagram, are replaced on the alchemical map by "chaos and not yet divided" (*hundun weifen* 混沌未分). The characters of the five agents in the middle part of the first map are replaced by the names of five alchemical ingredients: cinnabar, silver, mercury, lead and earth. The Zhou Dunyi diagram is itself an adaptation of a now-lost drawing attributed to the Taoist Chen Tuan 陳摶 (ca. 906–989), which was either titled "Diagram of the Anterior Heaven" (*xiantian tu* 先天圖) or "Diagram of the Non-Ultimate" (*wuji tu* 無極圖). While there is no definite proof that the diagram of Chen Tuan was a representation of the body and its alchemical processes, it is nevertheless very likely. Zhou Dunyi and Neo-Confucians would have extracted these maps from the alchemical context and integrated them into a general cosmological model. Furthermore, they would have modified a diagram using the alchemical and esoteric terms into one using cosmological terms such as yin and yang, the five agents, and so on.[14]

Although the different available versions of these diagrams carry different names, they have a number of common points. First, the schema is read from the top to the bottom, without indication of a hierarchy. It is composed of drawings mixed with inscriptions, among which the circle represents completeness and suggests the idea of unity. The bipolarity of yin and yang is represented by two colours, usually black and white, or red and black (see fig. 6.2). The encircled characters symbolize the element designated by the character. On the Zhou Dunyi diagram we have the five agents related to the five viscera and on other Taoist body maps the five ingredients used in Inner Alchemy (cinnabar, silver, mercury, lead, earth). The links between the different elements of the diagram (viscera or elements) are clarified by connecting lines. Nothing, neither in the title, nor in the form, suggests it is the body. We only know this through the written texts accompanying the drawings. This lack of precise contours is quite understandable because at some stage of alchemical transmutation the body becomes an entity free from the body of flesh. Consequently, the barriers between interior and exterior fade because the adept transforms into the cosmos or a sacred area depending on the context, or even both at the same time.

13 The main diagrams of this nature are *Taiji miaohua shenling hundong chiwenzhi tu* 太極妙化神靈混洞赤文之圖 inserted into two commentaries of the *Book of Universal Salvation*: Xiao Yingsou's 1226 preface in the *Yuanshi wuliang duren shangpin miaojing neiyi* (DZ 90, 6b) and Zhang Yuchu's (1359–1410) *Yuanshi wuliang duren shangpin miaojing tongyi* (DZ 89), 1.1a.

14 See Robinet 1990: 400.

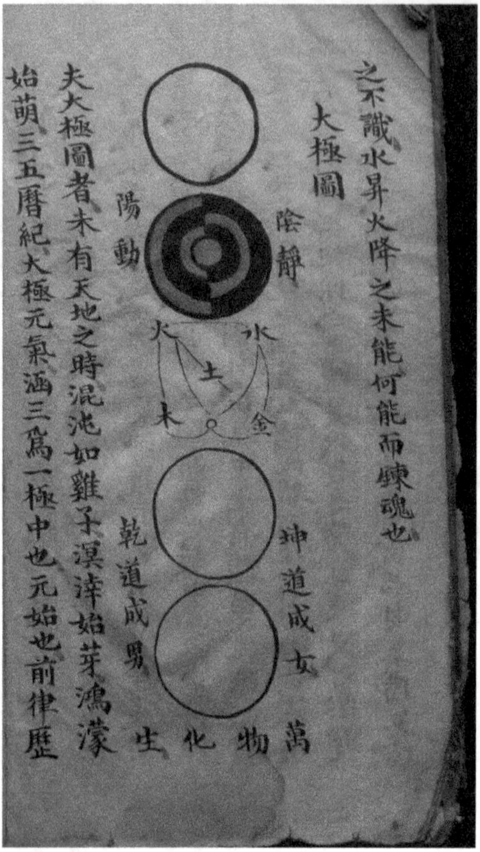


FIGURE 6.2
A Coloured Chart of the Great Ultimate. In *Lingbao taiji lianbi*, an eighteenth century manuscript belonging to Patrice Fava

This diagram, in fact, comprises the main elements involved in the alchemical process: the spatio-temporal disposition, the itinerary to be followed, the dynamic of the processes and the way to implement them. These charts are not easy to understand without an oral commentary or an accompanying text. Apart from the various inscriptions on these diagrams, the "Diagram on the Great Ultimate" by Zhou Dunyi and the representations of Inner Alchemy differ essentially in the way of reading them. The first must be read from the top to the bottom, while the alchemical representations are to be read from bottom to top. This is confirmed by the commentary of Huang Zongyan 黃宗炎 (1616–1686) to a drawing entitled "Diagram of Non-Ultimate" attributed to Chen Tuan, which emphasizes the reversal process (see fig. 6.3).[15]

15 See Huang Zongyan's 黃宗炎 (1616–1686) *Yixue bianhuo* 易學辨惑 [Debate on mistakes in learning mutations] in *Zhaodai congshu* 昭代叢書, 2.39b.

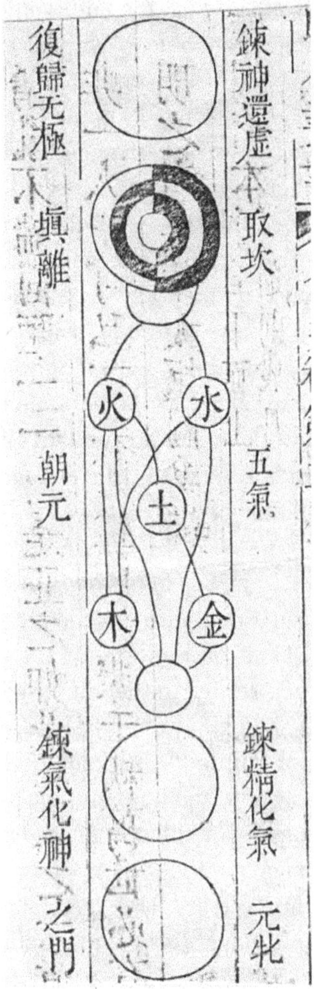


FIGURE 6.3
Meaning of the normal or reversal reading of the Great Ultimate. Huang Zongyan 黄宗炎, *Yixue bianhuo*, in *Zhaodai congshu* 昭代叢書, 2.39b

Regarding this way of reversal and the return to the origin, a text attributed to Zhang Sanfeng 張三豐, an eminent Taoist of the late fourteenth and early fifteenth centuries of Mount Wudang, describes this process as follows:

> First, make the yin contained in the yang of the superior orifice descend so that it enters the cauldron of metal of the "sea of breath" (i.e., abdomen) and joins to the perfected yang of the lower orifice. The perfected yin within the yang is the primordial spirit of the three *hun*-souls. The perfected yang of the lower orifice is the primordial breath of the body relating to the seven *po*-souls. Once these two breaths at the front and at the back of the body unite, *kan* [water] and *li* [fire] exchange and mingle,

> spirit and breath are knotted and condense, after which the embryonic breathing stabilizes. Therefore, each day an indescribable joy similar to that of sexual union floods into you and if you do not become attached to it, secretions and heat naturally form the hexagram *jiji* [combination of the trigrams *kan*, water, and *li*, fire]. This will spread into the four limbs and shine with brilliance as strong as an external fire. When water and fire are balanced, the fire phasing of the microcosmic orbit is regularized, the vapours rise, the breath of the throat reverses and returns to the primordial sea (i.e., abdomen). The external yang naturally penetrates inside and the true fire bursts into the upper part. The body becomes flexible, the adept tastes an infinite joy several times a day, he experiences the sensation of a swirling dragon, rising and falling in the abdomen, when, metaphorically, the young girl and the adolescent boy unite. This is the stage of gathering the yin to complete the yang, to cultivate and refine the jade liquor and to return it to the cinnabar field.[16]

This path of reversal movement leads the adept from the mundane world to the paradises. The myth of paradises is integrated into all the alchemical metaphors by the common image of the three islands of immortality; these images are included in the texts of a Taoist tradition related to the immortals Zhong Liquan 鍾離權 and Lü Dongbin 呂洞賓. The myth of these islands of the Eastern Sea, which would be the residence of immortals, harkens back to the Han dynasty. Writers transposed the islands onto the human body as metaphors for the three passes of the back. The passes are difficult to unlock but as the breath rises from the coccyx along the spine, they will open and become places of transmutations that lead to immortality. This metaphor suggests the link between psychophysiological changes inside the body following a specific itinerary, and specific changes in the state of mind. All of these changes happen in conjunction with physiological changes; the adept becomes calmer and calmer, until he or she reaches a supreme state of peace. Body and mind transformations go hand in hand and are indistinguishable.[17]

---

16 *Sanfeng zhenren xuantan quanji*, 4. Text inserted in *Daozang xubian* published in 1834 by Min Yide.

17 On these three islands, see Xiao Daocun's 蕭道存 *Xiuzhen taiji hunyuan tu* 修真太極混元圖 [Diagrams on the mystery of ultimate and primordial chaos for the cultivation of perfected nature] (DZ 149), 8a; French translation by Baryosher 1996: 73–77.

### 1.3 *The Three Chariots*

On the *Chart for the Cultivation of Perfection*, the backbone is depicted as three chariots pulled by three different animals. In the lower part, a chariot pulled by sheep; at the level of the kidneys, a chariot pulled by deer; at the level of the neck, a chariot pulled by buffalo. There are at least four other texts that, in addition to the *Chart*, include drawings of these three chariots.[18] The oldest representation is Yanluozi's diagrams (10th cen.) (see fig. 1.4, p. 16), followed by the drawing included in the commentary of the *Classic of the Difficulties* (13th cen.). Four centuries later, in the *Principles of the Tablets on the Innate Nature and the Vital Force* (17th cen.), there is a representation of the three chariots independent of all representations of the body inscribed alongside the legend "Accumulation of Fire and Transport of Metal."[19] Another seventeenth-century text comprising a representation of the body as a mountain depicts the three chariots along the backbone with the following caption: "The breath of the sheep is at the Caudal Pass, the breath of the deer follows the spine and the breath of the buffalo pulls the three chariots." According to Cao Yuanbai's 曹元白 (Yuyu zi 俞俞子) 1636 preface to the text, Cao received these drawings in Yecheng near Jinling (Nanjing) from Guo Shihao 郭士豪, a master of the Jingming 淨明 school whose byname was the "Taoist of Mount Longmian" (Anhui) (see fig. 6.4).[20]

These three chariots are a Taoist adaptation of a Buddhist metaphor. The integration of Buddhist elements was not a phenomenon occurring in the early expressions of Internal Alchemy. The incorporation of Buddhist ideas in Taoism is best understood a manifestation of the struggles and competition between Buddhists and Taoists in this era. Taoists have claimed that their way was superior because if Buddhists managed to transform and control their minds, Taoists transformed both mind and matter, including the body. Internal Alchemists had already adapted Buddhist methods of concentration and contemplation on the nature of the mind such as the Chan (Zen) methods, such as in the works of Zhang Boduan who is supposed to have been also a Chan monk; these Chan methods are also important in the Complete Perfection school. But gradually, Buddhist images or metaphors have been incorporated in the proper sense. In fact, a number of Inner Alchemical texts used Buddhist expressions to describe alchemical processes, involving both

---

18 The three chariots are represented on the drawings by Yanluozi (tenth century) in *Xiuzhen shishu* (DZ 263), 18.2–3; *Huangdi bashiyi nanjing zuantu jujie* (DZ 1024), 4a–b; *Xingming guizhi*, 3.16b and in Cao Yuanbai's 曹元白 (fl. 1636) *Daoyuan yiqi*.

19 *Xingming guizhi*, 3.16b.

20 Cao Yuanbai, *Daoyuan yiqi* 道元一炁.

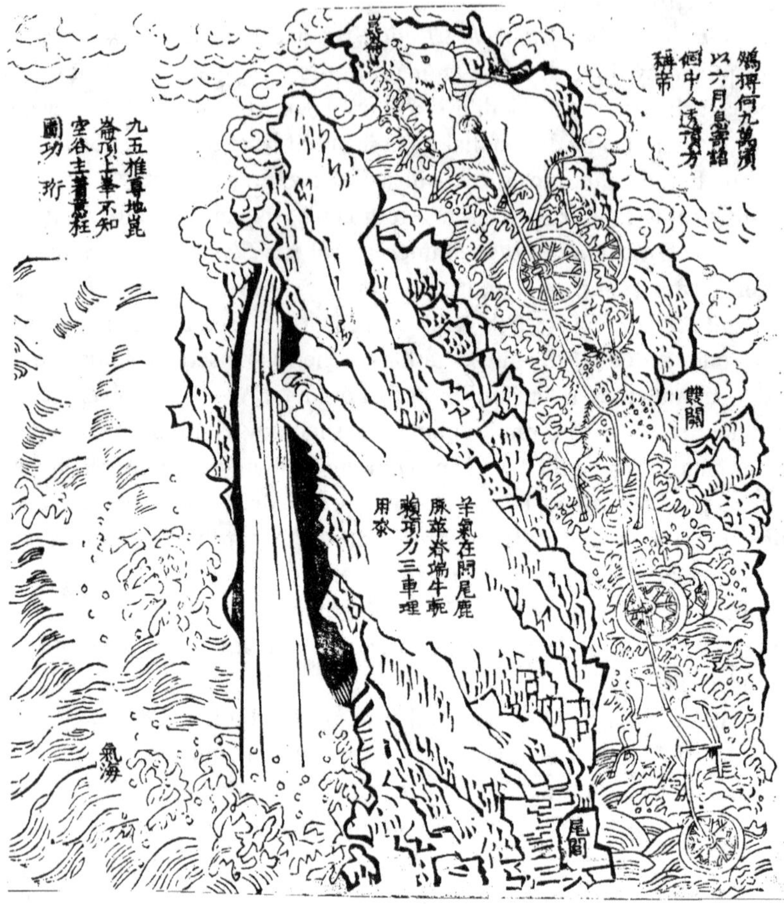


FIGURE 6.4 The three chariots according to the representation of *Daoyuan yiqi* 道元一炁 [Breath unifying the origin of the Way]

body and mind. Some terms referring to events in the history of Buddhism or to technical methods employed by this religion were diverted from their original meaning to evoke psychophysiological processes occurring inside the body. Locating these metaphors in parts of the body, on the one hand, enabled the adept to simultaneously transform body and mind and, on the other hand, to constitute an interior journey in the memory of the individual and for Taoism to appropriate elements of Buddhism.

This type of appropriation concerns only a few expressions. So far, we have identified four of them: two which are related to historical events of Buddhism and two others which are allegories used in the Buddhist context to express the path to enlightenment and the various methods proposed by different schools.

The first expression is "The Prince Shoots his Arrow on the Nine Bronze Drums," which appears in the text concerning the Caudal Pass in the *Chart for the Cultivation of Perfection*.[21] It is an allusion to an episode of the life of Prince Siddhartha, the historical Buddha, when he was about to be married. Siddhartha was subjected to several tests including archery, and defeated all his rivals after piercing seven successive drums with a single arrow. This story is reported in the *Lalitavistara*, a hagiography of Siddhartha for which there are several Chinese translations with variants.[22] In one translation, he only shoots the arrow through three drums.[23] In a later translation, it is said than his predecessor can only reach the eighth drum, suggesting that Siddhartha attains the ninth.[24] The number nine is the one that fits best in the Taoist context, because it is the number of supreme yang; but in the Buddhist context, it is the number seven that is predominant. This expression, therefore, provides another example of how the texts of Inner Alchemy reinterpreted Buddhist expressions from their original meaning.

"Shot through the Nine Bronze Drums" is an attested expression in the context of Inner Alchemy since at least the thirteenth century. It was a common expression by the Qing dynasty, and is found for example in a text attributed to Liu Huayang, the *Collection of Texts on Wisdom and Vital Force*: "The Worthy said: 'in one shot, an arrow pierces nine successive drums.'" The following commentary is appended to the passage: "The arrow is the [Original] Breath. The shot is the process that causes the spirit and the [Original] Breath to circulate at the same time. The nine drums correspond to the [three orifices of the] three passes of the back: the Caudal Pass, the one that surrounds the spine, and the Jade Pillow Pass. Each of these comprises two orifices on the left and right, as well as central orifice. The nine drums represent the three triads. It is necessary in the wonderful method to cross the passes to circulate the breath through the central opening; if one takes other paths, he will not be able to obtain the Way."[25] The prodigious strength of Prince Siddhartha becomes the inner strength of the adept, who uses his internal breath (the arrow) to unlock the three passes on the back.

The second example of borrowing a Buddhist event is the use of the term "Cao Stream" (Caoxi 曹溪) to designate the breath rising up from the coccyx. It

21 This metaphor is seen in *Baoyi zi Sanfeng laoren danjue* (DZ 281), 15b. This text was transmitted by Huang Gongwang (1269–1354) to his disciple Jin Yueyan 金月岩. See also the *Xingming guizhi*, 1.51.

22 See Jñānagupta's (523–600) translation in *Fo Benxingjijing* 佛本行集經, T. 190, 710c–711a.

23 See Dharmaraksa's (ca. 265–313) translation in *Puyao jing* 普耀經, T. 186, 501c–502a.

24 See Divākara's translation in *Fangguang da zhuangyan jing* 方廣大莊嚴經, T. 187, 564b.

25 *Jishuo huiming jing* 集說慧命經, attributed to Liu Huayang 柳華陽, p. 25.

is the name of the place where the sixth Patriarch of the Chan (Zen) Buddhism, Huineng 慧能 (638–713), would have experienced enlightenment. In Inner Alchemy, it designates the "watercourse" leading to enlightenment, i.e., the life water or [Original] Breath flowing up the spine. It is compared to a mountain stream flowing from the top (the brain) to the valley (lower body). This torrent leads to death if the water is allowed to flow down, and to immortality, if by using hydraulic chariots, we reverse its course to make it rise as far as the top of the head.

The metaphor of the three chariots is an adaptation of a famous parable of the *Lotus Sûtra*. This sutra preaches the doctrine of the unique vehicle, able to save all sentient beings, and including the three classic vehicles of Buddhism: the small vehicle or that of the Auditors, the median vehicle or that of the Buddhas themselves and the great vehicle or the vehicle of enlightened beings (bodhisattva). A father wants to save his numerous children who have remained in his flaming house. He promises to each of them, if they quickly rush out of the house, to give them a sheep chariot, a deer chariot or a buffalo chariot. These chariots respectively symbolize the small vehicle, the median vehicle and the great vehicle. The father symbolizes the Buddha, the burning house, our world of passions and the children, the sentient beings in ignorance.[26]

In Taoism, this metaphor attested from the tenth century onwards, represents the force in the body required to raise the breath along the length of the spine. In Inner Alchemy, the chariot, or more precisely the "hydraulic chariot" (*heche* 河車), allows the transport of water and fire, from the Caudal Pass located in the region of the coccyx to the Muddy Pellet at the top of the head. Many texts explain sometimes with notable differences, the meaning of this metaphor. From the Caudal Pass to the Spinal Handle Pass in the kidney area, the circulation is slow and relaxed; it corresponds to the speed of the chariot pulled by a sheep. From the Spinal Handle Pass to the Jade Pillow Pass at the neck, the circulation is faster; it corresponds to the deer chariot. From the Jade Pillow Pass to the Muddy Pellet, it takes a great strength to cross the pass, similar to that of a buffalo and it corresponds to the buffalo chariot.[27]

These three chariots correspond with the three steps of the alchemical work, and are also called: the "hydraulic chariot of the jade liquor" (*yuye heche* 玉液河車) corresponding to the small microcosmic orbit, the "chariot of the golden elixir" (*jinye heche* 金液河車) corresponding to the great microcosmic orbit, and the "purple hydraulic chariot" (*zi heche* 紫河車) corresponding to the

26 See Robert 1997: 93–126.

27 See the chapter "On the hydraulic chariot" in *Zhong Lü chuandao ji* (DZ 263), 15.19b–20a.

spirit leaving the body on its ascension to heaven. We also find terms such as "the small hydraulic chariot" (*xiao heche* 小河車), "the large hydraulic chariot" (*da heche* 大河車) and the "purple hydraulic chariot" (*zi heche* 紫河車) to designate these three levels in Inner Alchemical texts.[28] The small hydraulic chariot corresponds to the reversal of the cycle of the five agents, with the exchange of water and fire and the union of the tiger and the dragon forming the yellow sprout. The large hydraulic chariot is the technique called the "Golden Crystal Behind the Elbow" (*zhouhou jinjing* 肘後金晶) or the return of the crystal that enters the Muddy Pellet.[29] Lead is extracted and mercury added to form the great panacea. Once the yellow sprout is formed, there is coupling between lead and mercury to form the great panacea. The true breath is generated and the five breaths will pay homage to the Origin. Finally, the purple chariot corresponds to the Yang Spirit (*yangshen* 陽神) leaving the body.

## 2 The Union of Opposites

Alchemy is the art of uniting opposites, a union often compared to that of a couple. Just as a shaman had a sexual union with the numinous spirits who possessed him, there is a similar kind of sexual link in Internal Alchemy between the *hun* soul and the *po* soul.[30] The metaphors evoking this psychophysiological process focus mainly on the exchange between the various ingredients, an exchange sometimes expressed in terms of marital union, recalling the conjunction or the coitus well known to some western alchemists.[31]

The union of yin and yang breaths inside the body is expressed through the myth of the love story between a weaver and a cowherd. These two deities corresponded to two stars in the constellations of Lyra and of Capricorn; it is probably one of the oldest and best-known myths of China and Asia. There are many versions of this story, but the most common states the Weaver is the daughter of the Celestial Emperor and resided east of the Milky Way. She

28 There exist other names and interpretations of these three chariots. For exemple, Wang Qingsheng 王慶升 (ca. mid-thirteenth century), in his *Sanji zhiming quandi* 三極至命全蒂 [The three ultimates and the supreme destiny ensnared] (DZ 575, 17b) mentions the following three chariots: the chariot of the Yellow River, the hydraulic chariot, and the purple hydraulic chariot.

29 On these techniques, see Baldrian-Hussein 1984: 237.

30 See Kaltenmark 1960: 580.

31 See *Le rosaire des philosophes* 2008: 73–83.

was responsible for weaving the heavenly clouds, but was bored and alone. The Celestial Emperor allowed her to marry the cowherd abiding to the west of the Milky Way. After her marriage, however, the Weaver forsook her task and the Celestial Emperor ordered her to return to the east of the Milky Way. He allowed her to meet her husband once a year, the seventh day of the seventh month as a result of magpies forming a bridge over the Milky Way.[32] The seventh day of the seventh month is precisely the date in a year at which the proportion of yin and yang is equal.

In Internal Alchemy, the term "bridge of the magpie" (*xiqiao* 鵲橋) is used to designate two points respectively situated at the lower part of the trunk and at the upper part in the head, which should be connected by closing, below, the sexual orifices and above by using the tongue to join the Function Vessel (*renmai* 任脈) and the Control Vessel (*dumai* 督脈), two vessels in which yin and yang breaths circulate. The yang breath rises via these two bridges from the lower abdomen to the top of head and transforms into yin. After this, it goes down the front of body until it reaches the abdomen, where it again joins the Control Vessel thanks to the lower bridge. It is similar to the increasing and decreasing of yin and yang breaths in the cosmos. These allusions to the cowherd, the weaver and the Bridge of Magpies are already inscribed on the Yanluozi diagram (10th cen.). One example of the use of this metaphor is the following passage of the *Mirror to Enter the Art of Elixir by Master Cui*:

> Upper bridge of magpies, lower bridge of magpies,
> The stars move in the sky,
> The Earth is in unison with its ebb and rising tides.

Wang Jie 王玠 (14th cen.) wrote a whole paragraph to explain the meaning of these three verses. However, his explanations remain sealed to those who do not know the alchemical language, as the author uses metaphorical terms to explain these symbols. He writes:

> In the human body, the backbone is compared to the Milky Way. When the Milky Way forms an obstacle, magical magpies come to form a bridge, hence the term "bridge of magpies," which in the body designates the tongue. Indeed, in alchemical practice, the yellow matchmaker attracts the young boy who rises to the Muddy Pellet in the [head] and unites with the girl. This happens at the same time as the [upper] bridge of magpies is constituted. The yellow matchmaker waits, smiles and

32 On this myth, see Mathieu 1989: 34–35.

> encourages the young boy and the girl to go back into the bridal chamber, so they inevitably descend from the Muddy Pellet: at that time, the lower bridge of magpies is formed. The matchmaker, the young boy and the young girl do not really exist; they are metaphors that refer to nothing other than the heart, the kidneys and the creative thinking.[33]

### 2.1 *The Fire of the Heart and the Water of the Kidneys*

The manipulations used to unite opposites in the alchemical process are rooted in terminology from the *Classic of Changes* and the system of the five agents. It also extensively uses the vocabulary from myths such as the descriptions of the unity between the emotions rising from the heart and the vital force uprising from the sexual organs. Writers often use the terms "water and fire," the trigrams *kan* and *li*, the alchemical ingredients lead and mercury, as well as the symbols of the dragon and the tiger.

The dragon and the tiger refer also commonly to the four animals designating four constellations at the four directions: the Azure Dragon in the east,[34] the White Tiger in the west, a turtle entangled by a snake called the Dark Warrior in the north, the Vermilion Sparrow in the south. Two of them, the tiger and the dragon, are most often mentioned in alchemical texts. Their symbolism runs quite deep, as they are related to east and west, and therefore to the corresponding elements in the system of the five agents for the east (e.g., wood, the liver, the emerging yang) and west (e.g., metal, the lungs, the emerging yin). However, they are also metaphors with several meanings, referring to mobility, to a double character (the dragon is indeed related to both water and fire) and a large aptitude for metamorphosis. They are also well-known figures in folklore that often play a role in worship and festivals. These two animals may therefore refer respectively to the spirit and the breath, to fire and water, to man and woman, which are opposite but complementary elements, whose union is necessary in Internal Alchemy.

The fire of the heart typically moves upwards to fan the flame of passions and emotions. Instead, it must descend with the help of the gradual calming of the mind so that the innate nature can be revealed. The innate nature is located in a place near the heart called the Scarlet Palace. It is said in the *Chart for the Cultivation of Perfection* (fig. 3.6, text 13):

---

33 Cui Xifan's 崔希範 (ob. 940) *Cuigong ruyao jing rujie* 崔公入藥鏡註解 [Commentary on Master Cui's mirror to enter the art of elixir] (DZ 135), 3b.

34 On the symbolism of the dragon in China, see Diény 1987.

> The Cave of the Scarlet Palace is in reality the "innate nature" (*xing* 性) and is also designated as the trigram *li*, the "unique moment," the "Southern Palace," and the "chamber of the spirit." This is where purifications and transformations occur. It is also called "the maiden," the "true yin" or the "blue-eyed barbarian.[35] The corresponding direction is the south. The bone that physicians call the "doves tail" (xiphoid tip of the sternum) covers this region of the body. To evoke the spirit resulting from the thoughts of the posterior heaven, we say that the dragon comes out of the fire.

In the same way, the water of the kidneys typically moves down with the desires; it too must be reversed. The main functions of this water are described by a text near the drawing of the kidneys (fig. 3.6, text 16):

> The inner kidneys correspond to the two primary principles (yin and yang). Inside the kidneys there is a ring which represents the true essence,[36] wherein is contained both red and white breaths.[37] This cavity

---

35 The earliest attestation of the term we have found is in *Taishang jiuyao xinyin miaojing* 太上九要心印妙經 [Marvellous book of the nine essentials, heart seal of the most high] (DZ 225). This text is attributed to Zhang Guo 張果, a semi-legendary figure of the mid-Tang who became one of the famous eight immortals of China, but it most likely was composed in the Northern Song. On page 7b, the text reads, "In the body the embryo is the child of breath, breath is the mother of the spirit. How to keep the son and the mother together? By retaining the spirit and the breath. This breath is found inserted between *kan* and *li* in the form of a pestle and mortar. It looks like a lounging turtle, which is why he is called the 'divine turtle' (*shengui* 神龜), or the 'blue-eyed barbarian monk' (*biyan huseng* 碧眼胡僧)." This term is also used in *Zhenyi jindan jue* 真一金丹訣 [Explication concerning the elixir of the perfected one] (DZ 231), 4a. In Buddhism the "blue eyed barbarian monk" is a nickname for Bodhidharma, the first patriarch of the Chinese lineage of Chan Buddhism who hailed from India, thus a "barbarian" (*hu* 胡). Much like the tales involving the three chariots or the prince piercing the bronze drums with an arrow, this is another example how followers of Inner Alchemy reinterpreted Buddhist tales. See Despeux 2006: 291–314.

36 The only mention we found of a ring corresponding to the vital essence is in *Chen Xubai guizhong zhinan* (DZ 243, 2.4b): "Some say that (this mysterious orifice) is white and is shaped like a ring that measures 1.2 inches and contains the quintessence of the whole body."

37 *Taiqing daoyin yangsheng jing* (DZ 818) mentions two red and white breaths ascending the length of the spine. In Tantra, the left and right channels are respectively red and white. They correspond to the blood of the mother and the sperm of the father. The Chinese consider that at the moment of conception, the father's sperm and the mother's blood are mixed to form the embryo. Chu Cheng 褚澄, an early medieval physician, describes the conception as follow: "When man and woman unite, their passions must mingle harmoniously. If, at the time of fertilization, yin blood comes first, the yang seed penetrates it so that the blood of the woman envelops the seed of the man. In this way

> existed in the womb, and it is thanks to it that the body could develop. The left corresponds to the obscure (*xuan* 玄) which is yang, the right to the female (pin 牝) which is yin. The central cavity is actually the ocean of the essence posterior to heaven, the true lead.[38] Buddhists call it the "dog of Zhaozhou" 趙州,[39] Confucians call it the Great Ultimate and Taoists refer to as the dark water village, lead, or the correct breath of the North.[40] If the hydraulic chariot circulates in the normal direction, it allows procreation; if it circulates in reverse direction, it leads to immortality. It is also called the Cao Stream, i.e., the ancestral palace.[41] It sets up communication with the two eyes, after which it will move down to the Flowery Pond under the tongue to the Jade Spring.

The various secretions and body fluids are stimulated and, at the same time, their course is reversed, so that they flow not with passion, but diffuse harmoniously into the body. This is what is referred to in alchemical terms by the union and the exchange between the water of the kidneys and the fire of the heart. This process is often called the extraction of fire from water (i.e., the yang heat of the kidneys) and of water from fire (i.e., the yin coolness of the heart). In practice, this means that when the heart is appeased, the adept feels as if a fresh spring is flowing through the throat. His mind becomes quiet and this state of peace results in the appearance of heat in the region of the kidneys and the genitals; this will rise and gradually pervade the body. These sensations influence one another in an alternating manner, a process that is modelled on inhalation and exhalation. The adept should not be seduced by these physiological phenomena, which could lead him out of his concentration, out

the bones will grow and form the skeleton of the male embryo. If instead the yang seed comes first, the yin blood will mix with it and will find itself enveloped in semen, the blood will remain close to its origin, and there will be a female embryo." See *Chushi yishu* 褚氏逸書 [Documents bequeathed by Master Chu], in *Shuofu* 說郛, ed. Tao Zongyi 陶宗儀 (1321–1407), 74.14b.

38 We interpreted this text according to the Moli version; the other versions have Xianghai 相海, which could mean "double ocean" or "minister ocean."

39 That is to say enlightenment. This is an allusion to a "public case" (koan) in Chan Buddhism, reported for example in *Wumen guan* 無門關 (T. 2005), by Hui Kai 慧開 (1183–1260), p. 292c: "A monk asked the tutor Zhaozhou, 'The dog also have the Buddha nature?' Zhou replied, 'Wu' [none]." This is one of the most famous koan; later accounts indicate that many masters attained enlightenment by meditating on it.

40 See *Xingming guizhi*, 1.55: "This cavity is called by Buddhists 'perfect enlightenment,' by Taoists 'golden elixir,' and by Confucians 'Great Ultimate.'" This same phrase is repeated by the *Rushi wowen*, 2b.

41 Caoxi is a place name linked to the sixth patriarch of Chan Buddhism. It was yet another example of a Buddhist term reinterpreted in Inner Alchemy, as we have already explained.

of the central axis and out of the centre of his body. This latter would result in various unwanted mutations.

If the body is a sacred world inhabited by gods, with its paradises and hells, it is also a social world in which we find an organizational family structure, like the father and the mother, the husband and the wife who unite. It is said in the *Stanzas for Awakening to Perfection*:

> At the top of the flowery peak, the tiger roars,
> Near the Carrying Mulberry Tree, at the bottom of the ocean, the dragon whistles.
> Through the Yellow Matchmaker, they unite,
> And become husband and wife, vibrating in unison.[42]

For their union, this couple, designated by various metaphors (*yin* / *yang*, tiger / dragon, boy / girl) needs the intervention of the Yellow Matchmaker (*huangpo* 黄婆 or *huangmei* 黄媒), who is equated in these texts with intent or creative thinking. With the aid of this matchmaker, the adept will be able to enact unions and transformations of both body and mind at various stages of Internal Alchemy. Their union produces the holy embryo, which is nourished for ten months before reaching completion. The transformation of the adept undergoes a "renaissance" where a miniature replica of his being in the form of light called *yangshen* 陽神 [Yang spirit] is formed in the body. Once completed, this replica is born via the top of the head, called the "heavenly gate." It comes and goes from the body, according to the desire of the adept, by means of contemplation, as explained in the *Collection on the Zhong*[*li Quan*]*'s Transmission of the Way to Lü* [*Dongbin*]:

> By means of inner contemplation, collect the Yang Spirit,
> Refine your mind so that it rises above the Inner Court.
> It leaps up and out through the heavenly gate,
> And attains directly the stage of holiness.
> It comes, it goes, it comes and goes without error,
> It goes, it comes, without getting lost in the distance.
> If it wants to remain in the world,
> It remains united within the body.
> If it wants to become immortal, it will proceed to Penglai Islands.
> Only inner contemplation gives access to the deliverance.[43]

42 *Wuzhen pian zhushi* (DZ 145), 2.7a.

43 *Zhong Lü chuandao ji* 鍾呂傳道集, in *Xiuzhen shishu*, 16.22b.

In the context of Internal Alchemy, the reference to this union is foremost a cosmological one. The interior of trigram *kan* ☵ (the yang enclosed by two yin lines) corresponds to the fire in the water of the kidneys, and is exchanged with the yin line surrounded by two yang lines of the *li* trigram ☲; this corresponds to the water born of fire of the heart. Through this exchange, the trigram *kan* now has three yin lines and becomes the trigram *kun* ☷ symbolizing pure yin, while the trigram *li* is composed of three yang lines and becomes the trigram *qian* ☰, symbolizing the pure yang (see fig. 6.5). After this, metal is extracted from the kidneys water (i.e., the real tiger), and wood from the heart fire (i.e., the real dragon). It is said in the short text presenting the body at the upper part of the *Chart for the Cultivation of Perfection*: "The dragon goes out of fire" and it is an allusion to this stage of the alchemical work. By the union and exchange between the tiger and the dragon, is formed the yellow sprout, that is to say, the sprout of the plant of immortality which grows progressively; its colour is yellow because it grows at the centre of the abdomen and in the correlations system of the five agents, yellow is the colour corresponding to the centre.

The reference to the alchemy of metals compares principles drawn from parts of the body to lead and mercury, two basic ingredients for forming gold. One must extract lead from the kidneys and mercury from the heart to unite them; this will generate the great panacea. In the text presenting the kidneys (text 16), it is said that the true lead is the essence posterior to heaven.

On the *Chart for the Cultivation of Perfection*, two overlapping circles are located at the navel.[44] They most likely symbolize the union and the exchange between opposites (fire and water, *kan* and *li*), since we find two interlocking circles corresponding to this symbolism in a Taoist text of the end of the thirteenth century, the *Indications by Chen Xubai for Correctly Focusing the Centre*; this figure is accompanied by the following commentary: "Push the two breaths on the yellow way, reunite the three natures in the primordial palace. The dragon (lead) rises, and the tiger (mercury) descends; this relentlessly pushes these two animals. The union of *kan* and *li* is also called "the microcosmic orbit." When laying foundations for one hundred days,[45] the fire descends and the water rises in the central palace, yin and yang mingle in the alchemical pot. The clouds pile up, rain falls, the [Original] Breath is tied, the spirit condenses. This is what you must experience."[46]

---

44 On each side of the two interlocking circles appears as two horns; we didn't find any similar representation elsewhere.

45 Expression designating the first of the three stages of Inner Alchemy: supplementing energy loss and strengthening the essence during these hundred symbolic days.

46 *Chen Xubai guizhong zhinan* 陳虛白規中指南 [True central directions by master Chen Xubai] (DZ 243), 1.2b. Text by Chen Chongsu 陳冲素 nicknamed Xubai zi 虛白子

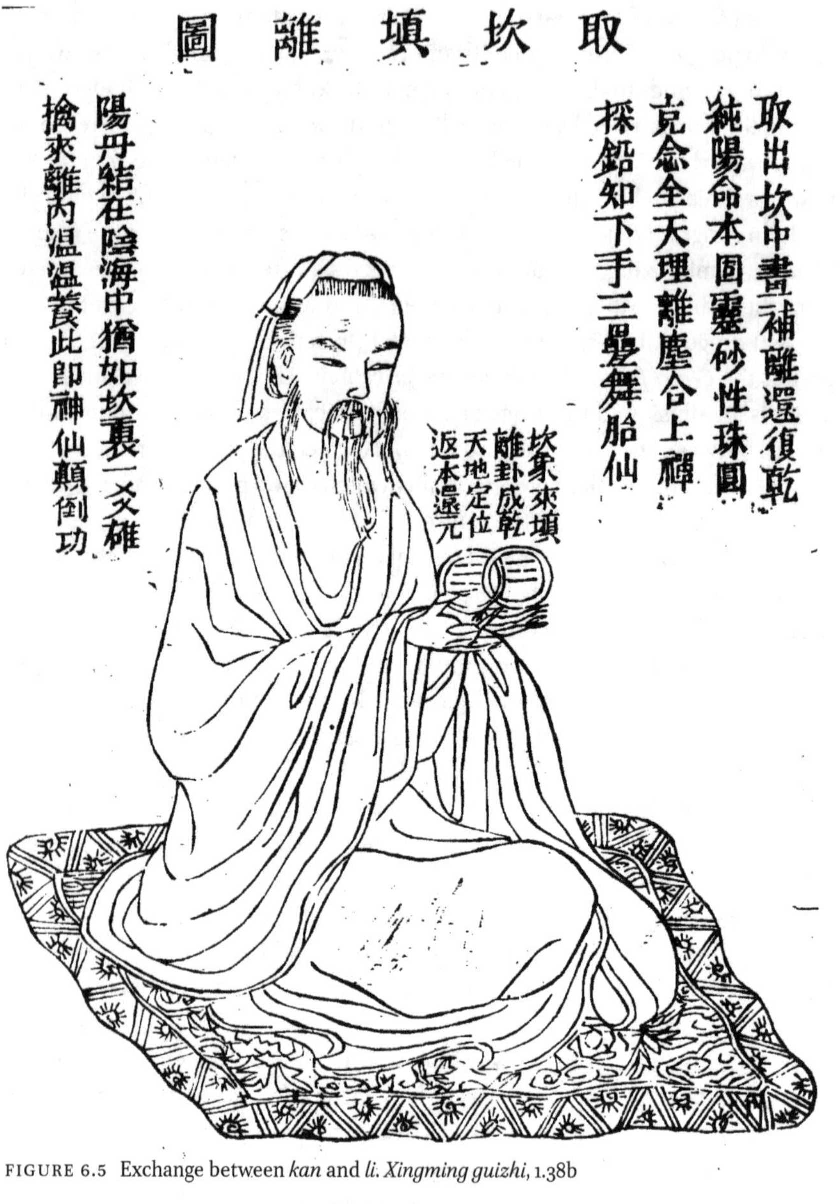
取坎填離圖
取出坎中畫補離還復乾
純陽命本固靈砂性珠圓
克念全天理離塵合上禪
採鉛知下手三疊舞胎仙
坎象來填
離卦成乾
天地定位
返本還元
陽丹結在陰海中猶如坎裏一爻雄
擒來離內温温養此即神仙顛倒功

FIGURE 6.5 Exchange between *kan* and *li*. *Xingming guizhi*, 1.38b

This drawing of two overlapping circles is also used in the *Alchemical Diagrams to Master Shangyang's Essentials of the Golden Elixir* (fourteenth century), to

(fl. 13th cen.) with an afterword by Yuxi zi 玉溪子, a byname of Li Jianyi 李簡易, the author of another text preserved in the Taoist Canon and prefaced 1264: Yuxi zi's *Yuxi zi danjing zhi yao* 玉溪子丹經之要 [Basic principles on alchemical texts] (DZ 245).

symbolize either the exchange of yin and yang or the formation of the hexagram Jiji ䷾ by the exchange between water and fire or the sevenfold reversal of the golden elixir.[47] The following inscription is found beside the circles: "In the black there is the white, the body becomes completely yang." This double circle is also represented in the *Chapters of the Cave by Master Qiaoqiao* (nineteenth century), where it symbolizes the alchemical furnace and the metal cauldron with the tiger and the dragon ascending and descending, the exchange between *kan* and *li*.[48]

### 2.1.1 The Iron Buffalo

As for the rising of the water of the kidneys, both the *Chart of the Inner Landscape* and the *Chart for the Cultivation of Perfection* use the metaphor of a buffalo to depict this movement. On the *Chart of the Inner Landscape* of the White Cloud Temple, we can see at the level of the abdomen the drawing of a ploughing buffalo, accompanied by the following poem:

> The iron buffalo ploughs the land where gold coins are buried,
> The boy who carves the stones strings them together.
> A grain of rice contains the whole universe,
> In a half-litre melting pot, mountains and rivers bubble.
> White-haired Laozi's eyebrows fall to the ground,
> The blue-eyed foreign monk raises his arms to heaven.
> Understanding is found within the mystery of the obscure,
> Only this obscure mystery can connect you [to the Dao].

The term "iron buffalo" refers primarily to an ancient Chinese custom of throwing an iron buffalo into a stream to appease their gods and prevent flooding. This is a custom that supposedly originated with Yu the Great.[49] In the Inner Alchemical context, the metaphor of the ploughing buffalo must be related to the water of the kidneys and the canalisation process with a rising upwards of the breath of the kidneys along the backbone. A text attributed to Zhongli presents the iron buffalo as follows: "Zhengyang zi 正陽子 (i.e., Zhongli) said: 'The iron buffalo is the breath of the kidneys, or the water corresponding to the celestial stems *ren* and *gui* connected to the North.'"[50]

---

47 *Shangyangzi jindan dayao tu* (DZ 1068), 2a.

48 See Liu Mingrui's 劉名瑞 (1839–1933) *Qiaoqiao dongzhang* 敲蹻洞章 [Chapters of Master Qiaoqiao], 2.8a.

49 See *Hanyu cidian* 漢語詞典, 11.1400.

50 See "Hundred Questions," in *Daoshu* 道樞 (DZ 1017), 5.20.

A passage of the *Stanzas on the Awakening to Perfection* (eleventh century),[51] reported in the *Alchemical Diagrams to Master Shangyang's Essentials of the Golden Elixir* and the *Chart for the Cultivation of Perfection*, describes the buffalo in more detail:

> The true iron buffalo has the appearance of an ugly child. By nature, bad and rebellious, he gallops in all directions. Everyone possesses this animal. Know how to domesticate it for ploughing and sowing: the golden buds will fill the courtyard; then you only need to water them with the divine water of the central palace. Without him, without the male and female energies of this infant, how could you find the true movement and the true rest? The production and the fulfilment of our lives depend on it.[52]

This passage is accompanied in the text of Master Shangyang by a drawing of a buffalo quite similar to that of the *Chart of the Inner Landscape* but with a difference: the buffalo is not shown ploughing (fig. 6.6). The *Spiritual Transmission of Taoist Rites* (14th cen.) presents the buffalo as follows:

> The iron buffalo ploughs the land for seeding golden lotus. You don't need to deploy any effort or to spend a penny, the water of the celestial river irrigates the fields spontaneously, the flowers bloom and diffuse their fragrance, heaven and earth are linked.[53]

The allusion to the stubborn nature of the buffalo galloping in all directions evokes a well-known metaphor in Chan Buddhism where the buffalo symbolizes our mind as a wild animal that should be tamed. The buffalo, that is the agitated and ignorant mind, can be tamed and purified by a graduated progression counting ten or twelve steps until enlightenment. Illustrations of this taming, usually in ten or twelve drawings, were a common fixture in texts from the Song onwards. They represent the taming of the buffalo and its purification from black to white. Eventually, it disappears completely, which represents the enlightenment of both the animal and its tamer.[54]

---

51 Text partially translated into English by Pregadio 2009. Also see an older translation in Tenney and Chao 1939: 97–117.

52 *Xiuzhen shishu* (DZ 263), 25.6b. Text included in *Shangyangzi jindan dayao tu* (DZ 1068), 9a.

53 See Wang Weiyi's 1294 preface to *Daofa xinchuan* (DZ 1253), 7b.

54 See Despeux 2015.

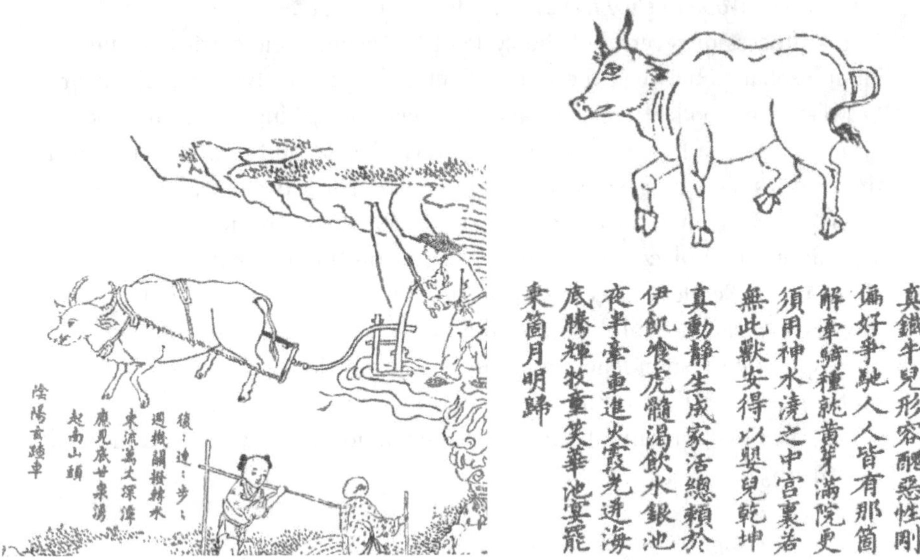
真鐵牛兒形容醜惡性剛
偏好爭馳人人皆有那箇
解牽騎種就黃芽滿院更
須用神水澆之中宮裏若
無此獸安得以嬰兒乾坤
真動靜生成家活總賴於
伊飢飡虎髓渴飲水銀池
夜半牽車進火霞光迸海
底騰輝牧童笑華池宴罷
乘箇月明歸

FIGURE 6.6 Iron buffalo in the *Chart of the Inner Landscape* (*Neijing tu* 內經圖) of the White Cloud Temple (1886) and in *Shangyangzi jindan dayao tu* (DZ 1068), 9a

In many Taoist contexts, the iron buffalo appears both as an ancient symbol to prevent flooding and as the wild animal from Chan Buddhism that must be tamed.[55] In Internal Alchemy, however, the iron buffalo not only represents the mind that must be tamed, but also the breath of the kidneys and sexual organs which, when purified and controlled, increase heat and brightness inside the body. This heat is often metaphorically cast as golden buds that are cultivated through calming the mind. The process, in turn, produces "divine water," the secretions descending from the head and mouth. There is a Taoist version of this taming allegory with a horse instead of a buffalo, which could explain the variant of the Sichuan version of the *Chart for the Cultivation of Perfection* produced by Duan Fu in 1922, which has a horse instead a buffalo.[56] It is further noted that on the versions representing a buffalo, the figure is that of a herdsman sitting on the back of the buffalo and playing a flute, the drawing situated beside the inscription "gate leading to immortality." However, this drawing is quite similar to the sixth Table of the Chan taming of the buffalo by Kuo'an, evoking a stage where the mind is calmed and already close to the goal: enlightenment in Buddhism, immortality in Taoism (see fig. 6.11).[57]

55 See *Daoshu* (DZ 1017), 5.20.

56 See Despeux 2015.

57 *Ibid.*

### 2.2 *The Wood of the Liver and the Metal of the Tiger*

In the process of reversal of the cycle of five agents, one carries out first of all an exchange between the water of the kidneys and the fire of the heart, between the wood of the liver and the metal of the lungs. The first heart-kidney exchange has a down-top trajectory. The second exchange between these opposites occurs between the right and left, or between wood and metal or the Blue Dragon of the liver (left) and the White Tiger of the lungs (right).[58] The union takes place, according to the text on the upper right part of the chart, in the Scarlet Palace cavity located just below the heart.[59] Two texts inscribed in the central region on the *Chart for the Cultivation of Perfection* develop the correspondences and the classical analogies in Taoism between on the one hand, the liver and the lungs, and on the other hand between the spirits, the directions and the alchemical metaphors (text 14 and 15, translated pp. 161–163).

### 2.3 *The Solar Crow and the Lunar Toad*

Most of the versions of the *Chart for the Cultivation of Perfection* have, below the petals of the lungs, on either side of the child, a representation of a horse and a monkey. This is an allusion to the expression "the heart is like a monkey, the intent like a horse" (*xinyuan yima* 心猿意馬). In other words, it is necessary to subdue one's thoughts and mind to achieve enlightenment or immortality. It is a well-known proverb in Chinese that describes the agitation of the mind. However, the Mount Wudang version of 1924 includes the drawings of the solar crow and the lunar toad instead of the crow and the horse, with a text explaining these two symbols in Inner Alchemy:

> The light of the toad is the light of the true yang. Who is able to understand that gold is produced by the moon? People see the gold produced by the moon, and they do not know that the light of the moon comes from the sun. The moon is a metaphor for the primordial nature. Water is a metaphor for the Kan Palace. The golden toad is a metaphor for this orifice of the true yang. The moon is a symbol for the primordial activity. When this nature begins to manifest itself, a glittering circle,

58 These should not be confused with the perfect tiger and the perfect dragon that we have mentioned above.

59 See the overview text on the body at the upper right of the *Chart for the Cultivation of Perfection*: "Below the heart is a cavity called the Scarlet Palace, which is the place of union and exchange between the tiger and the dragon." The meeting place is located in a conventional way below the heart in the Southern tradition. Cf. Zhang Boduan's (987–1082) *Yuqing jinsi qinghua biwen jinbao neilian danjue* (DZ 240).

> like a shooting star, appears while the nature of the substantial body disappears. The primordial yang, or the true nature, arises, like the full moon appearing when the clouds dissipate, or the sun appearing when the fog evaporates. At that precise moment, appear the signs of the production of the panacea that one must quickly gather.[60]

The sun and the moon are evoked here through their mythical elements: the hare and the toad for the moon, the raven and the Fusang Tree for the sun. In the moon resides a jade hare (*yutu* 玉兔) which grinds the elixir of immortality; or a toad, symbolizing the light from the yin breath, which at a certain stage of the process illuminates the whole body. In the sun sits a golden crow (*jinwu* 金烏) that carries this star in the sky.[61] These animals are symbols of regeneration and enlightenment. The solar crow and the lunar hare or toad, are well attested in antiquity and appear in ancient iconography. They are presented for example on the banner found in tomb No. 1 at Mawangdui (late 3rd cen. BCE) near Changsha in Hunan and are related to the paradise of the Queen Mother of the West, an important female divinity integrated to the Taoist pantheon. In Internal Alchemy, the golden raven represents the true breath originating from the heart secretions; the jade hare symbolizes the true water originating from the breath in the kidneys.[62] The *Stanzas on the Awakening to Perfection* gives the following recipe:

> Establish Qian [pure yang] and Kun [pure yin] as pots,
> In which you heat the hare and raven elixirs.
> Push them to move on the saffron orbit,
> And strive to produce the golden elixir.[63]

As for the "Carrying Mulberry Tree," it is a tree featured in an ancient mythical geography of China, most notably in the *Book of Mountains and Seas*[64] and on the banner of Mawangdui.[65] Situated at the top of the vibrant valley, ten suns rest on its branches, nine on the lower branches and one on the upper branches. In Internal Alchemy, it symbolizes the sunlight or the yang energy.

The Mount Wudang version seems closest to the alchemical symbolism, because these images of the solar crow and the lunar toad or hare are

60 See *Xingming guizhi*, 1.77.
61 On the solar bird and the lunar hare, see Loewe 1979: 127–133.
62 See "Hundred Questions," in *Daoshu* (DZ 1017), 5.30b.
63 *Wuzhen pian zhushi* (DZ 145), 2.3a.
64 *Shanhai jing*, 9.3a; Mathieu 1983: 45.
65 Loewe 1979: 50.

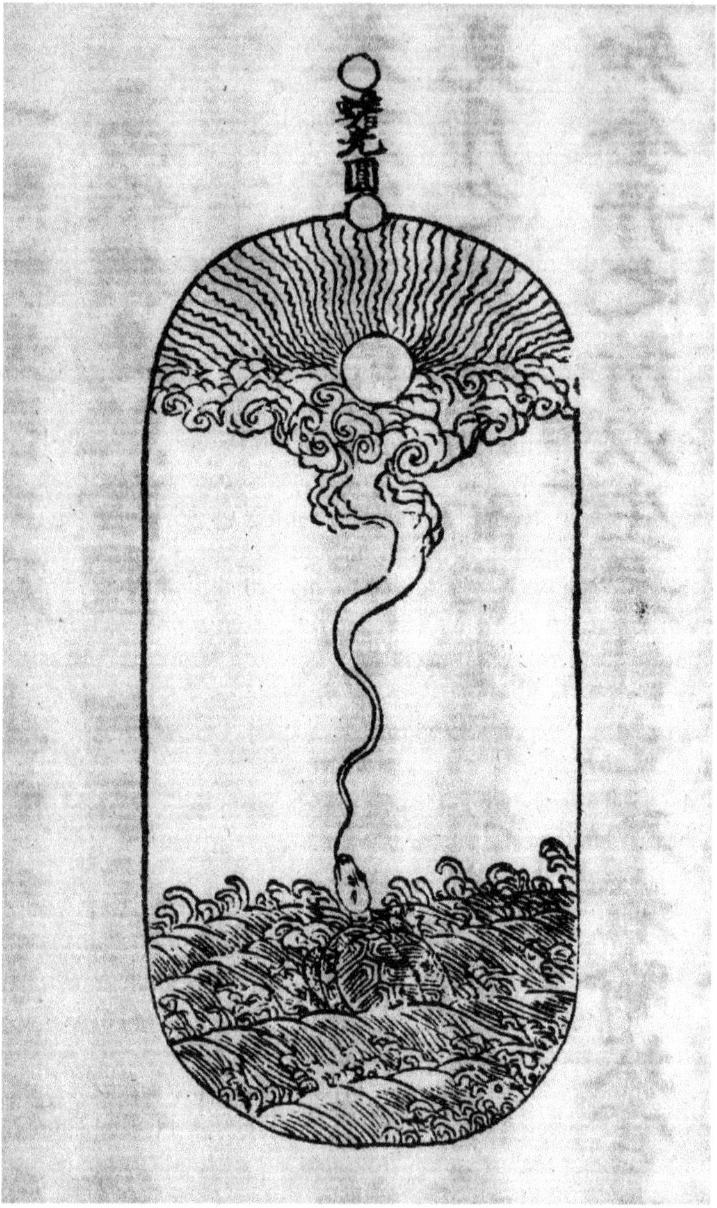

FIGURE 6.7 Light of the lunar toad. *Yuqing jinsi qinghua biwen jinbao neilian danjue* 玉清金笥青華祕文金寶內鍊丹訣 (DZ 240), 2.13a

fundamental in the writings of Inner Alchemy since the Song dynasty. They have resulted in several graphic representations, some emphasizing the light of the toad that illuminates the adept when his energies are collected (see fig. 6.7). Other texts focus on the couple of the lunar hare and the solar crow to symbolize the reversal of the production of the five agents, the manifestation of two different hues, one pale and the other golden. After these animals merge, the adept will bathe in a halo of light (see fig. 6.9). From the pictographic point of view, the drawing of the toad is similar to that of the *Principles of the Tablets on the Innate Nature and the Vital Force* (see fig. 6.8).

### 2.4 *The Elixir Spoon* (*daogui* 刀圭)

The different phases of union of opposites increase the inner brightness, or in alchemical terms, lead to a progressive transformation of metals into gold. The adept then experiences the apparition of sweet secretions, called the "elixir spoon" (*daogui*): "Tiger and dragon unite, the fire progresses across the constellations Niu, Wei and Dou.[66] It is when the sparkling and pure flower of the moon shines above the meandering river and when the crow flies, at this moment, you enjoy the elixir spoon."[67] *Gui* [Spoon] is an old measure of capacity corresponding to 64 grains of millet. The term *daogui* refers commonly to a "small spoon" (*gui*) shaped like a "knife" (*dao*) of an inch long, that physicians used as a measure for drugs powder. In Taoism, the gods are depicted as bringing the divine elixir to the alchemists in golden vessels and jade cups, and urging these adepts to take a small "knife shaped spoonful" to achieve immortality. For Internal Alchemists, the metaphor of the spoon refers not to the container but to the content, that is to say to the "divine cinnabar" (*shendan* 神丹) or the "clarified butter" (*tihu* 醍醐), a kind of sweet secretion that appears and drops from the head when the union of opposites is performed, and all the passes are unblocked, letting the whole body radiate bright light. This inner experience coming from an immersion in a subtle peace, is described by Zhang Boduan (fl. 10th cen.) in the following manner: "Hit the bamboo and make the turtle come out so that it absorbs the jade stamens, hit the lute and summon the phoenix so that it drinks from the elixir spoon. These days, all your body manifests a golden light. But do not talk about it to common people."[68]

This term *daogui* is in the centre of the *Chart for the Cultivation of Perfection* and represents the furnace. It can nevertheless take slightly different meanings according to the different internal alchemy traditions. It may denote the result of the union of breath and spirit, or that of the vital essence and the

66 Niu, Wei and Dou are three of the 28 constellations. It designates the cyclical revolution of the breath in the back and the front of the body.

67 *Lü Chunyang zhenren qingyuan chun danci zhujie* 呂純陽真人沁園春丹詞註解 [Explication of the alchemical lyric 'Spring in the Garden by the Qin' by the perfected Lü Dongbin] (DZ 136), 4b–5a.

68 See *Wuzhen pian zhushi* (DZ 145), 4.20b.

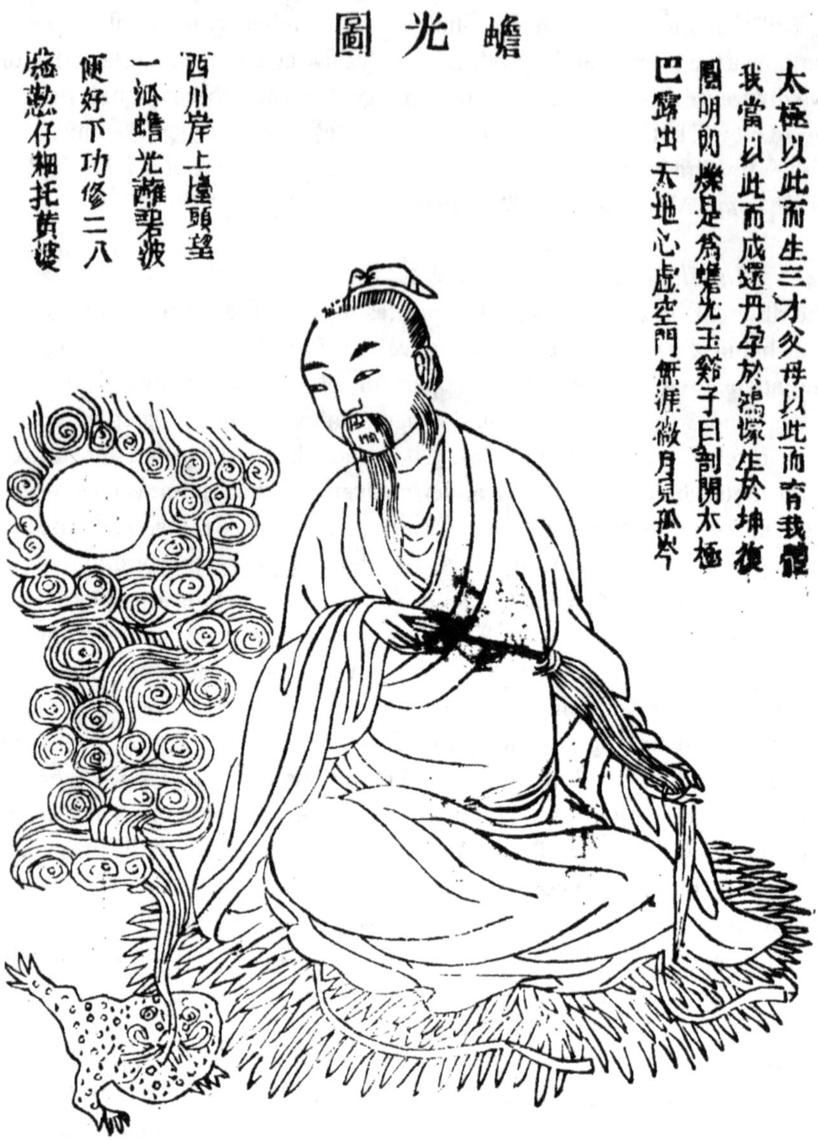


FIGURE 6.8 Light of the lunar toad. *Xingming guizhi*, 1.33b

Original Breath of the heart. In the *Correct Principles on Heavenly Immortality*, Wu Chongxu 伍冲虛 (1574–1644) explains as follows:[69]

69 Wu Chongxu 伍冲虛 was born in 1574 near the district of Nanchang in Jiangxi. In 1593, he met his principal master Cao Huanyang 曹還陽. In 1622, he wrote the first manuscript of the *Tianxian zhengli zhilun*.

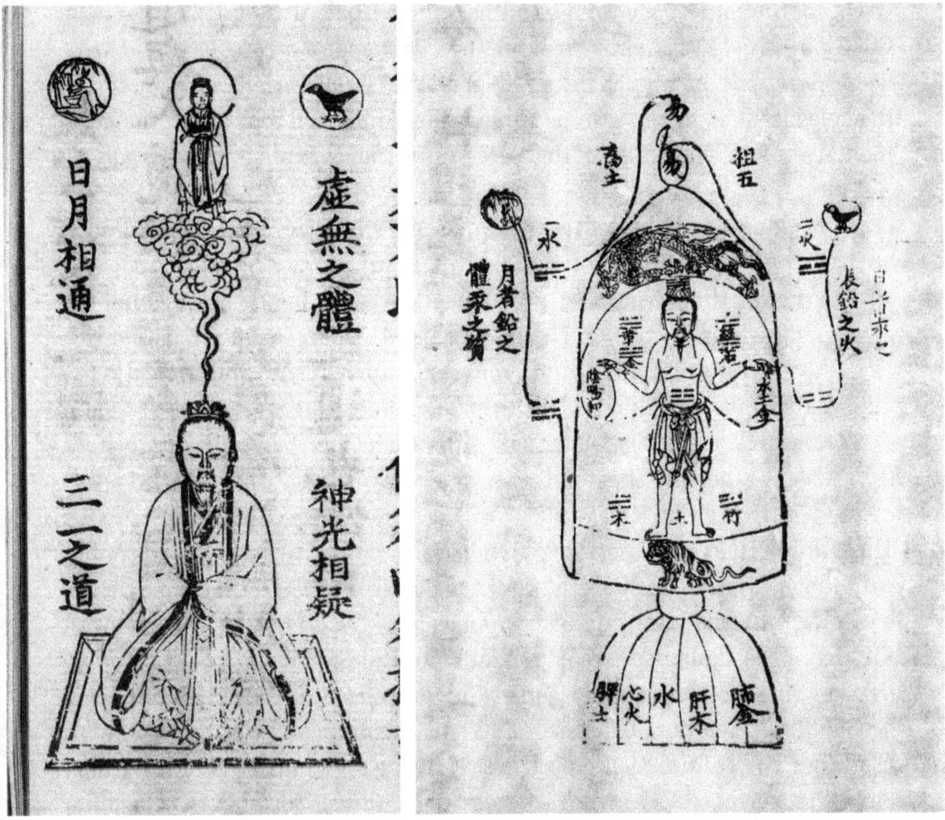


FIGURE 6.9 Two alchemical drawings with the crow in the sun and the hare in the moon
1. *Shangqing taixuan jiuyang tu* (DZ 154), 5a–b. Late twelfth century.
2. *Jinye huandan yinzheng tu* (DZ 151), 15b. Circa 1222

The trigram *li* represents the spirit in the heart known as the earth of *ji*. The trigram *kan* symbolizes the breath within the kidneys called the earth of *wu*. Both upper and lower earths (*tu* 土) are reunited to form the character *gui* 圭. The union of *wu* and *ji* is called the "elixir spoon," a metaphorical term for the union of the breath and the spirit. But in order to fulfil the elixir spoon by the meeting and the refinement of the two earths, it is important to know the favourable time to seize them and to unite them.[70]

70 See *Tianxian zhengli zhilun* 天仙正理直論, in *Wu Liu xianzong quanji* 伍柳仙宗全集 1962: 144.

One of the earliest occurrences of the term in Inner Alchemy is in a poem by Cui Xifan 崔希范 (ca. tenth century), the *Commentary on Master Cui's Mirror on the Admixture of Ingredients*, where it is said: "Drink the elixir spoon, spy on the celestial skill, distinguish new and full moon, dawn and dusk." The commentary by Wang Jie 王玠 (fourteenth century) makes explicit the term *daogui*:

> Drinking is to imbibe. The knife (*dao* 刀) symbolizes metal within water. *Gui* 圭 [Measure] is the double true earth *wu ji*. It means that when gathering the panacea for producing the cinnabar, one must gather the metal within the water. The metal cannot rise by itself, it must borrow the *wu* earth that transforms it into fire, which pushes and circulates the metal until the Muddy Pellet. At this point, it becomes true secretion sweet like ambrosia, which falls into the Yellow Court. The flavour we taste is exquisite. That is why we say that we drink the spoon of elixir.[71]

The *Chart for the Cultivation of Perfection* also contains the term "elixir spoon" with the inscription "flow at *wu*" (*liuwu* 流戊), as well as a sitting child on the lower left with the inscription "accomplish at *ji*" (*jiuji* 就己). The meaning of these terms is explained in a commentary of the *Book of Universal Salvation* by Xiao Yingsou 蕭應叟 (13th cen.): "*Kan* circulates until *wu*-period and *li* is accomplished at *ji*-period." These words are accompanied by a drawing similar to that of the central element of the *Chart for the Cultivation of Perfection*, but upside down.[72] We can also see inscribed at the top "during the exhalation we connect with the heavenly root" (*hu jie tiangen* 呼接天根) and at the bottom "during the inhalation we connect with the terrestrial root" (*xi jie digen* 吸接地根).[73] These two inscriptions summarize the various processes of comings and goings between the ascension from the terrestrial root during inhalation (i.e., psychic heat) and the descent from the heavenly root during exhalation (i.e., fresh fluids) by the reversal movement, and the union of the two elements at the centre, in the alchemical pot. The *Chart for the Cultivation of Perfection* here takes up elements that are given in another diagram of the *Collection on the Centre and the Harmony* by Li Daochun (ob. 1306) that we have already mentioned above (see fig. 6.10).[74] On the same way, as we already mentioned, the three phrases which are from bottom to top

71 *Cuigong ruyao jing zhujie* (DZ 135) by Wang Jie (ob. 1306), also named Wang Daoyuan and nicknamed Hunran zi 混然. He was originally from Xiujiang near Nanchang in Jiangxi, and was a disciple of Li Daochun.

72 *Yuanshi wuliang duren shangpin miaojing neiyi* (DZ 90), 4.26b.

73 *Xi jie digen* is only written on the Chengdu version.

74 *Zhonghe ji* (DZ 249), 2. 2a–3b.

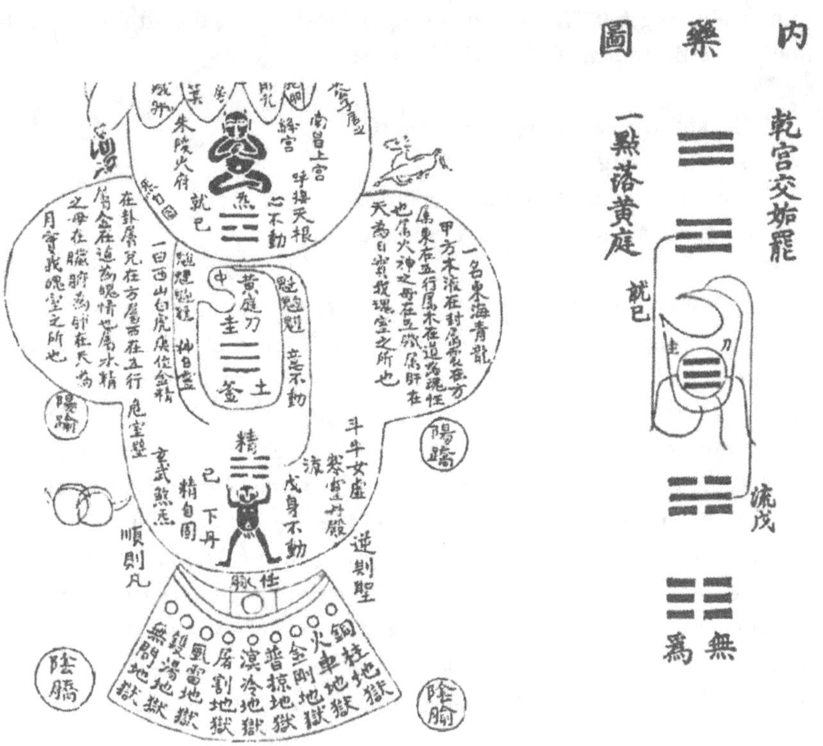


FIGURE 6.10 Analogy between the central part of the "Drawing of Internal Medicine" (*Neiyao tu* 內藥圖) in the *Chart for the Cultivation of Perfection* (Moli's one), and a diagram in *Zhonghe ji* (DZ 249), 2.3b

respectively on the right of the standing child "body does not move" (*shen bu dong* 身不動), at the right of the middle furnace "the creative thinking does not move" (*yi bu dong* 意不動) and on the right of the sitting child "the mind/heart does not move" (*xin bu dong* 心不動) are also explained with another diagram in the *Collection on the Centre and the Harmony.*

## 3 The Fire Phasing

### 3.1 *The Forge Bellows* (*tuoyue* 槖籥)

On the Chart, in the lower part of the body, just below the trapezium bearing the names of the underworlds, is a kind of pointed blade with the inscription "bellows" (*tuoyue* 槖籥). To the side, we can read these two inscriptions: "This is where an ordinary man moves towards death and the holy man takes flight," and "here is the orifice, the pivot of the mechanism, the gate leading to immortality (fig. 6.11)." This figure of the bellows evokes the fifth stanza of the *Book of the Way and its Virtue*, which reads:

> The space between heaven and earth,
> Isn't it like large bellows?
> Even though empty it is not vacuous,
> Pump it and more and more comes out.

This metaphor of the bellows borrows the terminology of laboratory alchemy, for which it was necessary to have a number of implements, such as the cauldron, the furnace in which burned a fire, with sometimes the need to fan the flames with a bellows. In internal alchemy, this term refers to the inner movement of the energies which provides the feeling of alternating between an opening (*kai* 開) of the body and the being in its entirety and a "closure" (*he* 合). This movement is associated with the rise and fall of breath that stirs up the inner fire. The northern and southern alchemical schools have different interpretations of this metaphor of the bellows. While the northern tradition considers that the bellows is activated between the heart and the kidneys, or between the spirit of the heart and the breath of the kidneys,[75] the southern tradition, however, places the bellows between the two kidneys:

> The left kidney is the kidney palace, the right kidney is the essence palace, once the water, once the fire, once the turtle, once the snake; thus, the bellows is activated between both kidneys. In the emptiness appears an orifice: the obscure female. The breaths of both kidneys are then connected and communication is established between the obscure (*xuan*) and the female (*pin*).[76]

This last description evokes the drawing of the *Chart for the Cultivation of Perfection* where in the kidney area there is a circle with two points inside it, connected by a line, which confirms our hypothesis that this chart manifests influences of the southern alchemical school. The "obscure" (*xuan*) and the "female" (*pin*) characters are also inscribed in the right and left kidneys. This

---

75 See *Taishang jiuyao xinyin xiaojing* 太上九要心印妙經 [Marvellous book of the nine essentials heart seal of the most high] (DZ 225) attributed to Zhang Guo 張果, but most likely dating of the Northern Song dynasty. According to Farzeen Baldrian-Hussein, it is a text of the Zhong-Lü tradition of Inner Alchemy (see Schipper and Verellen, 2004: 2.808–809).

76 *Yangsheng bilu* 養生祕錄 [Secret records on tending life] (DZ 579), 10a. This is a Yuan dynasty anthology which draws mainly upon sources of the southern alchemical tradition.

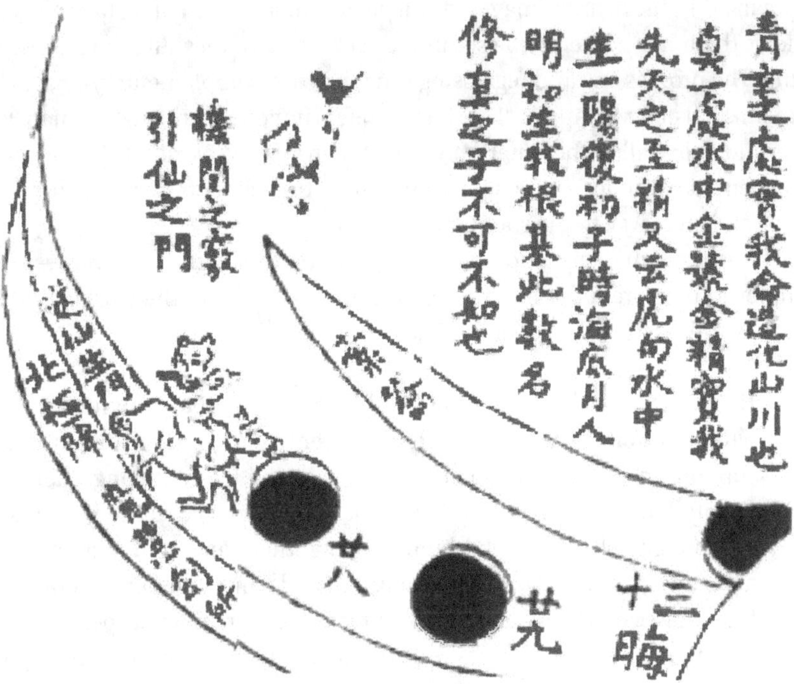


FIGURE 6.11 Forge Bellows. *Chart for the Cultivation of Perfection*

circle seems therefore to symbolize this orifice that appears when the bellows is activated, connecting the two kidneys.

### 3.2 *The Fire Phasing* (*huohou* 火候)

The refinement of substances occurs as the yang heat rises of and the yin secretions descend. The simultaneous rise and descent is regulated in accordance with the mechanisms of time, which follow the rhythm of time, the day, month, season, year and fanned by the bellows. The result is the formation of gold, or in Internal Alchemy the production of spiritual light, purple or violet, which corresponds to the colour of the best gold.

All the changes and transformations follow the lunar-solar calendar based on a sexagesimal system organised by the combination of cyclical signs, markers of time and space: a denary series of ten heavenly stems (*jia, yi, bing, ding, wu, ji, geng, xin, ren, gui*) and a duodenary series of twelve earthly branches (*zi, chou, yin, mao, chen, si, wu, wei, shen, you, xu, hai*). The pairs obtained by combining them form a sexagesimal cycle designating the years but also the month, day and hour. Time is thus formed by cyclical processes, like the course of the stars that revolve around the immutable Polar Star. By analogy, in the human body, the heart is imagined as a pivot similar to the Polar Star; the heart allows the inner heaven to be set in motion, for accomplishing the regressing time. The progressing and regressing times are two complementary phases, as explains Kristofer Schipper. "Fate 'in me' refers not only to the will of man, but also and above all to the inner universe of being, to the world of Chaos where fragmented existence regains its unity, where the perception of the duration stops and gives way to the spontaneous nature."[77]

These time markers and the hexagrams of the *Classic of Changes* are employed in express the inner time of the individual and the working of his inner world, as for example in the *Xiuzhen taiji hunyuan tu*:

> Heaven and earth, sun and moon obey principles that man must follow without error. Heaven and earth have twenty-four joint breaths in a year, sun and moon twenty-four revolutions. In the human being, there are twenty-four periods. Sky and earth have eight temporal knots, sun and moon eight phases; in the human being, there are eight trigrams. Sky and earth have spring, summer, autumn and winter; sun and moon have four phases of growth and decay, in man, there are the four periods *zi* 子 (11 pm–1 am), *wu* 午 (11 am–1 pm), *mao* 卯 (5 am–7 am); *you* 酉 (5 pm–7 pm). In macrocosm as in microcosm, everything is similar. As for man, he is the only one not aware of the laws of the sky and the earth, the sun and the moon. Who understands the ascending and descending of yin and yang specific to the sky and earth, knows the place where the breaths of the heart and the kidney unite in him. The one who perceives the codification of the sun and moon orbits knows himself the periods of communication between the [breaths of the] liver and the lungs. Regarding the breath of the heart considered as fire, it is based on the degrees of the solar revolution for increasing or decreasing it without error. For the breath of the kidneys considered as the essence, it complies with the rising and setting of the moon to add some or subtract some without error. The sky and the earth, the sun and the moon have no reason to be the only ones to prevail. Myself, I try to imitate them to become immortal.[78]

The alchemical transmutations are performed according to specific rhythms, the increasing and decreasing of yin and yang, as well as all other complementary elements such as water and fire, heat and cold. The fire phase differs according

77 Schipper 2008: 207.

78 *Xiuzhen taiji hunyuan tu* (DZ 149), 5b–6a.

to the different stages; it is modeled on the twelve time periods of a day, on the thirty moons in a month, or the twenty-four articulations of a year. This fire is generated by the concentration of the mind, of the spirit in a state of great concentration. Breathing seems to stop, the sun and the moon stop their course, the celestial mechanism stops, day and night are identical. This is the internal state that arises when the true yang manifests.

A diagram summarises the expression in alchemical terms of these different regimes: the "Drawing of the Fire Phasing and the Spiritual Mirror of Great Return" (*Dahuan xinjing huohou zhi tu* 大還心鏡火候之圖) which was drawn by Peng Xiao 彭曉 in 947 and was included in a commentary of the *Book of Universal Salvation* by Xiao Yingsou (see fig. 6.12).[79] According to the accompanying commentary, this includes the following elements from outside to inside:

1. First circle: The Eight Trigrams represent the earth, and engender phenomena through their interaction.
2. Second circle: Twenty-eight constellations representing the sky highlight the degrees of the sidereal revolution and key numbers of celestial origin.
3. Third circle: Thirty moons. In a month, the numbers of fire are in resonance with the action of sixty hexagrams.
4. Fourth circle: Black and white circles symbolize rest and motion; the passage of time is in resonance with the celestial mechanism of the evolution of yin and yang.
5. Fifth circle: Twelve hexagrams juxtaposed against the names of the twenty-four divisions of the year. These features progress and regress, as the tiger and the dragon rise and fall.
6. Sixth circle: Twelve periods of the day, it is the fire phasing, with the rise and fall according to the celestial cycle.
7. Seventh circle: The large numbers the sidereal revolution set in movement according to the four seasons and the five agents are matched with internal images.
8. Eighth circle: the yin-yang, the five agents and the ten thousand phenomena enter in the cauldron.

A similar drawing is also found in a text of Huang Gongwang 黄公望 preceding a paragraph entitled "Essential Principles of the Fire Phasing."[80] This "mirror" comprises only seven elements: 1) the twenty-eight constellations, 2) the twenty-four articulations of a year, 3) the characters indicating the thirty days of a lunar month, 4) the drawing of the thirty phases of the moon, 5)

79 *Yuanshi wuliang duren shangpin miaojing neiyi* (DZ 90), 9a–b.

80 Huang Gongwang, *Baoyi hansan bijue* (DZ 576), 23a.

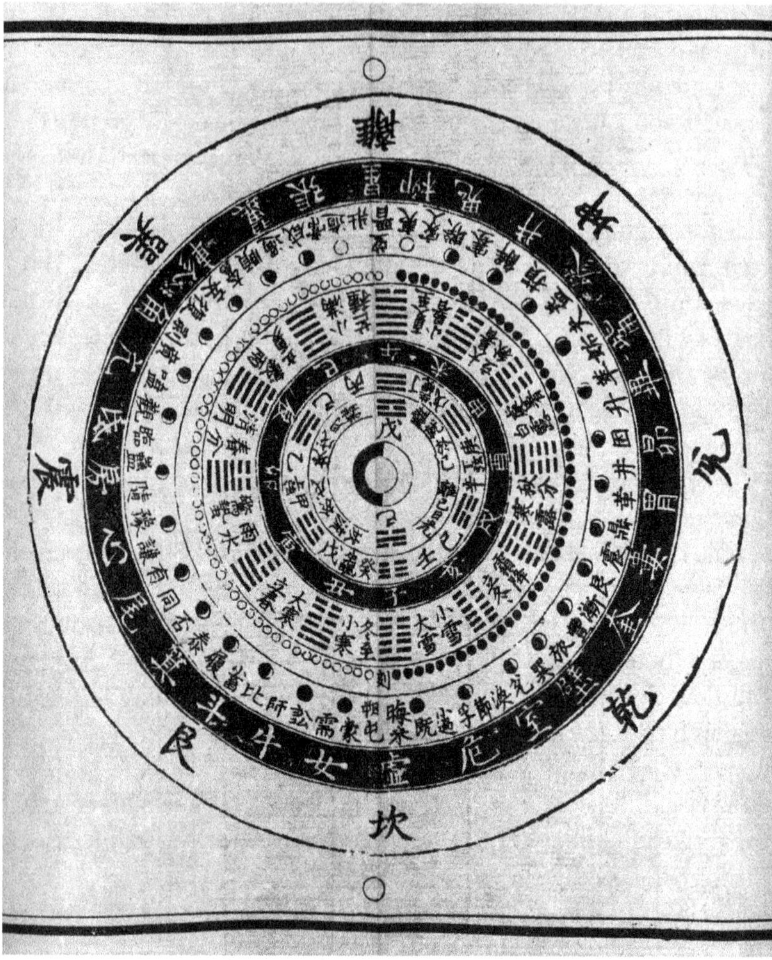


FIGURE 6.12 "Drawing of the the fire phasing of the spiritual mirror for the return". *Yuanshi wuliang duren shangpin miaojing neiyi* (DZ 90), 9a–b

the twelve hexagrams, 6) the names of these hexagrams, 7) a central circle. A similar representation, titled "Drawing of the Mirror for the Alchemical Way" (*Mingjing dandao tu* 明鏡丹道圖) contains the same elements, except for the inner circle. It is included in the *Alchemical Diagrams of the Golden Elixir* by Chen Zhixu (see Figure 6.13).[81]

1. First circle: Eight trigrams
2. Second circle: Twenty-eight constellations
3. Third circle: Thirty moons and numbers of thirty days
4. Fourth circle: Hundred black and white points

81 Chen Zhixu, *Shangyangzi jindan dayao tu* (DZ 1068), 7b.

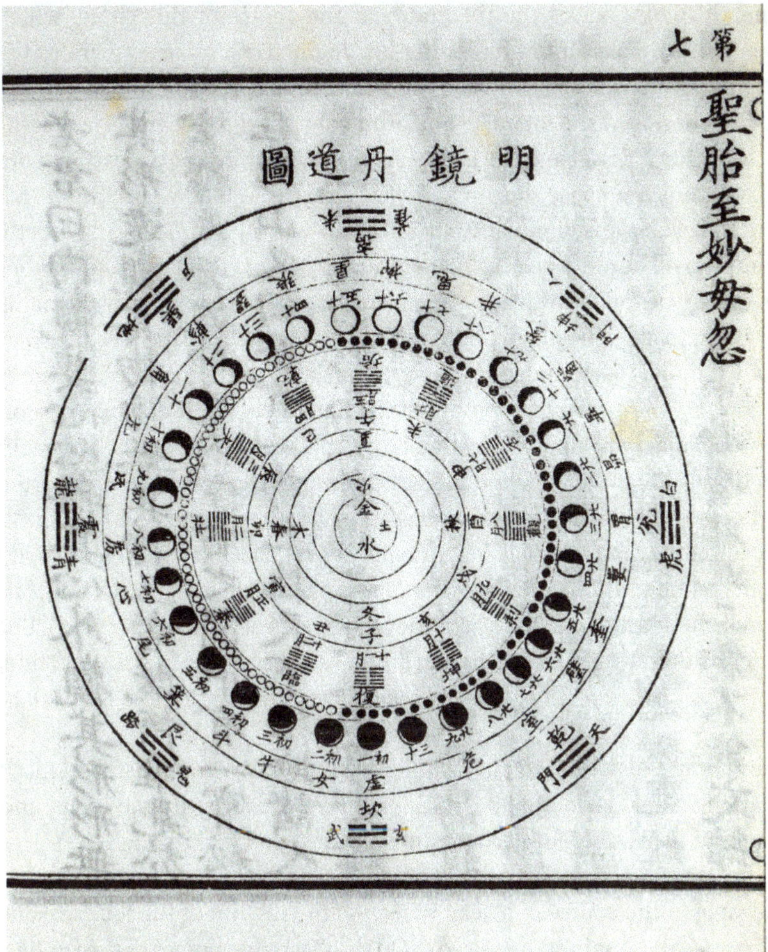


FIGURE 6.13 "Drawing of the alchemical path and the brighting mirror". *Shangyangzi Jindan dayao tu* (DZ 1068), 7b

5. Fifth circle: Twelve hexagrams and numbers of the twelve months of the year
6. Sixth circle: Twelve time periods
7. Seventh circle: Four seasons
8. Eight circle: Wood
9. Ninth circle: Fire
10. Tenth circle: Metal, water and earth

The majority of the illustrations on the fire phasing employ the circle which reflects the cosmic dimension of this metaphor: the model of the progress of yin and yang is the day and the night with its twelve time periods, the thirty phases of the moon or the twelve months of a year. A representation of a text on Inner Alchemy places the meditator at the centre of this circle, which suggests that he makes inner time turn, his microcosmic time accelerates the mutations (see fig. 6.14).

The fire phasing of the microcosmic orbit consists of propelling the breaths along the Control Vessel and the Function Vessel, establishing a closed circuit. This movement will cause the yin and yang breaths to follow a rhythm modelled on the evolutions of yin and yang in a day and a night. The yang breath, for example, will be at its peak at noon or in the body at the crown.

The *Chart for the Cultivation of Perfection* contains a number of elements similar to these alchemical mirrors symbolizing the fire phasing (see fig. 6.15). The body is indeed surrounded by thirty moons with the numbers of the thirty days below. On the drawings anterior to this chart, the thirty moons were, as on the Yanluozi diagram, simply mentioned by characters designating the main phases of this life cycle: new moon, first quarter, full moon and last quarter. However, the alchemical mirror of Master Shangyang represents the thirty moons, as on the *Chart for the Cultivation of Perfection.* On the latter, the body is also surrounded by six trigrams, *kun, zhen, gen, qian, xun, dui* (*li* and *kan* are represented inside the body, at the level of the heart and the kidneys). But the order of these trigrams is different to that of the mirror of the medicine, which is *kun, zhen, dui, qian, xun* and *gen.*[82] On the *Chart for the Cultivation of Perfection*, we also see the characters of the twenty-eight constellations.[83] These are inscribed inside the heart, the kidneys, the liver and the lungs, and the names of the twenty-four articulations breaths of a year on the spine.

The fire phasing of the macrocosmic orbit is modeled on the evolution of yin and yang in the course of a year, following the rhythm of the four seasons and of the twenty-four breaths of a year. On the Chart, the names of the twenty-four articulations breaths of a year are inscribed in hexagons symbolising the vertebra running the length of the spine. It begins with yin, at the bottom, corresponding to the "winter solstice" (*dongzhi* 冬至). These twenty-four

82 This order does not match the correspondances between trigrams and body parts in the *Xiuzhen taiji hunyuan tu*, 13a–b: the kidneys correspond to *kan*, the bladder to *gen*, the liver to *zhen*, the spleen to *xun*, the heart to *li*, the small intestine to *kun*, the lungs to *dui*, the large intestine to *qian*; neither it does not correspond to that of the *Yijing* 易經, chapter "Xici" 繫辭.

83 These twenty-eight constellations are also drawn in *Wushang sanyuan santian yutang dafa* (DZ 200), 22.2b around the character "centre" and the sun and the moon.

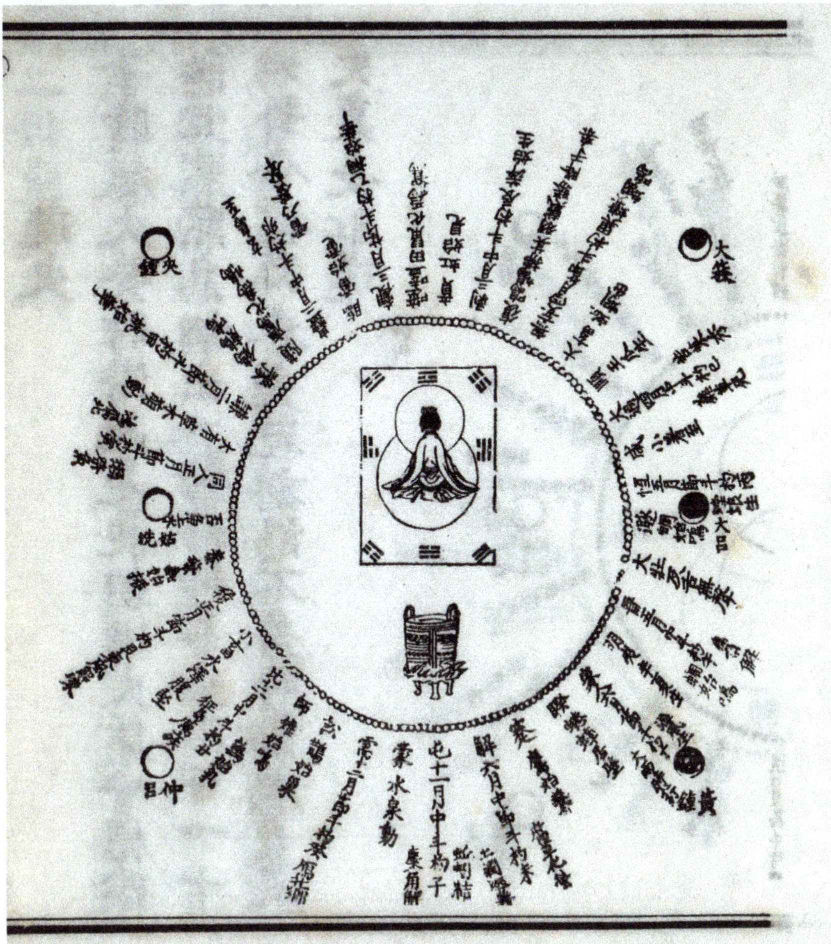

FIGURE 6.14 Drawing of the alchemical mirror of the "progression of fire" (*jin huo* 進火). *Jinye huandan yinzheng tu* (DZ 151), 10a

breaths are already represented on the Yanluozi diagrams and re-used by the commentary of the *Classic on Difficult Issues*.[84]

84 *Xiuzhen shishu* (DZ 263), 18.2a. They are also represented as dots in Qiu Changchun's *Dadan zhizhi* (DZ 244), 1.5a.

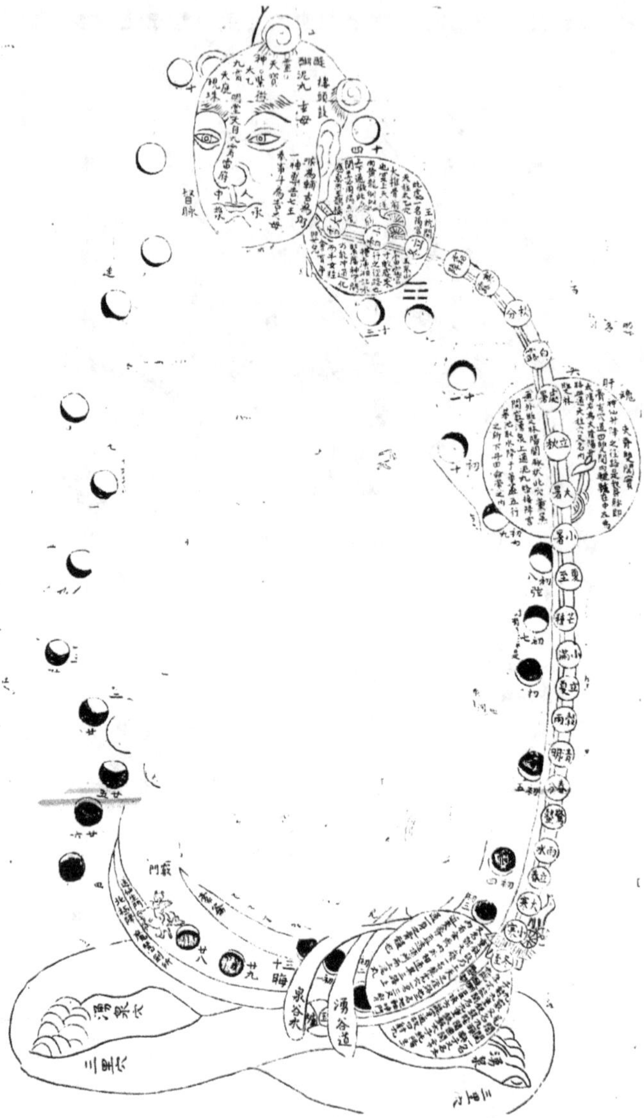

FIGURE 6.15 Alchemical Mirror. *Chart for the Cultivation of Perfection*

CHAPTER 7

# Thunder Processes Illustrated by the *Chart for the Cultivation of Perfection*

## 1 Schools Related to the Thunder Rites

Starting in the Song dynasty, several Taoist schools developed new ritual techniques called thunder rites. Individuals, especially in Jiangxi province, first experimented with these exorcistic and therapeutic rites in the beginning of the twelfth century. This is most clearly seen in the proponents of the Correct Method of the Heart of Heaven, who presented Emperor Huizong with scriptures detailing thunder rites in 1116.[1] While this school shared the closest affinity with the Heavenly Masters or the Correct Unity (Zhengyi 正一) Taoists, it is in fact related to four different scriptural traditions: Way and the Virtue, Numinous Treasure, Correct Unity and Upper Clarity.[2] The Heart of Heaven is the North Star. In this tradition, Zhang Daoling 張道陵 is deified as the marshal of the North Pole Court who exorcizes evil (*Beiji quxie yuanshuai* 北極驅邪元帥).[3] This court is presided over by the Northern Thearch or the Great Thearch of the Purple Tenuity (*Ziwei dadi* 紫微大帝). Other important deities of this current are the Perfected Warrior or the Dark Warrior (Xuanwu 玄武), the Black Killer (Heisha 黑煞), the deity of the seventh star of the Northern Dipper and the Sovereign Jade Emperor (Yuhuang dadi 玉皇大帝). All these names are mentioned on the *Chart for the Cultivation of Perfection* as residing in the head. The Correct Method of the Heart of Heaven is mainly based on three of the oldest talismans: the talisman of the Three Lights (*sanguang fu* 三光符), the talisman of the Celestial Net (*tiangang fu* 天罡符) and the talisman of the Dark Warrior (*xuanwu fu* 玄武符). It combines exorcist rituals and practices based on the meditative techniques of Internal Alchemy.[4] But this school did not survive long after the end of the Song dynasty.

1 See *Taishang zhuguo jiumin zongzhen biyao* (DZ 1227) compiled by Yuan Miaozong 元妙宗 (ca. 1086–1116). On this school and the related rites, see Schipper and Verellen, 2004: 1056–1079.

2 See Deng Yougong's 鄧有功 (1210–1279) preface to *Shangqing tianxin zhengfa* 上清天心正法 [Correct method of the heart of heaven of upper clarity] (DZ 566), 2a–b.

3 See *Taishang zhuguo jiumin zongzhen biyao* (DZ 1227), 2.6a–b.

4 The main texts of Taoist Canon belonging to this school are: *Taishang zhuguo jiumin zongzhen biyao* (DZ 1227) of Yuan Miaozong presented to Emperor Huizong in 1116. *Shangqing*

 | DOI:10.1163/9789004383456_009

During this same era, a similar tradition appeared, the Divine Empyrean (Shenxiao 神霄). This group introduced new methods cantered on the Five Thunders, received imperial sponsorship from Emperor Huizong. Their success was largely due to the Taoist Lin Lingsu 林靈素 who, from 1117 onwards, had great influence over the emperor.[5] This current was also integrated by the Heavenly Masters: the thirtieth Heavenly Master Zhang Jixian 张繼先 (1092–1127) and the fortieth Zhang Yuchu 張宇初 (1361–1410) were specialists of this tradition, which as we have seen, spread on Mount Wudang.

The third important current using thunder rites is that of the Pure Tenuity (Qingwei 清微), which arose in the thirteenth century. This lineage was accompanied by newly revealed scriptures, new forms of sacred writings incomprehensible to ordinary people, called "original revelations" (*yuanjiang* 元降). These Taoists also relied heavily on talismans imagined to have come from the Pure Tenuity Heaven, hence the name of this current. It recognizes *a posteriori* a woman as a matriarch, Zu Shu 祖舒 (ob. 904?), a native of Guangxi. It was, like the tradition of the Correct Method of the Heart of Heaven, composed of a synthesis of four traditions related to the Way and the Virtue, Correct Unity, Numinous Treasure and Upper Clarity lineages. The transmission was effected from master to disciple for nine generations Bai Yuchan's disciples, ending with Nan Bidao 南畢道 (b. 1196). A native of Meishan 眉山 in Sichuan Province, Nan cured Huang Shunshen 黄舜申 (b. 1224), an adept from Fujian who was the first prominent proponent of this current. Summoned to the court in 1286, Huang codified the thunder rites of this school.[6]

Although we lack historical evidence of the origins of the *Chart for the Cultivation of Perfection*, the analysis of its intrinsic elements allows us to bring to light a certain kinship with the thunder rites. The Inner Alchemical techniques of the schools practising the thunder rites come essentially from the southern tradition or from a syncretism between the southern and northern alchemical

---

*tianxin zhengfa* (DZ 566) by Deng Yougong 鄧有功 (mid twelfth century) of Huagai shan 華蓋山 in Jiangxi. *Shangqing beiji tianxin zhengfa* 上清北極天心正法 [Correct method of the heart of heaven of the northern pole] (DZ 567). *Wushang xuanyuan santian yutang dafa* (DZ 220) (after 1158) by Lu Shizhong 路時中 and *Wushang santian yutang zhengzong gaoben neijing yushu* 無上三天玉堂正宗高奔內景玉書 [Precious text of flying in the inner landscape, from the correct tradition of the jade hall of the supreme three heavens] (DZ 221). According to the preface of the *Shangqing tianxin zhengfa* by Deng Yougong, in 994, Rao Dongtian 饒洞天 dug the ground and found the records on the Method of the Heart of Heaven. On these texts, see Schipper and Verellen 2004.

5 See Strickmann 1975: 15–28.

6 See *Qingwei xianpu* 清微仙譜 [Chronology of the immortals of the pure tenuity heaven] (DZ 171) by Huang Shunshen 黃舜申, with a preface of 1293 by Chen Cai 陳菜.

tradition.[7] Bai Yuchan mastered the techniques of the Divine Empyrean, and signed himself as "Master of the Upper Clarity knowing the magical processes and military exorcisms of the North Star".[8] Zhao Yizhen 趙宜眞 (ob. 1382), who synthesized the northern and southern alchemical traditions, was a master of the Pure Tenuity tradition.[9]

From the Song dynasty onwards, Buddhist elements have influenced the theories and practices of Inner Alchemy. This is most evident in the writings of Zhang Boduan, who was influenced by Chan doctrines and wrote some poems on Chan.[10] The thunder rites, at least since Bai Yuchan, are full of Tantric influences such as the rituals associated with wrathful deities, whose external and internal aspects symbolise the anger that is used as a means of subduing evils. According to Buddhist conceptions, external and internal evils are principally illusions and the false thoughts of the follower. The notion of inner light was quite prominent in these methods, as well as other techniques and terms betraying the influence both of Chan and Tantric Buddhism.

In the schools using thunder rites, the universe was transposed into the human body, which included not only the physical world, but also the realms of gods and demons. These images are added to the classical vocabulary of alchemy and its inner processes. This synthesis of Taoist methods combines visions of the outer and inner worlds. These schools have integrated techniques of ingesting breath and saliva as suggested on the representation of the *Chart for the Cultivation of Perfection* in the text featured next to the throat. They used methods of visualization of body deities according to the Yellow Court tradition: the animal deities of the six viscera and the Perfected abiding in cranial palaces. They also use methods of the Numinous Treasure tradition, and the evocation of specific deities related to thunder rites and associated with certain parts of the body and their functions. The main psychophysiological techniques use the concentrations on certain body orifices and alchemical methods of the southern tradition. To these methods, there was a strong correlation between natural elements and areas of the body. For example, Bai Yuchan considers that the rain is the water in the kidneys:

7 The five patriarchs of the Southern School are Zhang Boduan, Shi Tai 石泰 (ob. 1158), Xue Daoguang 薛道光 (1078?–1191), Bai Yuchan (1194–1229?) and Chen Niwan (ob. 1213). It is from Chen Niwan onwards that a synthesis with the thunder rites of the Divine Empyrean tradition took place.

8 DZ 1220, 76.3a.

9 See Schipper 1987: 715–734.

10 See *Ziyang zhenren Wuzhen pian shiyi* 紫陽真人悟真篇拾遺 [Supplement to the essay of Ziyang zhenren's *Awakening to Truth*] (DZ 144).

> It is important to move the breath from its own ocean of yin, so that it fills the heaven and the earth and that rain occurs. The sunny weather corresponds to the fire of the heart. One imagines a large fire burning his body and opening into the great space of breath, bringing good weather.[11]

## 2 The Northern Dipper and the Setting in Motion of the Inner Heaven

A Song text probably written by a disciple of Zhang Boduan already compares the attitude of the alchemist to the North Star, a motionless centre in the sky around which all the stars move. He writes:

> The North Star, ever motionless, plays the role of central axis around which the surrounding stars move. This serves as an example on how the alchemist uses his mind. The persistence of immobility in the movement is how the man endowed with the aptitude to immobility uses his mind. To remain inert in the immobility is to be similar to wood or earth. The spirit abides in the centre, both eyes depend on it as do the two kidneys, and their mysterious use cannot be exhausted. The spirit obeys the orders of the mind, the breath obeys the openings, and the essence follows the calls of the spirit. These elements combine in a mysterious way.[12]

In the literature featuring the thunder rites, the North Star and the Northern Dipper play a fundamental role. The Dipper consists of nine stars: four stars located in the scoop, three in the handle and two invisible called Fu 輔 and Bi 弼. The stars of the handle are called Celestial Net (*tiangang* 天罡); in the human body, they correspond to the area of the heart, in which they play a crucial role. In the thunder rites, the thunder is summoned from the direction to which the handle points in order to expel demons. The Dipper also opens the way to heaven in both meditation and ritual. Wang Wenqing 王文卿 (1093–1153), specialist of the Divine Empyrean legacy, wrote in his *Song on the Obscure Pearl* that "the heart is the Celestial Net." Bai Yuchan (1194–1229) comments on this sentence as follows:

11 *Daofa huiyuan* (DZ 1220), 70.3b.

12 *Yuqing jinsi qinghua biwen jinbao neilian danjue* (DZ 240), 3b.

> The Celestial Net is the [original] breath of the killer. When the Celestial Net is at the direction of *chou*, the [original] breath bursts into the constellations *dou* 斗 and *niu* 牛. If anger arises in the heart, the [original] killer breath develops; it is maintained as much as possible and when the heart enters into a great fury. It is necessary to firmly clench the pass of the teeth by grinding them. Endure this breath until the anger appears through the [original] breath of the North. As soon as one exhales, the sky quakes, the earth cracks and the rain and thunder rage.[13]

On the *Chart for the Cultivation of Perfection*, the name Celestial Net is inscribed at the heart, between the representations of the seven stars of the Northern Dipper, the handle directed to the North. This disposition is similar to that shown on a diagram inserted in a text of Bai Yuchan where seven stars are surrounded by eight trigrams according to the precelestial disposition or Fuxi 伏羲 disposition, the whole being surrounded by a circle (see fig. 7.1). This drawing is explained by the following commentary:

> Mercury represents the heart where the spirit is purified, the innate nature or the red dragon. When inside and outside have merged in an indistinct chaos, not the slightest bit of yin remains. The lead represents the body, the concentration of the breath, the vital force or the white tiger. In the light bathing the ten thousand phenomena, the mirror reaches the Jade Purity.[14]

On the method for moving the Celestial Net, Bai Yuchan adds:

> The Celestial Net is the heart/mind; it is through it that we can move the different breaths. If we want to move the yang, the yang responds; it is the same for the yin. It is advisable to move the five agents that are constantly in audience with the Superior Thearch, to move the mechanism of the creations and transformations, to reverse the yin and the yang, to react according to the circumstances.

Thus, the North Star governs the movement of the sky and of the twenty-eight constellations, whose names of twenty-one of them in groups of seven, those

13 *Xuanzhu ge*, in *Daofa huiyuan* (DZ 1220), 70.8a.

14 *Xiuzhen shishu* (DZ 263), 1.1a, "Formula on the fire phasing in the golden elixir" (*Jindan huohou jue* 金丹火候訣).

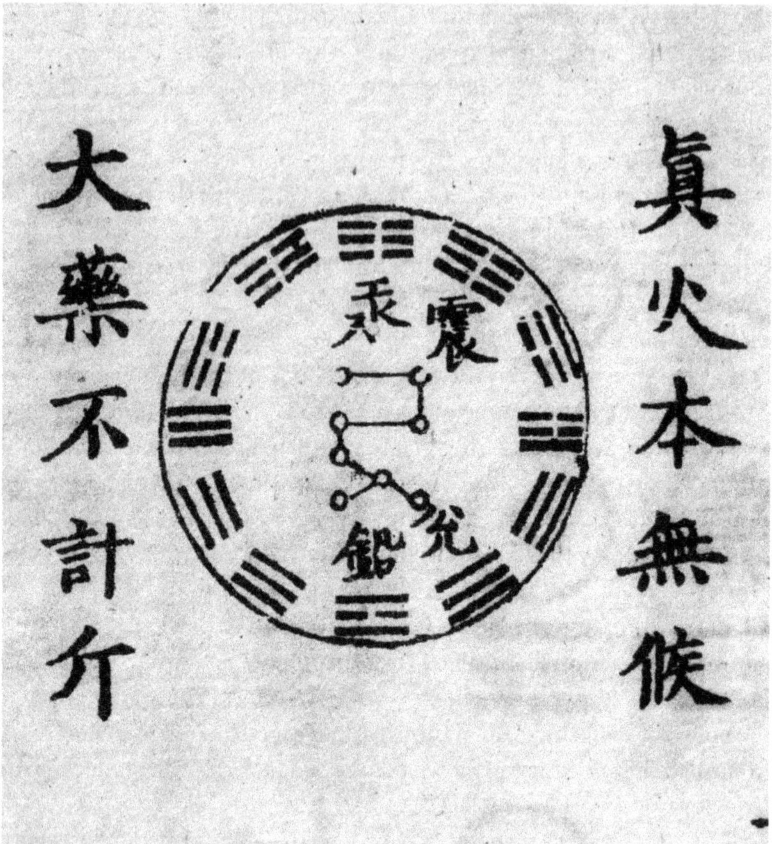


FIGURE 7.1 "Drawing of the fire phasing for the golden elixir according to Master Bai" (*Bai xiansheng jindan huohou tu* 白先生金丹火候圖). In *Xiuzhen shishu* (DZ 263), 1.1a

corresponding to the south, east and west, are inscribed on the *Chart for the Cultivation of Perfection* around the design of the seven stars. The names of the eastern stars (*jiao, kang, di, fang, xin, wei, ji*) are written in the two leaflets representing the liver and the gallbladder, those of the West (*chou, wei, mao, bi, zi, shen*) in the two leaflets representing the lungs and those of the South (*jing, gui, liu, xing, zhang, yi, chen*) around the seven stars in the heart. The seven constellations corresponding to the North have their names inscribed below, at the level of the standing black child, surmounted by the character *jing* [Essence], and are related to the kidneys. In Inner Alchemy, the stillness of the adept is necessary for the moving of all the powers and breaths inside the body according to the fire phasing and this motion is in harmony with the outer world.

Several centuries later, a prominent Taoist of the Dragon Gate tradition, Liu Yiming 劉一明 (1734–1821), reporting the teachings of the Ming adept Zhang Sanfeng 張三豐, gives a more accurate description of the way of moving the inner heaven:

> Rotate the Northern Dipper by the handle. In the furnace, purify the sun and the moon, which will sweep away completely the thirty-six thousand phenomena. In the way (path) of the cultivation of perfection, we must know the progression of the Northern Dipper around the North Star in order to reverse the process of transformations, to rotate around the axis of *qian* and *kun*, to clearly understand yin and yang, instead of letting the yin and yang play with us. The North Star is the seventh star of the Northern Dipper [...] It is the assistant minister of the North Pole, it maintains the balance between life and death, it controls the handle of transformations and evolutions, it moves the five agents, makes the four seasons follow one another, it generates the ten thousand beings, governs the constellations, it is the axis of the cycles of breaths. Its responsibility is immense, and its merit is great.[15]

On the left cheek on the representation of the *Chart for the Cultivation of Perfection*, is the following inscription: "The throat is the star Fu, the tongue, the star Bi. Only one worthy divinity governs the seven princes who serve the Northern Dipper. The heart is the mother of the tongue." This last assertion is consistent with the theory of traditional Chinese medicine that the tongue is the external manifestation of the heart. Moreover, the *Taoist Methods, United in Principle* states: "The tongue is the fire official in correspondence with the heart, which is the Northern Dipper."[16] Fu and Bi, respectively the eighth and ninth stars of the Northern Dipper, intended to protect from calamities and chase evil influences. They are considered as the assistants of the North Star. In the *Classic on Military Techniques Related to the Northern Dipper*, we find the following passage: "The eighth star, Fu, has the surname of Jingchang 精常, the secret name of Shangkai 上開 and the social name of Zhengyan 正延. Its main function is to keep an eye to the great ministers of the nine provinces of all the kingdoms in the empire, to examine their crimes and their merits."[17] The same book gives a similar description of the function of the star Bi.

---

15 Liu Yiming (1734–1821), *Xiuzhen biannan canzheng* 修真辯難參證 [Examination and resolution of the difficulties in the cultivation of perfection], ed. Min Yide 閔一得, p. 118.

16 *Daofa huiyuan* (DZ 1220), 72.1ab.

17 *Beidou zhifa wuwei jing* (DZ 870), 3a.

Furthermore, in the central part of the *Chart for the Cultivation of Perfection* is a visual representation of the seven characters corresponding to the secret names of the deities of the seven stars of the Northern Dipper. In thunder rites, these seven characters serve as incantations for the destruction of hells. In the texts setting out the Northern Dipper rituals, it is mentioned that these stars are the seat of deities presiding in the world of happiness and calamities, of life and death. Note that the secret name (*hui* 諱) is often used in talismans where it is regarded as the replacement or the representative of the designated individual.

Therefore, the light of the North Star illuminates the world and destroys evil. It directs the course of the twenty-eight constellations and, in rituals, the twenty-eight lamps arranged on the four sides of the altar symbolize these twenty-eight constellations.[18] In Inner Alchemy, it is the light of the heart / mind that destroys the evil within.

## 3 Processes Associated with the Thunder

### 3.1 *The Thunder*

The *Classic of Changes* states: "Beings are stimulated by means of thunder and lightning, they are made to move with wind and rain."[19] Thunder was revered as a deity in ancient times, but under the Tang Dynasty, it became an important deity in Taoist practice. This was especially the case during the reign of Emperor Xuanzong who in the fifth year of the *tianbao* reign (746) promulgated an imperial edict proclaiming that thunder is the wake-up call for all sentient beings.[20]

The thunder is linked to the North and the North Star.[21] In the human body, the thunder deity is deemed as the Primordial Spirit (*yuanshen* 元神). Bai Yuchan writes:

> The thunder deity is also a transformation by resonance of the Primordial Spirit. When the adept discerns movement from rest, he communicates perfectly with heaven and earth. He can call the wind, summon the

18 *Wushang xuanyuan santian yutang dafa* (DZ 220), 22.2b–3a: drawing of the 28 constellations preceded by a text titled "The Celestial Net controls the twenty-eight constellations."

19 "Xici," *Yijing*, 2.1.

20 Qin Huitian 秦蕙田, *Wuli tongkao* 五禮通考 (SKQS), 36.32; Doré 1914: 685.

21 See *Daofa huiyuan* (DZ 1220), 67.24.

> thunder to behead the pernicious elements and the seductive demons, to hunt and enslave demons and divinities, there is no offering or gift that he cannot give. That is the way of "using the Primordial Spirit."[22]

In other words, outside are the thunder and the lightning that repel all troubles, inside are the true thought and the Primordial Spirit, as is explained by a great Master of the Divine Empyrean, Zhang Jixian 張繼先 (1092–1127): "Where do we begin to tame the demons? Within you lies the Primordial Spirit that remains stable and calm. When the sword of wisdom goes into action, demons and deities are tamed, troubles and calamities are eliminated."[23]

Zhang Yuchu distinguishes between the thunder (*lei* 雷) and the lightning (*ting* 霆). He writes: "The thunder is the axis (*shu* 樞) of Heaven, it has a good nature and governs life. Its essence is yang, but its appearance resembles yin. This is the reason why the celestial stems *jia, bing, geng, ren* correspond to the yang thunder. The lightning is the pivot (*ji* 機) of the earth, it has a bad nature and governs destruction, its essence is yin, its appearance is yang. Therefore, the celestial stems *yi, ji, ding, xin* correspond to the yin lightning."[24] We remember that on the *Chart for the Cultivation of Perfection*, the term *shuji* 樞機 [Axis/pivot], is written below the circle with two dots representing the obscure (*xuan* 玄) and the female (*pin* 牝) or the yin and yang of the internal kidneys.

The thunder appears in the calm of the alchemical transmutations, it is a supreme luminous force that eliminates all yin within the adept and serves outside in the rites. The correlation between thunder rites and alchemical practices is explained well in Zhang Jixian's poem "The Breath of the One Connects all the Passes:"

> The thunder is accomplished by the transformation of the precelestial Breath,
> The holy men and the heavenly immortals are similar to Perfection.

---

22 *Daofa huiyuan* (DZ 1220), 70.6a.

23 *Mingzhen powang zhangsong* (DZ 979), 2b–3a. Zhang Jixian, the thirtieth master of the School of Heavenly masters, lived at the time of Emperor Huizong, who summoned him to the Court. He received the nickname of Master Xujing (Xujing xiansheng 虛靖先生). His works reflect an influence of Chan Buddhism, of the alchemical school of the South, of the Zhong-Lü tradition and that of Chen Tuan. According to *Yuxi zi danjing zhiyao* (DZ 245) by Li Jianyi, he received the alchemical formulas from Liu Haichan 劉海蟾, the first master of the southern alchemical school. He is considered as a great master of the Divine Empyrean tradition.

24 *Yuanshi wuliang duren shangpin miaojing tongyi* (DZ 89), 1.2a.

> The [original] breath of the One connects all passes
> The Ancestors are reborn and close to me.[25]

In thunder rites, if the heart plays an important role, the gallbladder remains the predominant organ, because it is directly associated with the thunder. Wang Wenqing writes: "The [Original] Breath of the gallbladder is the thunder." Bai Yuchan comments:

> The gallbladder is inside the liver, which contains the blue-green breath. If anger rises in the gallbladder, the red breath accumulates, the five breaths turn in circles and enters the palace of the gallbladder, water and fire enter into conflict, and the thunder resounds. The heroism of the gallbladder and the anger of the liver generate thunder. The angry heaven emits a rumble of thunder shaking all.[26]

This association of thunder and gallbladder was already mentioned in the *Book of the Yellow Court*.[27] In Inner Alchemy, the five thunders are the breaths of the five agents and of the five viscera in the human body. The basic idea of these schools is the union of the internal practices and external rites. Without Inner Alchemy, it is not possible to efficiently perform rites for removing disease or demons, to make it rain or to obtain any other efficiency. In other words, it is necessary to practice Inner Alchemy to write talismans, to pronounce incantations, to perform effective rites, to cure diseases.

### 3.2 *The Mysterious Pearl*

The Mysterious Pearl is an ancient term commonly used in Inner Alchemical texts, but receives a particular explication in the context of the thunder rites. The access to knowledge, according to a Chinese myth, is favoured by the possession of an obscure or mysterious pearl (*xuanzhu* 玄珠), that a model sage of China, the Yellow Emperor, had once lost. The pearl symbolizes the Way and is sometimes referred to as the pearl of nine meanders (*jiuqu zhu* 九曲珠).[28] It is similar to a grotto-womb or a labyrinth evoking the birth and the origin of things. A myth associates the pearl and the Yellow Emperor, in a legend reported by Zhuangzi, a great thinker of the fourth century BCE:

---

25 *Mingzhen powang zhangsong* (DZ 979), 1b.
26 *Xuanzhu ge*, in *Daofa huiyuan* (DZ 1220), 70.7a.
27 *Huangting neijing yujing zhu* (DZ 402), 2.3a.
28 See Kaltenmark 1981: 480–481; trans. Despeux 1979: 69–70.

> As he was walking to the north of the Red River, the Yellow Emperor climbed Mount Kunlun. With his gaze, he took in the south, thinking of his return; and in this way, he lost his obscure pearl. He charged Knowledge to search for it, but in vain. He tasked Piercing-View to bring it to him, but in vain. He ordered Dispute to find it for him, but in vain. He instructed Indistinct Images to seek it, and Indistinct Images found it. 'Strange, he said, that only Indistinct Images could find it.'[29]

In Inner Alchemy, the Mysterious Pearl symbolizes the beginning of production of the elixir of immortality. It is like the pearl in the oyster that is gradually growing. It is generated by the union of two opposite principles, the yin and yang breaths, metaphorically called at a certain stage of the process the tiger and the dragon. Zhang Boduan (987–1082) writes:

> In the obscure cavity, the medicine appears,
> In the yang furnace, the fire blazes at a suitable fire phasing.
> The tiger and the dragon are united,
> In the metal cauldron, the Mysterious Pearl is born.[30]

He writes also in his *Stanzas on the Awakening to Perfection*:

> The tiger leaps, the dragon spins,
> The waves break under the wind.
> In the centre, the axis keeps its uprightness,
> And the Mysterious Pearl is born.[31]

More than a century later, a text attributed to the famous Yuan Taoist Qiu Chuji (1148–1227), clarifies the mystical state corresponding to the onset of the Mysterious Pearl:

> The tiger and the dragon do not refer at this stage to the emblems of the liver and the lungs, but to the true yin and the true yang of the heart and the kidneys. The two mingle in one, indistinctly. When, with the creative thinking, the adept is attentive to the *zi* period [the manifestation of yang in the body], something of the size of a grain of millet appears naturally. Every day a grain is produced. The monk calls it the "grain-relic," the

29 See "Heaven and Earth" in *Zhuangzi jijie* 莊子集解, 3.71.
30 *Jindan sibai zi* 金丹四百字 [The elixir explained in four hundred words] (DZ 1081), 7a.
31 *Wuzhen pian zhushi*, DZ 145, 1.3a–b.

> Taoist, "the mysterious pearl." Every day, the true breath increases by ten feet, and longevity becomes incalculable. After three hundred days, the breath is transformed into the cinnabar of the size of an orange musket-ball, and one can quite naturally live long and not die.[32]

On most versions of the *Chart for the Cultivation of Perfection*, the inscription describing the internal kidneys mentions the "village of the dark water" (*xuanshui zhi xiang* 玄水之鄉), the Mount Wudang version instead mentions the Mysterious Pearl: "Inside the cavity between the two kidneys is the true postcelestial essence or the true lead. The Confucian calls it the "Great Ultimate" (Taiji), while Taoists [call] it the "Mysterious Pearl."

This term is also used in the writings on thunder rites. Wang Wenqing wrote a "Song of the Mysterious Pearl" that has a commentary by Bai Yuchan. The general ideas of Inner Alchemy are included in it, and we perceive a primordial importance of the stars, as well as a correlation between certain body elements and the thunder rites elements. This song begins as follows:

> Ineffable is the great way.
> Practice breath retention and contemplate inside,
> Make the Celestial Net move,
> The seven stars shine in the cold.
> The five stars are connected,
> And gather at the Muddy Pellet.
> Water and fire are fighting,
> Metal and wood dominate,
> Metal and water generate each other,
> Fire and wood meet.
> Earth is the spirit of intent,
> Following [Original] Breath, it creates or controls.
> Wind, fire, thunder, lightning rage;
> Rain, fine weather, snow, hail follow one another,
> Since the [original] breath of the One circulates everywhere.
> In the chaos, the elements confront one another,
> In the dispersion, the ten thousand phenomena appear.
> In the accumulation, it becomes the infant
> Who transforms himself in the Thunder deity.[33]

---

32 Qiu Chuji (Changchun 長春) (1148–1227), *Dadan zhizhi* [Clear directions on the great elixir] (DZ 244), 1.8a.

33 *Daofa huiyuan* (DZ 1220), 70.1a–4a.

### 3.3 *The Celestial Eye and the Spirit Light*

On the *Chart for the Cultivation of Perfection*, the space between the eyebrows bears the inscription "celestial eye" (*tianmu* 天目), a place from where a wire leads to a circle in which is inscribed "spirit light" (*shenguang* 神光). These are two typical notions of the thunder rites. The term "celestial eye" evokes the Buddhist term *tianyan* 天眼 [Celestial eye], which designates one of the five or six supernatural faculties (*liutong* 六通), i.e., seeing anything, even at a vast distance. It is also called "wisdom eye" (*huiyan* 慧眼), and is, as here, located in-between the eyebrows. The light of the spirit is used in the schools related to thunder rites to write talismans, especially those used for healing. One method of the Pure Tenuity tradition is described in a chapter of the *Methods of the Tao, United in Principle*:

> Enter the meditation chamber and burn incense. Sit upright, grind your teeth, then incant the following three times with a pure mind. Concentrate your spirit, steady your breath, and focus your vision as described in the rules. After a while, when your mind is calmed, move the spirit light upwards from the ancestral palace to between the eyebrows. Grabbing the brush, attract this divine light from the celestial eye to the brush tip, and write the talisman.[34]

The spirit light appears and develops when the mind is devoid of any delusion, when it is perfectly quiet and clear. Therefore, only masters who have attained a high level of practice in Inner Alchemy can control the light of the spirit and use it to write talismans. These practices too, varied over time. We give here, by way of example, a method described in a text claiming to belong to the Numinous Treasure tradition and included in the *Methods of the Tao, United in Principle*:

> Imagine that, from the red heaven, the spirit is stabilized, either by walking, sitting, standing or lying down. Stay quietly in a dark room, the half-closed eyes letting just a ray of light pass, and the look directed towards the nose. Gradually the impression grows that the light goes directly in between the eyebrows, in the cavity of the Cavern Chamber (*Dongfang xue* 洞房穴), the place where the spirit enters and exits, a place also called the Bridge of the Magpies. Then it penetrates the Muddy Pellet and the top of the head until the mind enters into a deep concentration. The light collected at the top of the head is directed to reach the Obscure Pass. The adept will then stop and start again as before.

---

34 *Daofa huiyuan* (DZ 1220), 13.1a.

> This is called 'harmonisation.' Harmonise the spirit for eighty-one days, after which a light will glow, and the concentration of the mind increases. The whole body until the Muddy Pellet consists of light. The adept lives in the present moment and masters his thoughts. After one hundred and twenty-eight days, the divine light is as intense as those of the sun and the moon; barely visible, it begins to take shape. One has the feeling to be like an infant who moves and exits from the top of the head. When this concentration is very strong, a divine light will appear that is similar to yellow clouds. Suddenly the adept feels that the light passes outside and sees his own body as motionless as a corpse. He must quickly think that the large cave filled with red light becomes his own body. Then, after a certain time, he begins again as previously.[35]

Another text by Wang Qizhen 王契真 (ca. 1250), belonging to the Numinous Treasure tradition describes the basic practices that can work for the weal of the living and the dead. He mentions this light of the spirit:

> Sit up straight, so that the ears are in the plane of shoulders, and the nose in the same line as the umbilicus. Collect the six senses,[36] concentrate the force of the spirit in the eyes, the eyes being turned neither outward nor inward, and contemplate the divine light. After three days, in the secret chamber appears a point of divine light, and the spirit is stabilized. After four days, the divine light gradually invades the chamber. In this state of concentration, things are not yet apparent. But after seven days you can see all the demons and numinous spirits.[37]

These descriptions are stamped by Buddhist elements, such as the classical correlation between the concentration of the mind (*dhyāna*) and the wisdom (*prajñā*), an insight that grows with concentration, also described as the spiritual light. They also evoke the tantric methods of the transfer of consciousness allowing the conscious principle to go out of the body by the crown.

---

35 *Daofa huiyuan* (DZ 1220), 244.33a–b.

36 The five sense organs and the mind, considered in both Buddhist and Taoist traditions as the sixth sense.

37 *Shangqing lingbao dafa* (DZ 1221), 4.8ab.

## 4 Elements of the *Chart for the Cultivation of Perfection* Linked to the Correct Method of the Heart of Heaven

### 4.1 *The Ancestral Breath and the Breath of the Three Lights*

The depiction of the kidneys on the *Chart for the Cultivation of Perfection* has seven- or eight-turn spiral topped by three characters carrying the radical of rain. Beside the spiral is the inscription "Jasper Pond."[38] Below, we can see the caption "Lapis Lazuli Pond," the name of one of the ponds of the Land of Supreme Joy in the western paradise over which the Buddha Amitābha reigns.[39] The use of this expression here reflects the syncretism of Taoist texts in the late Qing dynasty where writers readily combine Buddhist and Taoist expressions. Below the spiral, in the gourd-shaped pocket, we can see on the Mount Wudang version and that of Guangzhou the following inscription: "The embryo is constantly irrigated and fed, it is the ocean where I take root." The author of the tenth century *Manuscript on the Cultivation of Cinnabar and the Wonderful Way of the Perfected Origin* also represents this as a spiral.[40] The illustration contains the following inscription: "This is the representation of the accomplishment of the embryo into a human being, it is the representation of the accomplishment of the elixir into the spirit." The following explanation is given further on: "*Tai* 胎 [Embryo] is synonymous with *tai* 泰 [Stability]. In the chaos, the embryo is the space between heaven and earth: for human beings, the embryo is the fusion of essence and blood."[41]

The spiral is also an element that often appears in thunder rites. It symbolizes the motion of thunder, and the evocation of the corresponding deities who should act during the rites. That is why it is particularly present

38 The Jasper Pond is mentioned in a poem attributed to Donghua shangfang lingfei 東華上房靈妃: "In the Moon Palace is born the Medicine Spring, in the sun there is the Jasper Pond." See *Zhen'gao* (DZ 1016), 3.15a; *Xuanzhu ge* 玄珠歌 (Song of the Mysterious Pearl) (tenth century) by Tongxuan xiansheng 通玄先生, DZ 573.3b. In *Yunji qiqian*, 96.4b, we find this sentence: "In the sun is the Jasper Pond." In contrast, a "jasper embryo" (*qiongtai* 瓊胎) is mentioned in *Daofa huiyuan* (DZ 1220), 244. 31a.

39 It is described in particular in T. 360 *Wuliang shoujing* 無量壽經, 1.271b.

40 *Zhenyuan miaodao xiudan liyan chao* 真元妙道修丹歷驗鈔 attributed to Caoyi zi 草衣子 or Dongzhen zi 洞真子, in *Yunji qiqian* (DZ 1032), 72.31b. Another version of this text is in the DZ 152 with the title *Xiuzhen liyan chaotu* 修真歷驗鈔圖 [Copy of diagrams of attested methods for the cultivation of perfection] with no attributed author, but this version does not include the representation of the spiral. We don't know who is designated by this nickname, nor the era at which he lived. Several fragments of writings relating essentially to external alchemy are cited in the *Yunji qiqian* (1024) and the *Daoshu* by Zeng Zao (1150). On this topic, see Ch'en 1975: 287–289.

41 *Yunji qiqian* (DZ 1032), 72.31b–32a.

in the talismans that the ritual master draws. For example, the *Taoist Methods, United in Principle* comprises a series of eight turn spirals drawn in the inward or outward direction with a line heading out in different directions designated by the name of one of the eight trigrams (fig. 7.2). These set in motion the officials of thunder and lightning, those of the celestial and terrestrial thunder, of water, the king of thunder of the twelve periods and the twenty-four breaths of a year.[42] Another passage of this same compilation containing a form of Divine Empyrean rite by Wang Wenqing 王文卿 (1093–1153) explains how, while tracing the spiral, the officiant mentally pronounces a mantra: "Reciting the mantra of the thunder of five thearchs, he moves the brush in twelve inwardly spiralling movements and then makes it go out from the inside by a line."[43] It also appears that each turn of the spiral corresponds to a particular efficiency if we are to believe a Song writing stating that at the first spiral, thunder and lightning are initiated, at the second, the starlight, at the third, the generals, at the fourth, the gods and demons come to the tip of the brush, and so on.[44] On the *Chart for the Cultivation of Perfection*, the spiral probably indicates the setting in motion of thunder inside the body, which, according to Zhang Jixian, comes from the fiery celestial breath posterior to heaven.[45] This spiral is topped by three characters bearing the radical of rain. We find these three characters in only one document of the Taoist Canon, the "Great Rites for the Prayers to the Five Thunders of the Precious Pearl Governed by the Emperor." This text is included in the *Taoist Methods, United in Principle* and transmitted by Zhu Meijing 朱梅靖 of the Jixian yuan Academy to Li Xianyun 李閑雲, a high court official, the thirty-sixth Heavenly Master Zhang Zongyan 張宗演 (d. 1292) and others.[46]

The term "precious pearl" (*baozhu* 寶珠), which appears in the title of the process, suggests a kinship with the Numinous Treasure tradition, because it is in a "precious pearl" that the Celestial Worthy of Original Commencement preaches the *Book of Universal Salvation*.[47] However, the main process is

42 *Daofa huiyuan* (DZ 1220), 114.4b–5b.

43 *Daofa huiyuan* (DZ 1220), 117.2b. We can also see in the *Daofa huiyuan* (111.16b) an eight-turn spiral and above the four characters for lightning, rain, cloud, thunder and wind.

44 *Taishang zhuguo jiumin zongzhen biyao* (DZ 1227), 4.6b.

45 *Mingzhen powang zhangsong* (DZ 979), 1b. Most of the literature about thunder rites makes the same association. For example, it is said in *Daofa huiyuan* (DZ 1220), 111.1: "The non-igneous breath fills the Cinnabar Field, the thunder starts to move in the outbreath, it goes out quickly and rumbles in the sky."

46 See Schipper and Verellen 2004: 1108.

47 See *Yuanshi wuliang duren shangpin miaojing sizhu* (DZ 87), 1.14a: "The Worthy of the Origin suspended a precious pearl of the size of a grain of millet in the Darkness of space, at a distance of fifty feet from the ground. He sent up the celestial Perfected, the great

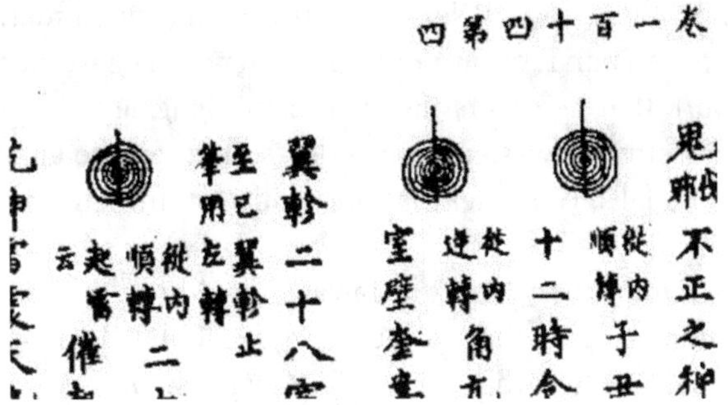

FIGURE 7.2 Thunder talismans in *Daofa huiyuan* (DZ 1220)

presented as originating from Wei Huacun 魏華存, reflecting the link with the Upper Clarity tradition, in accordance with the syncretism observed in the currents using thunder rites. Furthermore, this method which would have been transmitted to the thirty-sixth Heavenly Master Zhang Zongyan 張宗演 (1244–1292), a specialist of the Divine Empyrean legacy, was in the possession of a certain Zhu Meijing 朱梅靖, who lived at Mount Qingcheng 青城 in Sichuan.

In this method, the three characters are described as corresponding to the movements of the Celestial Net, that is to say, the stars of the Northern Dipper around the North Star, of the Supreme Yang (Taiyang) and of the Supreme Yin (Taiyin).[48] These characters, which share with many others the radical of rain were traced by the officiant during the ritual also included incantations, hand gestures, stepped movements, inner visualizations and invocations. The semantic character "rain" is above the characters and is used for the secret name (*hui* 諱) of a deity. It is a celestial element that spreads over the name and is like a canopy protecting, hiding, or imprisoning it.[49] The three above mentioned characters are accompanied by an order that the officiant should

deities, the superior holy men, the Perfected of the meritorious deeds, the supreme gods and the Perfected of the Wuji and of the ten directions. An immeasurable crowd entered this precious pearl in which the primordial Beginning delivered this writing from beginning to end." This passage is adapted from the eleventh chapter of the *Lotus Sutra* where a jeweled stupa appears in space, and Śākyamuni explains that a Buddha of the past has vowed to appear whenever the *Lotus Sutra* would be exposed. Śākyamuni then enters the stupa and continues his sermon.

48 This method is the "Diling baozhu wulei qidao dafa" 帝令寶珠五雷祈禱大法, in *Daofa huiyuan*, 111.11a, 111.12b–14b.

49 Berthier-Baptandier 1993: 9.

recite: "When we first shake the Celestial Net, we emit the following order: "That the general officer of the Thunder Court obey the order of the governor general of the Yanhuo Court, that he orders the great deity Dengxie 鄧燮 to very quickly make the northern and western winds rise, so that on the altar the clouds amass and the rain falls. The order must be applied at the lightning speed.'"[50]

The Celestial Net, the Taiyin (moon) and the Taiyang (sun) are the three lights that play an important role in the Correct Method of the Heart of Heaven, both in rituals and in meditative practice. The *Correct Method of the Heart of Heaven of the Upper Clarity* of the twelfth century indicates a process for ingesting these three breaths:

> Ingesting the Taiyang breath. When the sun is three feet high, turn towards it, pray to the Lord of the Sun, the Sovereign Emperor of Taiyang, to make the true breath descend from its radiant light that floods your whole body. Then through the nose inhale the blue-green breath nine times and swallow it. Repeat the operation nine times (the same process is applied for the breaths of the Taiyin and of the Celestial Net that eliminate evil elements.[51]

The second character, comprising below the radical of the rain elements of the sun and of constancy, is accompanied by the following order: "Order to the Taiyang. The officer of the Thunder Court receives orders from the great general of the Thunder Court to control the iron brush and to order the great deity Xinzhen 辛貞 to make the northern and western winds rise so that they bring rain over the altar. The order must be executed at lightning speed."[52]

The third is accompanied by the following order: "First call to the Taiyin: the officer of the Thunder and Wind Court prepares himself to order his servant, the white tiger Zhang Hou 張后, to quickly assemble the killer wind of the five directions, to sweep and purify the altar and that black clouds amass and spread the rain. The order must be applied at lightning speed."[53]

---

50 *Daofa huiyuan* (DZ 1220), 111.11a.

51 *Shangqing tianxin zhengfa* (DZ 566), la–3a. This text (3.20a) mentions the thirtieth heavenly master Zhang Jixian (1092–1127), a specialist of Divine Empyrean methods.

52 *Daofa huiyuan*, 111.12b.

53 *Daofa huiyuan*, 111.14b.

### 4.2 *The Breaths of the Three Treasures*

On the head, there are three spirals and three points on the forehead linked by a line. These elements are similar to those of a talisman entitled "True talisman of the three pneumas of emptiness and of the jade light of the nine yang, which, by its brightness, destroys the underworld." (See fig. 7.3). This talisman belongs to a rite intended to save beings from the suffering of the nine hells, and is included in a text of the Correct Method of the Heart of Heaven tradition.[54] The three breaths represented by the three spirals are the [original] breath of the Jade Sovereign (*yuhuangzhi qi* 玉皇之炁) or the light of the celestial treasure (*tianbaozhi guang* 天寶之光), the breath of the jade emptiness (*yuxuzhi qi* 玉虛之炁) or the light of the Numinous Treasure (*lingbaozhi guang* 靈寶之光), and the [Original] Breath of the jade flower (*yuhuazhi qi* 玉華之炁) or the light of the divine Treasure (*shenbaozhi guang* 神寶之光). On the *Chart for the Cultivation of Perfection*, three characters are inscribed on the forehead, *ling* 靈, *shen* 神 and *tian* 天with below the character *bao* 寶, and they should be read as three two characters words, "the numinous treasure" (*lingbao* 靈寶) the "celestial treasure" (*tianbao* 天寶) and the "divine treasure" (*shenbao* 神寶),[55] which confirms the link we have established between the three spirals on the head and their symbolism as the light of the Three Treasures presented in the text of the tradition of the Correct Method of the Heart of Heaven cited above (see fig. 7.3).

### 4.3 *The Constellation of the Three Terraces (Santai 三台)*

The three points on the forehead are the representation of the constellation of the Three Terraces. These are three groups of two stars located below the Northern Dipper that cover the Polar Star; they are the canopy of the world and maintain all things at their place. They are the object of multiple rituals and have a protective function of human life.

Their evocation is also characteristic of the texts from the Correct Method of the Heart of Heaven. It is said for example in the *Secret Essentials of the Principal Perfected Assisting the Country and Saving the People*: "Whenever you want to write talismans, you should use the formula related to the Northern Dipper, the shape of the stars of the Three Terraces which drives the stars to transmit the breath which concentrates and flows through the brush. From the top of the upper terrace a yellow breath comes out, from the top of the

54 *Wushang xuanyuan santian yutang dafa* (DZ 220), 15.9b.

55 The Mount Wudang version has "a moxa on the celestial bone" (*jiu tiangu*) and below the character "Treasure" (*bao*).

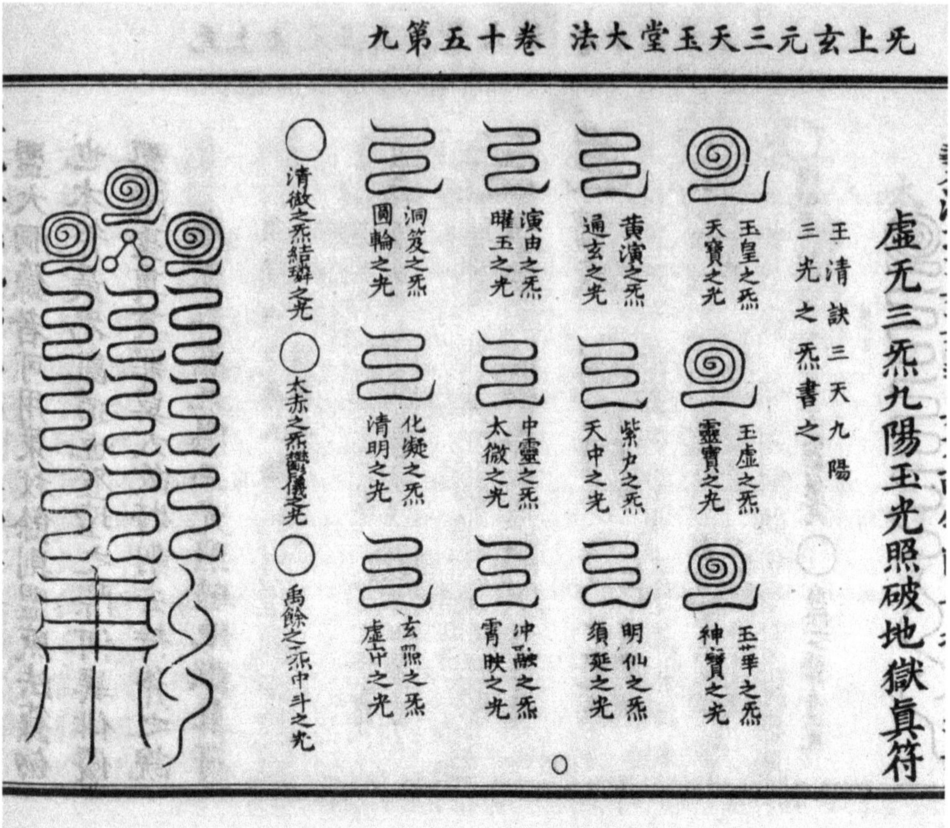


FIGURE 7.3 Talisman of three radiances. *Wushang sanyuan santian yutang dafa* (DZ 220), 15.9b

median terrace, a white breath and from the top of the lower terrace, a blue-green breath."[56] According to the *Great Rites of the Numinous Treasure and of the Highest Purity*, the Three Terraces are [a] the upper terrace which is the stellar sovereign, i.e., the essence of emptiness developing efficient power, [b] the median terrace which is the stellar sovereign Liuchun Sikong, and the [c] lower terrace which is the stellar sovereign Qusheng silu, the worthy of the stars and of the twenty-eight constellations who harmonizes yin and yang and rules over the ten thousand beings.[57] These three points represent the Three Terraces that often appear in the talismans of the Correct Method of the Heart

56 DZ 1227, 2.lob.

57 Wang Qizhen 王契真 (fourteenth century), *Shangqing lingbao dafa* (DZ 1221).

of Heaven.[58] Taking the example of the *Wushang xuanyuan yutang dafa*, the title of the talisman is "Perfected Talisman of the Jade Light of the Nine Yang and of the Three Breaths from the Void that Illuminate and Destroy the Hells" (*Xuwu sanqi jiuyang yuguang zhaopo diyu zhenfu* 虛無三炁九陽玉光照破地獄真符) (fig. 7.4). The explanation of the decomposition of the talisman indicates in each case the names of the breaths and of the lights represented by the spirals and the sinuous lines. The three spirals represent the three lights of the three jewels whose name is inscribed on the forehead of the human body of the *Chart for the Cultivation of Perfection*, corresponding respectively to the Yuhuang, Yuxu and Yuhua breaths. The nine winding lines correspond to the nine yang lights.

The light of the Three Terraces is mentioned in the earliest known texts describing methods of Internal Alchemy, at least in the Southern tradition, since they are mentioned in the *Stanzas on the Awakening to Perfection* of Zhang Boduan, where it is said: "The adept should carefully protect the furnace, accumulate his [breath] in the three [cinnabar] fields, to accomplish the treasure in resonance with the Three Terraces."[59]

### 4.4 *The Destruction of Hells*

As mentioned earlier, hells and paradises are both transposed into the human body. Therefore, given the resonance between inside and outside in these schools, the officiant must also destroy the hells that are in him when he meditates, for him and during rituals for the salvation of souls. By a journey in his body, he destroys all yin within. In this way, he expels any demonic form and at the same time frees others, be it a sick patient, a deceased person or other circumstances. This journey passes through the various palaces discussed in Chapter 4 such as the Fire Palace of the Vermilion Mound and the Cinnabar Hall of the Spirits of the Cold.

Besides the three lights the officiant ingests and the Three Terraces mentioned above, on the *Chart for the Cultivation of Perfection*, we note the presence in the median part of seven characters having the demon radical. These are the secret names of the Stellar Lords of the Northern Dipper's Seven

58 See *Daofa huiyuan* (DZ 1220), 118.14b–16a, in a method of the Divine Empyrean tradition, where the talisman is formed by the three points and, below the head, the body of the talisman drawn with sinuous lines. Or *Lingbao wuliang duren shangjing dafa* (DZ 219), 36.28b, including the drawing of three points and the incantation on the Three Terraces. This method aims to control demons and comprises elements of the Divine Empyrean literature.

59 See *Wuzhen pian zhushi* (DZ 145), 2.28a.

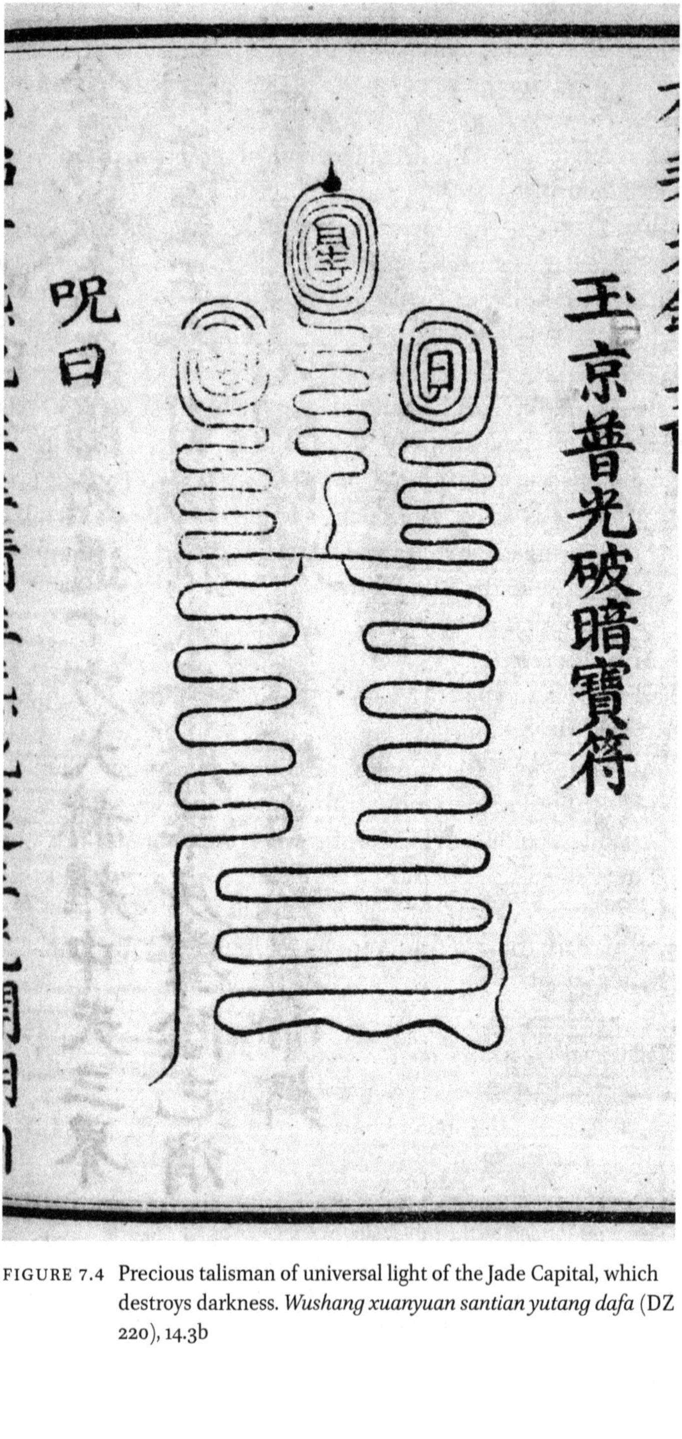


FIGURE 7.4 Precious talisman of universal light of the Jade Capital, which destroys darkness. *Wushang xuanyuan santian yutang dafa* (DZ 220), 14.3b

Origins (*Beidou qiyuan xingjun* 北斗七元星君).[60] They form an incantation that opens the door of the city of hells and allows the wandering spirits to be saved.[61] These secret names are also used for exorcist and therapeutic purposes. For example, they are pronounced in a therapeutic ritual and the writing of talismans to cure in particular the epidemics of fever malaria[62] or in a method of incantations and writing talismans that originated with Lei Shizhong 雷時中 (1121–1295) and Lu Shizhong 路時中. These two Taoists who have had many disciples are associated with the creation of the rites of the Jade Hall (Yutang 玉堂). These are essentially meditative practices close to those of internal alchemy even though the function is mainly exorcist. This method includes an incantation intended to cure the intrusion of evil elements and to protect the body.[63]

Parallel to the external rites, the practitioner should therefore practice visualizations destroying hells in his body, as in this type of practice described in the *Summary Principles on the Internal Process for Refining according to the Great Ultimate Principle* (thirteenth century):

> Sublimation when sitting in silence. The day that we practice sacrifices and refinement, write a cinnabar yang talisman and the precious registers. In the evening, before the food offerings, burn incense, arrange a bamboo stick, a bowl of pure water and another bowl of pure water to serve as a purification basin. Burn the cinnabar yang talisman and throw it in the purification basin, then burn the precious registers in the furnace. When all the preparation is finished, sit in meditation and do not move until the end of the practice. After completing the ritual of inner purification, think that the Worthy Great One (Taiyi) saving all suffering beings is sitting in your Niwan palace [head]. He makes a great genuflection, recites the secret incantation and spreads an infinite light destroying all the hells of the underworld. Then, visualize the Worthy Great One spreading an infinite light which originates from the Niwan and moves towards the North [downwards], crosses the eighteen degrees [of the spine], until the Spinal Handle Pass, and continues into the region below the two kidneys called the City of darkness; all the hells are illuminated by the

---

60 See *Daofa huiyuan* (DZ 1220), 121.8b, "Talisman of the ice pond" (bingchi fu 冰池符) used to diminish fever in a patient and with these names: *fu, xing, huan, bi, piao, kui, shao*.

61 See *Daofa huiyuan* (DZ 1220), 207.2a.

62 See *Daofa huiyuan* (DZ 1220), 211. 5b.

63 See *Daofa huiyuan* (DZ 1220), 154.19b.

> dazzling light shining on this triple world, its sufferings, and emptying the hells.[64]

Zhang Yuchu (late fourteenth century) gives a more hermetic and more succinct description:

> Below the kidneys is found the labyrinthic palace of the yin sources, the Luofeng, infernal city of the North. With my true light, I completely dispel the darkness, I move the true water of Taiyin [kidneys] to the *dong* 東 and *jing* 井 constellations to wash and purify the wandering spirits, then I save them with the fire of Li in the South, of Taiyang [heart], with which I refine them.[65]

A document of the Correct Method of the Heart of Heaven tradition states that it is the light of the Celestial Net that destroys evil and the hells:

> The Master said: "Use the true light of the great mighty virtue of the Celestial Net to illuminate and destroy the evil and the demons and transform pain into happiness. The method consists of using the twenty-eight constellations distributed to the four sides, during the twelve periods of the day, and to control them with the Celestial Net."[66]

It is probable that the reference in the centre of the *Chart for the Cultivation of Perfection* to the seven stars of the Northern Dipper, to the Celestial Net and to the twenty-eight constellations, alludes to the inner sky which will destroy the hells, in conjunction with the external rituals performed by the officiant. This *Chart for the Cultivation of Perfection* includes a number of key elements of this practice: the reference to the Great One (Taiyi) at the level of the head, the secret incantation opening the door of the hells in the central region near the heart, the mention of the City of Darkness and of the nine hells in the region below the kidneys. These elements are therefore mnemonic benchmarks for the follower who has to perform a process similar to that described in the

64 Zheng Sixiao 鄭思肖 (Suonan 所南) (1241–1318), *Taiji jilian neifa* (DZ 548), 1.5ab. This can be compared with the description of the inner cultivation of the adept, as described in *Lingbao dalian neizhi xingchao jiyao* 靈寶大煉內旨行持機要 [Summary for the practices of the esoteric instructions of the great numinous treasure sublimation rite] (DZ 407); English translation by Lagerwey 1987: 233–234).

65 See *Yuanshi lingbao wuliang duren jing zhu* (DZ 89), 2.14b.

66 *Wushang xuanyuan santian yutang dafa* (DZ 220), 22.2a–b.

text above. The essential idea is the union of the interior and the exterior, the transparency and the luminosity from the top to the bottom of the body and of the universe. In one thought, the light flashes up to the Nine Empyreans, it destroys the hells below, and the follower loses the perception of the existence of his body.[67]

67 See the *Erlan Xinhua* 二懶心話 [Spiritual words of the two lazy] in the collection of the *Daozang xubian*, lb: "When applying this practice for a long time, i.e., the practice of *neizhao* 内照 [Inner illumination], it seems that pure light flashed up to the Nine Empyreans and destroyed the nine lower sources. At this point, the adept loses the feeling of his body."

# Conclusion

Analysis of the *Chart for Cultivation of Perfection* demonstrates this Taoist representation of the body dates from the Qing dynasty, probably not earlier than the eighteenth century. Yet, it resonates with the drawings of the body and alchemical processes which have developed since the drawings of Yanluozi (tenth century) under the Song, Yuan and Ming dynasties. Most of its visual elements are richer than those of Yanluozi; they are inspired by diagrams found in alchemical texts of Song and Yuan. Moreover, in spite of this evolution, the drawings, even though they present variants, nevertheless display a remarkable continuity.

The place and the date of creation of the original *Chart for Cultivation of Perfection* remains uncertain. All the known copies come from temples belonging to the Dragon Gate lineage, which in many places have developed alchemical techniques linked to the cultivation of perfection and to thunder rites. The known versions show a broad diffusion of the chart.

The alchemical techniques mentioned in the form of symbols, captions, texts or drawings, correspond to texts from the Ming and Qing dynasties. The symbolic language of these charts is not as heavily influenced by laboratory terms as was the case in the Song dynasty. Rather, its language makes reference to the natural world, the animal world, and the heavens. The exchange and union process between opposites such as yin and yang, water and fire, are described in poetic terms. It is likewise for the process of transmutation of the three basic ingredients (the spermatic essence, the breath and the spirit), or the five agents (wood, fire, earth, metal, water). These changes occur in three steps suggested by the symbolism of three chariots represented along the spine, drawings already present on the Yanluozi diagrams (tenth century).

There is also emphasis on specific elements of the southern alchemical tradition linked to Zhang Boduan, such as the representation of orifices as places of transition from one reality to another, places of transmutation and access points to reality. Similarly, the kidneys are of paramount importance. It is the subject of several diagrams and inscriptions consisting of terminology found in the alchemical texts of the southern tradition. Here is situated the pivot of transformations, the root of life, the place from where springs thunder. But the unique feature of this body map is the close link established between Inner Alchemy and the thunder rites, combining inner meditation, visualizations and rituals in a simultaneous action on the inner world of the officiant and the outside world.

 | DOI:10.1163/9789004383456_010

The body itself is not drawn according to visual reality, but as a cosmological place and a sacred area. It is the perfected state (*zhen* 真) of the body, just as the charts of the Five Peaks are the real and efficient representations of the five mountains. In the empty space of the sheet, the representations by lines are only there to evoke the places for the realization of the Way or of alchemical process. If Yanluozi had drawn two representations more anatomical in style next to the alchemical representations, these types of representations have completely disappeared in later Taoist works, especially when the charts underwent simplification. Indeed, if the depictions of the six viscera remained on the *Chart for the Cultivation of Perfection*, would it not be even more important to highlight the central representation of the "alchemical pot." This pot was the trapeze with above the cruciform flower and its centre, the lines being there to contain the inscriptions about the transformations in five viscera and the five directions, and evoke the image of the athanor, place of transmutations.

The image of the body, an oval outline from which the limbs are absent, is a stylistic form that first appeared in the Song dynasty. Indeed, if the lower limbs are represented, crossed in lotus posture in accordance with the meditation technique commonly used, they appear more like a support for the central oval than an integral part of the body. The more the body is refined, the more its contours disappear until reinstatement to the Way, to emptiness.

Even more than in the other representations, the circle dominates, or at least the idea of circular motion. It is suggested by numerous circles: the circle crowning the head, the central circles forming a flower, the circles of the three passes, the circle inside the kidneys, without forgetting the encircled characters. This habit of drawing circles for representing the unity that comprise the phenomena or the movement probably goes back to the school of Chan Buddhism. A nested circle of black and white rings, a probable model of representation of the "Chart of the Great Ultimate" (*Taiji tu*), represents the Ālayavijñāna, the eighth cognitive faculty of Buddhism called "storehouse consciousness," support of all knowable, receptacle of the seeds of all phenomena.[1] This diagram is integrated into a text on the history of Chan Buddhism written by Zongmi (780–841), a specialist in both Chan and Flower Ornament (Avatamsaka) Buddhist schools. It also exists in the Buddhist context

1 On this drawing, cf. Michael Lackner, "Die Verplanung am Beispiel der Denkens of T'u", 1990. The drawing of the *ālayavijñāna* is in the Taisho 2015 *Chanyuan zhuquan ji duxu* by Zongmi (780–841), p. 413, its authenticity is disputed however, because the drawing is not only on later editions.

representations by five black or white circles of the "Map of the Five Positions" (*Wuwei tu* 五位圖) representing schematically five positions of the mind in its relation to the world, or five forms of relationship between the noumenal and the phenomenal, the universal and the personal, the one and the many, according to the Cao Dong school (ninth century) of Chan Buddhism.[2] He also recalled the use of the circle by two masters of one of the five main schools of Chan Buddhism: the Guiyang school. Guishan Lingyou 溈山靈佑 (775–853) and Yangshan Huiji 仰山慧寂 (807–883) used the circle in their teaching, to express the totality, the relations between the one and the multiple, and the simultaneous understanding of the noumenal and the phenomenal.[3] But in the Taoist context it also bears the connotation of a magical place, a place of passage called hole, cavity, pass, a locus of transmutation, of all possibilities. It is also the delimitation of a space, and the control of the object: when a Taoist adept draws a character in a circle, he fixes and controls the object or the god represented.

In the *Chart for the Cultivation of Perfection*, we find the semantic component of "rain" representing the breath of Supreme Yin (Taiyin), the Supreme Yang (Taiyang) and the Celestial Net. One essential difference between this *Chart* and other known body maps is the representation of the thirty lunar phases around the body, which strongly evokes the dynamism, the waxing and waning cycle of yin and yang, and the phases of the sun and of the moon, in both the microcosm and the macrocosm. While characters designating the phases of the new moon, full moon and the moon quarters are inscribed on the representation of the *Book for Universal Salvation*, they are replaced here by drawings and we cannot truly say that there has been an amalgam with the representation of the alchemical mirror of Xiao Peng. We note that in any case, under the Qing Dynasty, the lunar phases tend to be represented by drawings.[4]

The *Chart for the Cultivation of Perfection*, while continuing the body maps examined since the Song, stands out from the fact that, contrary to the drawings of Yanluozi or the *Chart of the Inner Landscape* which essentially represent the internal work of cultivation of Self through alchemical processes, it concerns an internal cultivation for an external use and an exteriorization during the rituals. These are in this case rituals linked to the Thunder rites. The history of the dissemination of the Chart in the various regions of China, Chengdu,

2 The Cao Dong school is named after its two founders masters Dongshan Liangjie 洞山良价 (807–869) and Caoshan Benji 曹山本寂 (840–901). Of these five positions, consult Lu 1971: 127–163.

3 See the biography of Yangshan Huiji in *Wudeng huiyuan*, 9.532–533.

4 See Liu Mingrui's drawings in *Qiaoqiao dongzhang* (2.3a); Wu Chongxu, *Tianxian zhengli zhilun nei jindan xinfa mizhi*, in *Daozang jinghua*, 19.

Mount Wudang, Baiyun Guan of Beijing and various places on the East Coast, does not allow us to link it to a particular school of the thunder rites. The intrinsic study of the palaces invoked, the divinities, the talismans, the references to paradises and hells, the terminology, suggests that they are rites which belong to a school linked to the Correct Method of the Heart of Heaven and to the rites of the Jade Hall developed by Lu Shizhong (after 1138) and Lei Shizhong. The rites of the Jade Hall are defined as the "internal secrets" of the Correct Method of the Heart of Heaven.

Lei Shizhong (1121–1295) gravitated to the Mount Wudang area and had many disciples. Even if the existing copies of the *Chart for the Cultivation of Perfection* do not give that of Mount Wudang as the oldest, it is not impossible that it is nevertheless the place of origin of this chart. As regards palaces and alchemical terminology, the *Chart for the Cultivation of Perfection* is a continuation of the Universal salvation scripture's comments and is also based on the *Combined Scriptures of the Founding Acts of the Jade Emperor on High* (13th century), an important text for the current of the Pure Subtility, but also in the Dragon Gate tradition and other currents employing the thunder rites.

This representation of the body is a "diagram" (*tu* 圖), or a "diagram and register" (*tulu* 圖籙). It is related to other famous diagrams of Taoism, especially the Numinous Treasure and alchemical traditions. One Song text, the *Representations of the Original Chaotic Great Ultimate in the Culture of Perfection* by Xiao Daocun, makes great use of the drawings, notably the circles. From the Song onwards, the habit to illustrate the methods for the cultivation of perfection became more and more numerous. The question arises, as with most of maps: how should we read them?[5]

An overall reading of this diagram is comparable to "creative thinking" (*yi* 意), the internal image that allows the efficient implementation of any act and empowers creation.[6] The role of a register, as is suggested by the name given on the version of the Dragon and Tiger Altar, the magical aspect, talismanic, one could even say exorcist, is certainly present. We know only the circumstances of the etching of the stele of the Wudang Mountains, created at the anniversary of Lü Dongbin, and we have found that commemorative steles of an almost talismanic value were often engraved on the occasion of important cultural ceremonies. Laszlo Legeza mentions this talismanic value of the steles. While Zhejiang Province was often affected by fires, an official had engraved a "Diagram for the Perfected Warrior to Push away the Fire" ("Zhenwu bihuo tu" 真武避火圖). He says: "I instructed Chen Jijin, Deputy Director of Studies, to copy and ... to oversee how it would be engraved on stone to be implemented

5 See Lackner 1990.
6 See Berthier-Baptandier 1993: 59–92.

across provincial towns, in order to expel evil influences originating from the site, while remaining available those wishing to make prints."[7] This *Chart for the Cultivation of Perfection* is reminiscent in many ways of talismans, especially those drawn with a head and representating a god's body,[8] a sacred geography.

One finds in the *Great Method of the Jade Hall of the Three Heavens, of the Supreme Mysterious Origin* a series of six talismans having a human form and representing a body, which are intended to purify the body of different elements: the three corpses and the seven *po*; they eliminate the fatigues of the heart due to the passions, to sex, to avidity, the wilting of the complexion, the fatigue of the body (see fig. 7.5).

Talismans are the body of primordial breath allowing the access to the sacred world, they are the "perfected form" (*zhenxing* 真形) and the revelation of Reality. Likewise, the *Chart for the Cultivation of Perfection* is made of primordial breath, it guides the adept who, at different states creates this inner landscape and becomes efficient.

In Taoism, the relationship between the diagrams (*tu*), the talismans (*fu* 符), and the registers (*lu* 籙), has already been noted; Brigitte Baptandier has even translated the term *tu* as a "talismanic table,"[9] an expression which is well suited to our representation, actually built as a talisman. We find similar components, such as circled characters, trigrams, spirals, pictographic parts, symbolic system, and inscriptions. The body of the follower himself is a talisman, in the sense that it includes only half of the elements, its counterpart being in the celestial world or the world of the Perfection (*zhen* 真). According to the *Book of the Abyssal Perfection* (*Dongzhen jing*), "the gods of the body command 18,000 deities. When man concentrates his mind on them, the 18,000 deities do not disperse, in this case, the heavens bring down 18,000 other deities to complete the interior of the body, which made 36,000 deities in all, which together raise the whole body and make it ascend to the three heavens. Then the man becomes a divine immortal, his transformation is flawless."[10] Thus this *Chart for the Cultivation of Perfection* is not a representation of the body, it is a double of the body, a sort of grimoire. In fact, it is at the same time by its exploration and suddenly in its totality that, like a mirror, this diagram reveals the organization and the operation of the world of the meditator, which is that of his body, the universe and of the world of the gods.

---

7 Legeza 1976: 121.

8 See *Wushang xuanyuan santian yutang dafa* (DZ 220), 10.5b–6b. Or *Dongxuan lingbao wuliang duren shangpin jing dafa* (DZ 219), 68.23a 68.24a.

9 See Berthier-Baptandier 1993.

10 *Wushang biyao* (DZ 1138), 5.12b–14b.

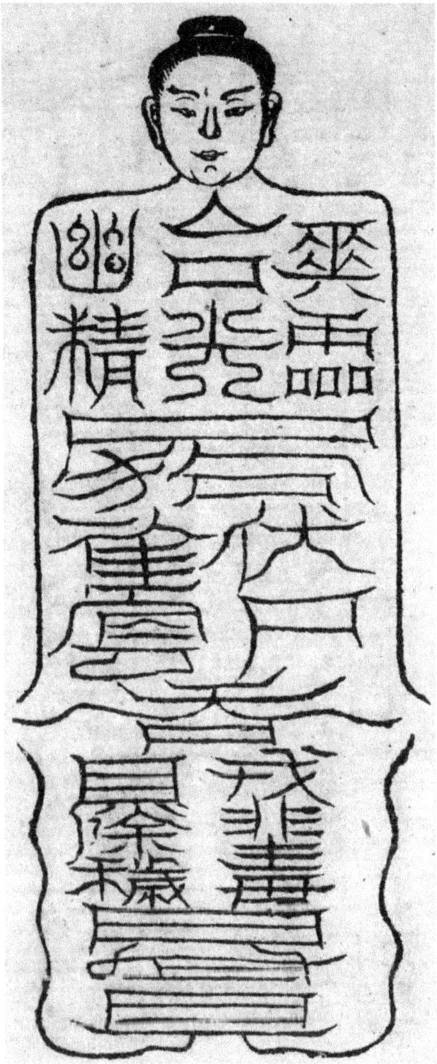

*Wushang xuanyuan santian yutang dafa*, 20.12b

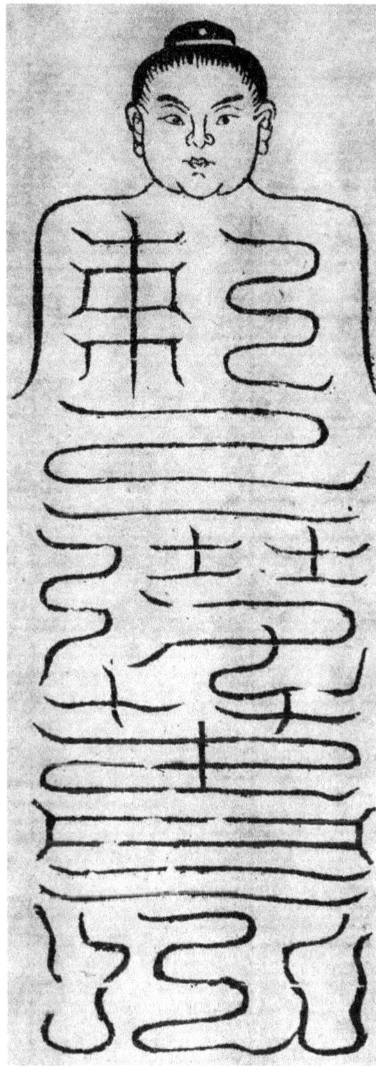

*Wushang xuanyuan santian yutang dafa*, 20.13a

CONCLUSION Talismans evoking the shape of the human body. *Wushang xuanyuan santian yutang dafa* (DZ 220), 20.12b–13a

# Bibliography

## Abréviations

DZ: Daozang (Taoist Canon)
T.: Taisho (Buddhist Canon)
BEFEO: Bulletin de l'École francaise d'Extrême-Orient
EFEO: École française d'Extrême-Orient
SKQS: *Siku quanshu* 四庫全書 (Wenyuange 文淵閣)

## Primary Sources


*Baoyi hansan bijue* 抱一函三秘訣 [Secret instructions on holding the One and encasing the three]. Eds. Jin Yueyan 金月巖 and Huang Gongwang 黃公望 (1269–1354). DZ 576.

*Baoyi zi Sanfeng laoren danjue* 抱一子三峰老人丹訣 [Alchemical instructions of the old man three peaks, the master holding the One]. Eds. Jin Yueyan 金月巖 and Huang Gongwang 黃公望 (1269–1354). DZ 281.

*Beidou zhifa wuwei jing* 北斗治法武威經 [Scripture of martial power, of the method of ruling from the Northern Dipper]. DZ 870.

*Bichuan Zhengyang zhenren lingbao bifa* 祕傳正陽真人靈寶秘法 [Secret transmission of Master Zhengyang's complete methods of the Numinous Treasure]. A Song text attributed to Zhongli Quan 鍾離權. DZ 1191.

*Binhu maixue. Qijing bamai kao* 瀕湖脈學奇經八脈考 [Pulses according to Li Shizhen]. Study on the eight marvelous vessels]. Li Shizhen 李時珍 (1518–1593). Beijing: Zhongguo zhongyiyao chubanshe, 2007.

*Bintui lu* 賓退錄 [Records after the guest has left] by Zhao Yushi 趙與時 (1175–1231), ed. *SKQS*.

*Chanyuan zhu quanji duxu* 禪源諸詮集都序 [Preface to the collected writings on the source of Chan]. Zongmi 宗密 (780–841). T. 2015, vol. 48.

*Chen Xubai guizhong zhinan* 陳虛白規中指南 [True central directions by Master Chen Xubai]. Chen Chongsu 陳冲素 nicknamed Xubai zi 虛白子 (1279–1368). DZ 243.

*Chuci zhangju* 楚辭章句 [Elegies of Chu, semantic and syntaxic analysis], ed. Wang Yi 王逸. *SKQS*.

*Chunqiu fanlu* 春秋繁露 [Luxuriant gems of the Spring and Autumn]. Dong Zhongshu 董仲舒 (195/179–115/104). *Hanwei congshu* 漢魏叢書.

*Chushi yishu* 褚氏逸書 [Documents bequeathed by Master Chu]. Attributed to Chu Cheng 褚澄 (Six Dynasties). In *Shuofu* 說郛, ed. Tao Zongyi 陶宗儀 (1321–1407), j. 74.

*Cuigong ruyao jing zhujie* 崔公入藥鏡註解 [Commentary on Master Cui's mirror to enter the art of elixir]. Cui Xifan 崔希範 (ob. 940); commentary by Wang Jie 王玠 (14th century). DZ 135 and *Xiuzhen shishu* 修真十書 [Ten books on the cultivation of perfection] (DZ 263), 13.1a.

*Cunzhen huanzhong tu* 存真環中圖 [Chart on the cycles for maintining the Perfection]. Yang Jie 楊介, preface by Jia Weijie 賈偉節 (1113). Lost.

*Dacheng jiejing* 大成捷徑 [The path to the great accomplishment]. Ed. Liu Huayang 柳華陽 (1736–?). Taibei: Zhenshanmei chubanshe, 1967.

*Dadan zhizhi* 大丹直指 [Clear directions on the great elixir]. Attributed to Qiu Chuji 邱處機 (Changchun 長春) (1148–1227). DZ 244.

*Dadong yujing* 大洞玉經 [The scripture of the great cavern] (DZ 7).

*Da Ming Xuantian shangdi ruiying tulu* 大明玄天上帝瑞鷹圖錄 [Illustrated album on the auspicious miracles performed by the supreme the arch of the dark heaven]. DZ 959.

*Daode jing* 道德經 [The scripture on the way and its virtue]. Attributed to Laozi 老子.

*Daofa huiyuan* 道法會元 [Taoist methods, united in principle]. DZ 1220.

*Daofa xinchuan* 道法心傳 [Spiritual tradition of Taoist rites]. Wang Weiyi 王惟一 (ob. 1294). DZ 1253.

*Daoji lingxian ji* 道迹靈仙記 [Annals of numinous transcendents from the traces of the Tao]. DZ 597.

*Daomen shigui* 道門十規 [Ten rules for Taoists]. Zhang Yuchu 張宇初 (1361–1410). DZ 1232.

*Daoshu* 道樞 [Pivot of the way]. Zeng Zao 曾慥 (ca. 1145). DZ 1017.

*Daoyuan yiqi* 道元一炁 [The breath of the One, origin of the Tao]. Cao Heng 曹珩 or Cao Yuanbai 曹元白 (1636), preface by Guo Shihao 郭士豪. Reprint Beijing: Beijing Normal University Press, ed., 1990.

*Daozang* 道藏 [Taoist Canon]. A Ming printing reproduction of 1444. Taibei: Xinwenfeng chubanshe, ed., 1977.

*Daozang jinghua* 道藏精華 [Quintessence of the Taoist canon]. Xiao Tianshi 蕭天石, ed. Taibei: Ziyou chubanshe, 1956–979.

*Daozang jiyao* 道藏輯要 [Essentials of the Taoist canon]. Edited during the *kangxi* era (1662–1722) by Peng Dingqiu 彭定求 at the Qingyang Tenoke in Chengdu. Reprint in 1820 by Jiang Yuanting 蔣元庭 and in 1906 by He Longxiang 賀龍襄.

*Daozang xubian* 道藏續編 [Sequel to the Taoist canon], 1834. Ed. Min Yide 閔一得.

*Dayue Taiheshan zhi* 大嶽太和山志 [Monograph on the mountain of the great harmony]. Ren Ziyuan 任自垣 (1431). In *Daojiao wenxian* 道教文献 (FB 784:7.4–5) (http://www.lib.cam.ac.uk/mulu/fb78407.html).

*Dengzhen yinjue* 登真隱訣 [Secret instructions for the ascent to Perfection]. Tao Hongjing 陶弘景 (456–536). DZ 421.

*Dongtian fudi yuedu mingshan ji* 洞天福地嶽瀆名山記 [Record of the cavern-heavens, auspicious sites, holy mountains, and marshes, and famous mountains], Du Guangting 杜光庭 (850–933). DZ 599.

*Dongxuan lingbao zhenling weiye tu* 洞玄靈寶真靈位業圖 [Table of the ranks and functions in the pantheon]. Tao Hongjing 陶弘景 (456–536). DZ 167.

*Dongzhen Taishang daojun yuandan shangjing* 洞真太上道君元丹上經 [Superior scripture of the mysterious cinnabar]. DZ 1345.

*Dongzhen Taishang suling dongyuan dayou miaojing* 洞真太上素靈洞元大有妙經 [The marvelous scripture of the unadorned spirituality and the vast possessions]. DZ 1314.

*Dongzhen Taiyi dijun taidan yinshu dongzhen xuanjing* 洞真太一帝君太丹隱書洞真玄經 [Mysterious scripture of Dongzhen and hidden documents on the supreme elixir according to the Lord Emperor and the Great One]. DZ 1330.

*Erlan xinhua* 二懶心話 [Spiritual sayings of the two lazy men]. Ed. Min Yide 閔一得. In *Daozang xubian* 道藏續編, 1834.

*Fangguang da zhuangyan jing* 方廣大莊嚴經 [Lalitavistara]. Translated by Divākara (613–688), T. 187, vol. 3.

*Fo benxing jijing* 佛本行集經 [Lalitavistara]. Trans. Jñānagupta (523–600). T. 190, vol. 3.

*Gaoshang shenxiao yuqing zhenwang zishu dafa* 高上神霄玉清真王紫書大法 [Great magic from the purple book of the perfected king of the highest divine empyrean jade purity]. DZ 1219.

*Gaoshang Yuhuang benxing jijing* 高上玉皇本行集經 [Combined scriptures of the founding acts of the Jade Emperor on high]. DZ 10.

*Gaoshang Yuhuang benxing jingsui* 高上玉皇本行經髓 [Essentials of the combined scriptures of the founding acts of the Jade Emperor on high]. Liu Chuyuan 劉處元 (Yuan). DZ 12.

*Gezhi congshu* 格致叢書 [Collectaneum of thorough investigation]. Ed. Hu Wenhuan 胡文煥 (ca. late 16th century). 1603.

*Hailu suishi* 海錄碎事 [Some crumbs from the oceanic writings]. Ye Tinggui 葉廷珪 (*ca.* 1115). Shanghai: Shanghai guji chubanshe, 1989.

*Han Wudi neizhuan* 漢武帝內傳 [The Inner story of the Emperor Wu of the Han]. DZ 292.

*Huainan zi zhushi* 淮南子注釋 [Commentary on the works of the prince of Huainan]. Liu An 劉安 (*ca.* 179–122), commentary by Gao You 高誘 (*ca.* 168–112). Taibei: Hualian chubanshe, ed., 1973.

*Huandan bijue yang chizi shenfang* 還丹秘訣養赤子神方 [Divine recipes for nourishing the infant according to the secret process of returned cinnabar]. Xu Mingdao 許明道 (ca. late 12th century). DZ 232.

*Huangdi bashiyi nanjing zuantu jujie* 黃帝八十一難經纂圖句解 [Phrase-by-phrase glosses of the eighty-one difficulties of the Yellow Emperor's canon], 1269. Li Jiong 李炯. DZ 1024.

*Huangdi bashiyi nanjing zhushi tuxu lun* 黃帝八十一難經注釋圖序論 [Treatise with illustrations and commentaries on the eighty-one difficulties of the Yellow Emperor's canon], 1269. Li Jiong 李駉. DZ 1024.

*Huangdi neijing Lingshu jing* 黃帝內經靈樞經. See *Lingshu*.

*Huangdi neijing suwen* 黃帝內經素問 [Inner canon of the Yellow Emperor, basic questions]. Taibei: Xuanfeng chubanshe, ed., 1974.

*Huangdi yinfu jing zhu* 黃帝陰符經註 [Commentary on the *Huangdi yinfu jing*]. Ed. Tang Chun 唐淳. DZ 121.

*Huangting dunjia yuanshen jing* 黃庭盾甲緣身經 [Book of the hidden period and the causal karma body of the yellow court]. In *Yunji qiqian* [Seven lots from the bookcase of the clouds]. DZ 1032, 14.

*Huangting neijing yujing zhu* 黃庭內景玉經註 [Commentary on the precious book of the inner landscape of the yellow court]. Commentary by Liangqiu zi 梁丘子 (Tang). DZ 402.

*Huangting neijing wuzang liufu buxie tu* 黃庭內景五藏六府補瀉圖 [Chart on the procedures of tonification and purgation of the six receptacles and five viscera according to the inner landscape of the yellow court]. Ed. Hu Yin 胡愔. DZ 432; and *Xiuzhen shishu* (DZ 263), 54.

*Huangting neiwai yujing jingjie* 黃庭內外景玉經解 [Commentary on the precious book of the outer landscape of the yellow court]. Commentary by Liangqiu zi 梁丘子. DZ 407.

*Huangting waijing jing* 黃庭外景經 [Precious book of the outer landscape of the yellow court]. DZ 403.

*Hua Tuo xuanmen neizhao tu* 華陀玄門內照圖 [Drawings of the interior of the body by Hua Tuo]. 1095; reproduced by Sun Huan 孫煥 in 1273. Reprint in *Daozang jinghua*, vol. 14–2. Taibei: Ziyou chubanshe, ed., 1976.

*Jianwuji* 漸悟集 [Gradual enlightenment]. Ma Danyang (1123–1183). DZ 1142.

*Jindan dacheng ji* 金丹大成集 [Collected works on the great accomplishment of the elixir]. Xiao Tingzhi 蕭庭芝. In *Xiuzhen shishu* 修真十書, DZ 263, 9–13.

*Jindan sibai zi* 金丹四百字 [The elixir explained in four hundred words]. Attributed to Zhang Boduan 張伯端. DZ 1081.

*Jin'gai xindeng* 金蓋心燈 [Spiritual lamp of the golden canopy]. Min Yide 閔一得 (1749–1836), Yunchao gushu yinlou cangban. Reprint, 1876. In *Zangwai daoshu* 藏外道書, vol. 31.

*Jingang jing* 金剛經: an abbreviated title. See T. 235, vol. 8 *Jingang boruo boluomi jing* 金剛般若波羅密經, translated by Kumārajīva.

*Jingudong zhi* 金鼓洞志 [Monograph on the Metal Drum Grotto] (1807). In *Zangwai daoshu*, vol. 20.

*Jinye huandan yinzheng tu* 金液還丹印證圖 [Illustrations of the return of the liquified gold to the cinnabar field]. Longmei zi 龍眉子, preface of 1218. DZ 151.

*Jishuo huiming jing* 集說慧命經 [Collection of texts on wisdom and vital force]. Liu Huayang 柳華陽. In *Wu Liu xianzong quanji* 伍柳仙宗全集.

*Laozi Xiang'er zhu jiaozheng* 老子想爾註校證 [The Xiang'er Commentary to the Laozi. Critical Edition]. Rao Zongyi 饒宗頤, ed. Shanghai: Shanghai guji chubanshe, 1991.

*Lidou weiyi* 禮斗威儀 [Magnificent ceremonial rites of Northern Dipper]. In *Huangshi yishu kao* 黃氏遺書考 [Study of the lost books by Master Huang]. Huang Shi 黃奭 (1809–1853). Shanghai: Shanghai guji chubanshe, ed., 1996.

*Liexian zhuan* 列仙傳 [Biographies of famous transcendents]. Liu Xiang 劉向 (Han). DZ 294.

*Lingbao bifa* 靈寶秘法. See *Michuan zhengyang zhenren* 秘傳正陽真人.

*Lingbao dalian neizhi xingchi jiyao* 靈寶大煉內旨行持機要 [Summary for the practices of the esoteric instructions of the great Lingbao sublimation rite]. Lin Lingzhen 林靈真 (1239–1302). DZ 407.

*Lingbao guikong jue* 靈寶歸空訣 [Lingbao instructions for returning to the void]. Zhao Yizhen 趙宜真 (d. 1382). DZ 568.

*Lingbao lingjiao jidu jinshu* 靈寶靈教濟度金書 [Golden book of salvation according to the Lingbao tradition]. Transmitted by Ning Quanzhen 寧全真 (1101–1181), compilation attributed to Lin Lingzhen 林靈真 (1239–1302). DZ 466.

*Lingbao taiji lianfa* 靈寶太極煉法 [Method of sublimation of the taiji in the numinous treasure tradition]. Ed. He Huaide 何懷德. From private holdings of Patrice Fava.

*Lingbao wuliang duren shangpin dafa* 靈寶無量度人上品大法 [Great rites of the book of universal salvation]. DZ 219.

*Lingbao wuliang duren shangpin miaojing futu* 靈寶無量度人上品妙經符圖 [Talismans and charts of the *Book of Universal Salvation*]. DZ 147.

*Lingshu jing* 靈樞經 [Pivot of numinous spirits]. In *Sibu beiyao* 四部備要, Taibei: Zhonghua shuju, 1969.

*Lishi zhenxian tidao tongjian houji* 歷世真仙體道通鑑後記 [Continuation of the comprehensive mirror of transcendents who embodied the Tao through the ages]. Ed. Zhao Daoyi 趙道一. DZ 298.

*Lü Chunyang zhenren qinyuan chun danci zhujie* 呂純陽真人沁園春丹詞註解 [Explanation of the alchemical lyric 'Spring in the Garden by the Qin' by the perfected Lü Dongbin]. Commentary by Yu Yan 俞琰 (1258–1314). DZ 136.

*Lüzu quanshu* 呂祖全書 [Complete book of the patriarch Lü Dongbin]. Edition of 1868 by the Chongshantang in Hunan. Taibei: Ziyou chubanshe, ed. 1967.

*Lüzu zhi* 呂祖志 [Monograph on the patriarch Lü Dongbin]. DZ 1484.

*Mengqi bitan* [Brush talks from the dream brook]. See Hu Daojing.

*Mingshi* 明史 [History of the Ming dynasty]. Beijing: Zhonghua shuju, 1974.

*Mingzhen powang zhangsong* 明真破望章頌 [Stanzas of understanding truth and refuting error]. Zhang Jixian 張繼先 (1092–1127). DZ 979.

*Nanjing tuyi* 難經圖義. See *Huangdi bashiyi nanjing*.

*Neiwaigong tushuo jiyao* 內外功圖說輯要 [Illustrated principles on inner and outer practices]. Ed. Xi Yukang 席裕康. Taibei: Ziyou chubanshe, 1920.

*Panxi ji* 磻溪集 [Panxi collection]. Ed. Qiu Chuji 丘處機 (Changchun 長春) (1148–1227). DZ 1159.

*Puyao jing* 普耀經 [*Lalitavistara*]. Translated by Dharmarakṣa. T. 186, vol. 3.

*Qianlong jiyuan xianzhi* 乾隆济源縣志 [Monograph of the district Jiyuan from the Qianlong era].

*Qiaoqiao dongzhang* 敲蹻洞章 [Cavern chapters of Master Qiaoqiao]. Liu Mingrui 劉名瑞 (1839–1933). 1892; Taibei: Zhenshanmei chubanshe, 1965.

*Qijing bamai kao* 奇經八脈考 [A study on the eight marvellous vessels]. Ed. Li Shizhen 李時珍 (1518–1593). See *Binhu maixue*.

*Qingwei danjue* 清微丹訣 [Instructions for the practice of inner alchemy of the pure tenuity school]. DZ 278.

*Qingwei xianpu* 清微仙譜 [Chronology of the transcendents of the pure tenuity heaven]. Ed. Huang Shunshen 黄舜申 (ca. 1224–1287). DZ 171.

*Rixia jiuwen kao* 日下舊聞考 [Hearsay of old matters from under the sun]. Ed. Yu Minzhong 于敏中 (1714–1779). Beijing: Beijing guji chubanshe, 1985.

*Rushi wowen* 如是我聞 [Thus I have heard]. In *Daozang xubian* 道藏續編.

*Sanfeng zhenren xuantan quanji* 三峰真人玄譚全集 [Collection of the mysterious words of the perfected three peaks]. In *Daozang xubian*.

*Sanji zhiming quandi* 三極至命筌蹄 [The three ultimates and the supreme destiny ensnared]. Wang Qingsheng 王慶升 (ca. mid-13th century). DZ 275.

*Shangqing beiji tianxin zhengfa* 上清北極天心正法 [Correct method of the heart of heaven of the northern pole]. DZ 567.

*Shangqing dadong zhenjing* 上清大洞真經 [Perfected scripture of the great cavern of the upper clarity]. Ed. Jiang Zongying 蔣宗瑛 (ob. 1281). DZ 6.

*Shangqing huangting wuzang liufu zhenren yuzhou jing* 上清黃庭五藏六府真人玉軸經 [Precious scroll of the perfected being on the six receptacles and five viscera of the yellow court of upper clarity]. DZ 1402.

*Shangqing lingbao dafa* 上清靈寶大法 [Great rites of the numinous treasure and the upper clarity]. Ed. Wang Qizhen 王契真 (14th century). DZ 1221.

*Shangqing lingsu shangpian* 上清靈素上篇 [Unadorned spirituality, upper chapters]. DZ 1371.

*Shangqing qusu jueci lu* 上清曲素訣辭籙 [Registers for the instructions on the emanations from the labyrinth, an upper clarity text]. DZ 1392.

*Shangqing Taixuan jiuyang tu* 上清太玄九陽圖 [Upper clarity illustrations of yang-nine by Master Taixuan]. Hou Shanyuan 侯善淵 (ca. late 12th cen.) or Taixuanzi 太玄子. DZ 154.

*Shangqing tianguan santu jing* 上清天關三圖經 [Three limits scripture on the passes of heaven]. DZ 1366.

*Shangqing tianxin zhengfa* 上清天心正法 [Correct method of the heart of heaven, of the upper clarity tradition]. DZ 566.

*Shangshu* 尚書 [Documents]. In *Shisanjing zhushu* 十三經註疏. Beijing: Zhonghua shuju, 1979.

*Shangyangzi jindan dayao* 上陽子金丹大要 [Master Shangyang's essentials of the elixir]. Ed. Chen Zhixu 陳致虛 (ob. 1331). DZ 1067.

*Shangyangzi jindan dayao liexian zhi* 上陽子金丹大要列仙志 [Record of famous transcendents in Master Shangyang's essentials of the elixir]. Ed. Chen Zhixu 陳致虛 (ob. 1331). DZ 1069.

*Shangyangzi jindan dayao tu* 上陽子金丹大要圖 [Alchemical diagrams to Master Shangyang's essentials of the elixir]. Chen Zhixu 陳致虛 (ob. 1331). DZ 1068.

*Shangyangzi jindan dayao xianpai* 上陽子金丹大要仙派 [Lineage pertaining to Master Shangyang's essentials of the elixir]. Ed. Chen Zhixu 陳致虛 (ob. 1331). DZ 1070.

*Shanhaijing* 山海經 [Classic on mountains and seas]. Taibei: Qiye shuju, 1975.

*Shilin guangji* 事林廣記 [Guide through the forest of events]. Ed. Chen Yuanqing 陳元靚. 1478.

*Shisan jing zhushu* 十三經注疏 [Commentaries and annotations on the thirteen classics]. Beijing: Zhonghua shuju, 1980.

*Shizhou ji* 十洲記 [Records on the ten continents]. In *Yunji qiqian* (DZ 1032), 26.1.

*Shunzhi Huaiqing fuzhi* 順治懷慶府志 [Monograph of the Huaiqing prefecture from the shunzhi Era (1644–1661)] Eds. Peng Qingdian 彭清典 and Xiao Jiazhi 蕭家芝.

*Siku quanshu*. See *Yingyin wenyuange siku quanshu*.

*Songshu* 宋書 [History of Liu-Song]. Beijing: Zhonghua shuju, 1976.

*Suwen*. See *Huangdi neijing suwen*.

*Taiji jilian neifa* 太極祭鍊內法 [Inner method of taiji for sacrificing to and sublimating the Spirits of the Deceased]. Ed. Zheng Sixiao 鄭思肖 (Suonan 所南) (1241–1318). DZ 548.

*Taiping jing* 太平經 [Book of the great peace]. DZ 1101a.

*Taiqing daoyin yangsheng jing* 太清導引養生經 [Book of the great clarity on gymnastics and nourishing life]. DZ 818.

*Taishang chu sanshi jiuchong baosheng jing* 太上出三尸九蟲保生經 [Scripture of the most high for the protection of life through the elimination of the three corpses and the nine worms]. Five Dynasties? DZ 871.

*Taishang cibei daochang xiaozai jiuyou chan* 太上慈悲道場消災九幽懺 [Water litany for the remission of sins, a ritual for the mercy of the most high]. Attributed to Ge Xuan 葛玄. DZ 543.

*Taishang dongxuan lingbao wuliang duren shangpin jingfa* 太上洞玄靈寶無量度人上品經法 [Scriptural method of the book of universal salvation]. Ed. Chen Chunrong 陳春榮. DZ 93.

*Taishang huangting neijing yujing* 太上黃庭內景玉經 [Jade scripture of inner effulgences of the Yellow court]. DZ 331.

*Taishang huangting waijing yujing* 太上黃庭外景玉經 [Jade scripture of outer effulgences of the yellow court]. DZ 332.

*Taishang jiuyao xinyin miaojing* 太上九要心印妙經 [Marvelous book of the nine essentials heart seal of the most high]. DZ 225.

*Taishang Laojun xuanmiao zhenzhong neide shenzhou jing* 太上老君玄妙真中內得神呪經 [Divine spells of inner virtue, from the mystical pillow of the most high Lord Lao]. DZ 872.

*Taishang Laojun zhongjing* 太上老君中經 [The most high Lord Lao's book of the centre]. DZ 1168.

*Taishang Lingbao wufu xu* 太上靈寶五符序 [The five talismans, powerful treasure of the most high]. DZ 388.

*Taishang suling dongyuan dayou miaojing* 太上素靈洞淵大有妙經 [The marvelous scripture in the unadorned spirituality and vast possessions of the most high]. DZ 1314.

*Taishang zhuguo jiumin zongzhen biyao* 太上助國救民總真秘要 [Secret essentials of the most high principal perfected assisting the country and saving the people]. Ed. Miaozong 元妙宗. DZ 1227.

*Taixi jingzhu* 胎息經註 [Commentary on the book of embryonic breathing]. DZ 130.

*Taiyi jinghua zongzhi* 太乙金華宗旨 [Main principles of the golden flower of the great one]. In *Daozang xubian*.

*Tianxian zhengli zhilun* 天仙正理直論 [Direct treatise on the correct principles of the celestial immortality]. Ed. Wu Chongxu 伍冲虛 (1574–1644). In *Wu Liu xianzong quanji* 伍柳仙宗全集 [Collection of the works of Wu Chongxu and Liu Huayang]. Taibei: Zhenshanmei chubanshe, 1962.

*Ton-isho* 頓醫鈔 [Manuscript on medicine]. Ed. Kajiwara Seizen 梶原性全 (1266–1337). Manuscript in the Waseda University Library.

*Wangwushan zhi* 王屋山志 [Monograph on Mount Wangwu] by Li Guiyi 李歸一.

*Wudang fudi zongzhen ji* 武當福地總真記 [Comprehensive collection of true [facts] concerning the land of bliss of Wudang]. Ed. Liu Daoming 劉道明. DZ 962.

*Wudeng huiyuan* 五燈會元 [Uniting to the origin of the five lamps]. Eds. Puji 普濟 and Su Yuanlei 蘇淵雷. Beijing: Zhonghua shuju, 1984.

*Wuliangshou jing* 無量壽經 [Sutra of the buddha of infinite life]. Trans. Samghavarman. T. 360, vol. 12.

*Wuli tongkao* 五禮通考 [Study on the five rites]. Ed. Qin Huitian 秦蕙田. *SKQS*.

*Wu Liu xianzong quanji* 伍柳仙宗全集 [Collection of the works of Wu Chongxu and Liu Huayang]. 1896; Taibei: Zhenshanmei chubanshe, ed., 1962.

*Wumen guan* 無門關 [The Gateless Gate]. Ed. Huikai 慧開 (1183–1260). T. 2005, vol. 48.

*Wushang huanglu dazhai licheng yi* 無上黃籙大齋立成儀 [Standardized rituals of the supreme yellow register retreat]. DZ 508.

*Wushang santian yutang zhengzong gaoben neijing yushu* 無上三天玉堂正宗高奔內景玉書 [Precious text of flying in the inner landscape, from the correct tradition of the jade hall of the supreme three heavens]. Ed. Lu Shizhong 路時中. DZ 221.

*Wushang xuanyuan santian yutang dafa* 無上玄元三天玉堂大法 [Great method of the jade hall of the three heavens, of the supreme mysterious origin]. Ed. Lu Shizhong 路時中. DZ 220.

*Wuxing dayi* 五行大義 [Compendium on the five agents]. Ed. Xiao Ji 蕭吉. *Congshu jicheng chubian*. Shanghai: Shangwu yinshuguan, 1932.

*Wuzhen pian zhushi* 悟真篇註釋 [Explication of the stanzas on awakening to perfection]. Ed. Zhang Boduan 張伯端 (984–1082). DZ 145.

*Xiang'er zhu*. See *Laozi xiang'er zhu jiaozheng*.

*Xingming guizhi* 性命圭旨 [Principles of the tablets on the innate nature and the vital force]. Manuscript of the Baoren tang 寶仁堂. Kangxi era (1654–1722).

*Xishan qunxian huizhen ji* 西山群仙會真集 [Records of the transcendents of the Huizhen Hall on Xishan]. DZ 246.

*Xiuzhen biannan canzheng* 修真辯難參證 [Revision of the discussions on the cultivation of perfection]. Eds. Liu Yiming 劉一明 (1734–1821) and Min Yide 閔一得. In *Qigong yangsheng congshu* 氣功養生叢書 [Collection of books on *qigong* and nourishing life]. Shanghai: Shanghai guji chubanshe, 1989.

*Xiuzhen liyan chaotu* 修真歷驗鈔圖 [Copy of diagrams of attested methods for the cultivation of perfection]. DZ 152.

*Xiuzhen shishu* 修真十書 [Ten books on the cultivation of perfection]. DZ 263.

*Xiuzhen taiji hunyuan tu* 修真太極混元圖 [Diagrams on the mystery of ultimate and primordial chaos for the cultivation of true nature]. Ed. Xiao Daocun 蕭道存. DZ 149.

*Xiuzhen zhixuan pian* 修真指玄篇 [Essay indicating the mystery in the cultivation of perfection]. Ed. Bai Yuchan 白玉蟾 (early 12th cen.). In *Xiuzhen shishu* 修真十書, DZ 263, 1–8.

*Xuantian shangdi qisheng lu* 玄天上帝啟聖錄 [Records of the epiphany of the supreme ancestor of the dark heaven]. DZ 958.

*Xuanzhu ge* 玄珠歌 [Song on the mysterious pearl]. Ed. Wang Wenqing 王文卿 (1093–1153). In *Daofa huiyuan* 道法會元 (DZ 1220), 70.

*Xuanzhu ge* 玄珠歌 [Song of the mysterious pearl]. DZ 573.

*Yangsheng bilu* 養生祕錄 [Secret records on tending life]. DZ 579.

*Yangxing yanming lu* 養性延命錄 [Records concerning tending life and the lenghthening of life]. Ed. Tao Hongjing 陶弘景. DZ 838; and in *Yunji qiqian* 雲笈七籤 (DZ 1032), 32.

*Yanxia fangyan* 巖下放言 [Unstrained words from the foot of a precipice]. Ed. Ye Mengde 葉夢得 (1077–1148). *SKQS*.

*Yijing* 易經. See *Zhouyi zhengyi* 周易正義.

*Yimen guangdu* 夷門廣牘 [Extensive archives from Yimen]. Ed. Zhou Lüjing 周履靖 (late 16th cen.). *Congshu jicheng* 叢書集成.

*Yingyin wenyuange siku quanshu* 影印文淵閣四庫全書 [Photofacsimile reprint of the erudite literature pavilion's copy of the books of the four stores]. Ed. Ji Yun 紀昀 (1724–1805). Taipei: Shangwu, 1983–1986.

*Yiwen leiju* 藝文類聚 [Classified collection based on the classics and other literature]. Ed. Ouyang Xun 歐陽詢 (557–641). Shanghai: Shanghai guji chubanshe, 1965.

*Yixue bianhuo* 易學辨惑 [Debates on mistakes by learning mutations]. Ed. Huang Zongyan 黃宗炎 (1616–1686). In *Zhaodai congshu* 昭代叢書 [Collection of the glorious period]. Ed. Zhang Chao 張潮.

*Yongjia xianzhi* 永嘉縣志 [Monograph on the Yongjia district], Zhang Baolin 张宝琳. Wuhan: Hubei sheng tushuguan chubanshe, 2010.

*Yuanshi wuliang duren shangpin miaojing neiyi* 元始無量度人上品妙經內義 [Esoteric interpretation of the book of salvation]. Ed. Xiao Yingsou 蕭應叟 (ca. 13th cen.). DZ 90.

*Yuanshi wuliang duren shangpin miaojing sizhu* 元始無量度人上品妙經四註 [Four commentaries on the wonderful superior book of universal salvation from the canon of the numinous treasure]. DZ 87.

*Yuanshi wuliang duren shangpin miaojing tongyi* 元始無量度人上品妙經通義 [Comprehensive interpretation on the book of salvation]. Ed. Zhang Yuchu 張宇初 (1361–1410). DZ 89.

*Yuanshi wuliang duren shangpin miaojing zhujie* 元始無量度人上品妙經註解 [Commentary on the book of salvation]. Ed. Chen Zhixu 陳致虛 (ob. 1331). DZ 91.

*Yuhan bizhi* 玉函秘指 [Secret indications of the jade case]. Ed. Zhou Lüjing 周履靖. In *Yimen guangdu* 夷門廣牘.

*Yunji qiqian* 雲笈七籤 [Cloudy bookcase with seven labels]. Ed. Zhang Junfang 張君房. DZ 1032.

*Yuqing jinsi qinghua biwen jinbao neilian danjue* 玉清金笥青華秘文金寶內鍊丹訣 [Alchemical formula for the inner purification of the gold treasure; secret writings from the golden box of the jade purity heaven, transmitted by the transcendent Qinghua]. Ed. Zhang Boduan 張伯端 (987–1082). DZ 240.

*Yuqing wuji zongzhen Wenchang dadong xianjing zhu* 玉清無極總真文長大洞仙經註 [Commentary on the great cavern scripture according to Wenchang]. DZ 103.

*Yuxi zi danjingzhi yao* 玉溪子丹經之要 [Basic principles on alchemical texts by Yuxi zi]. Ed. Li Jianyi 李簡易 (ca. 1264). DZ 245.

*Zang wai daoshu* 藏外道書 [Taoist texts outside the canon]. Chengdu: Bashu shushe, 1992.

*Zhang ziyang bamai jing* 張紫陽八脈經 [The book on the eigth marvelous vessels by Zhang Ziyang]. In *Wu Liu xianzong quanji*, 60a–b.

*Zhen'gao* 真誥 [Declarations of the perfected]. Ed. Tao Hongjing 陶弘景 (456–536). DZ 1016.

*Zhenjiu jiayi jing xiaoshi* 針灸甲乙經校釋 [Modern translation and annotations on the basic classic of acupuncture and moxibustion]. Ed. Huangfu Mi 皇甫謐 (205–281). Beijing: Renmin weisheng chubanshe, 1979.

*Zhenling weiye tu* 真靈位業圖 [Table of the ranks and functions in the pantheon]. Ed. Tao Hongjing (456–536). DZ 167.

*Zhenyi jindan jue* 真一金丹訣 [Explication concerning the elixir of the perfected one]. Ed. Wang Chang 王常. DZ 231.

*Zhenzhong jing* 枕中經 [The book in the pillow]. DZ 1422.

*Zhizhenzi longhu dadan shi* 至真子龍虎大丹詩 [Poems on the great elixir of the dragon and the tiger]. Ed. Zhou Fang 周方. DZ 269.

*Zhonghe ji* 中和集 [Collection of the centre and the harmony]. Ed. Li Daochun 李道純 (ob. 1306). DZ 249.

*Zhong Lü chuandao ji* 鍾呂傳道集 [Collection on the Zhong Liquan transmission to Lü Dongbin]. In *Xiuzhen shishu* (DZ 263), 14–16.

*Zhouyi zhengyi* 周易正義 [Correct meaning on the rites of Zhou]. *Shisan jing zhushu*. Beijing: Zhonghua shuju, 1979.

*Zhuangzi jijie* 莊子集解 [Commentaries on the Zhuangzi]. In *Zhuzi jicheng* 諸子集成. Shanghai: Shanghai shuju, 1986.

*Zhuzhen shengtai shenyong jue* 諸真聖胎神用訣 [Divinely efficacious holy wombs methods of the host of perfected]. DZ 826.

*Ziyang zhenren Wuzhen pian shiyi* 紫陽真人悟真篇拾遺 [Supplement to the stanzas of Ziyang Zhenren's awakening to perfection]. Ed. Zhang Boduan. DZ 144

*Ziyang zhenren wuzhen pian zhushu* 紫陽真人悟真篇註疏 [Commentary on the stanzas on awakening to perfection by the perfected of the purple yang]. Ed. Zhang Boduan. DZ 141.

*Zuanxiu Longmen fapai puxu* 纂修龍門法派譜序 [Introduction to the genealogy of the Dragon Gate school]. Ed. Chen Kongsheng 陳孔升 (ca. 1909).

*Zuozhuan* 左傳. *Shisan jing zhushu*, vol. 2, 1980.

## Secondary Sources

An. 2008. *Le rosaire des philosophes*. Ed. Étienne Perrot. Paris: La Fontaine de Pierre.

Andersen, Poul. 1985. "The Transformation of the Body in Taoist Ritual". In *Religious Reflections on the Human Body*. Ed. Jane Marie Law. Bloomington and Indianapolis: Indiana University Press. 186–208

Andersen, Poul. 1989–90. "The Practice of *Bugang*." *Cahiers d'Extrême-Asie* 5: 15–53.

Baldrian-Hussein, Farzeen. 1984. *Procédés secrets du Joyau Magique. Traité d'alchimie taoïste du XIe siècle*. Paris: les Deux Océans.

Baldrian-Hussein, Farzeen. 1985. "Yüeh-yang and Lü Tung-pin's Ch'in-yüan ch'un: A Sung Alchemical Poem." In *Religion und Philosophie in Ostasien. Festschrift für Hans Steininger*. Eds. K.H. Pohl and H.H. Schmidt. Naundorf, Würzburg: Königshausen and Neumann. 19–31.

Baldrian-Hussein, Farzeen. 1989–1990. "Inner Alchemy: Notes on the Origin and the Use of the Term *neidan*." *Cahiers d'Extrême-Asie* 5: 163–190.

Baptandier, Brigitte. 2016. "Les *mudra* du Lüshan pai, le battement de la vie." In *Empreintes du tantrisme en Chine et en Asie orientale: imaginaires, rituels, influences*. Ed. Vincent Durand-Dastès. Louvain: Peeters. 139–157.

Baryosher-Chemouny, Muriel. 1996. *La quête de l'immortalité en Chine: Alchimie et paysage intérieur sous les Song*. Paris: Dervy.

Berling, Judith. 1980. *The Syncretic Religion of Lin Chao-en*. New York: Columbia University Press.

Berthier-Baptandier, Brigitte. 1993. "Le tableau talismanique de l'Empereur de Jade. Construction d'un objet d'écriture." *L'Homme* 126: 59–92.

Bokenkamp, Stephen. 1983. "Sources on the Ling-pao Scriptures." In *Tantric and Taoist Studies*, Volume 2. Ed. Michel Strickmann, Bruxelles: Mélanges de l'Institut Belge des Hautes Études Chinoises. 434–486.

Bokenkamp, Stephen. 1986. "The Peach Flower Font and the Grotto Passage." *Journal of Oriental and Asiatic Studies* 106: 65–77.

Boltz, Judith. 1983. "Opening the Gates of Purgatory: A Twelfth-Century Taoist Meditation Technique for the Salvation of Lost Spirits." In *Tantric and Taoist Studies in Honour of R. A. Stein*, Vol. II. Ed. Michel Strickmann. Bruxelles: Institut Belge des Hautes Études Chinoises. 487–511.

Boltz, Judith. 1985. *Taoist Rites of Exorcism*. Ph.D. diss. University of California, Berkeley.

Boltz, Judith. 1987/1995. *A Survey of Taoist Literature, Tenth to Seventeenth Centuries*. Berkeley: Institute of East Asian Studies and University of California Press.

Bray, Francesca, Vera Dorofeeva-Lichtmann and Georges Métailié, eds. 2007. *Graphics and Text in the Production of Technical Knowledge in China. The Warp and the Weft*. Leiden: Brill.

Brook, Timothy. 1993. "Rethinking Syncretism: The Unity of the Three Teachings and their Joint Worship in Late-Imperial China." *Journal of Chinese Religions*, 21.1: 13–44.

Carré, Patrick. 1999. *Le Livre de la Cour Jaune*. Paris: Seuil.

Chao, Shin-yi. 2009. "Summoning the Thunder Generals. Internal Alchemy in the Thunder Rites." In *Internal Alchemy*. Eds. Livia Kohn and Robin R. Wang. Magdalena, NM: Three Pines Press. 104–120.

Ch'en, Kuo-fu 陳國符. 1949. *Daozang yuanliu kao* 道藏源流考 [Studies on the origins and development of the Taoist Canon]. Shanghai: Zhonghua shuju.

Chenivesse, Sandrine. 1996. “Écrit démonifuge et territorialité de la mort en Chine. Étude anthropologique du lien.” *L'Homme* 36: 61–86.

Chenivesse, Sandrine. 1998. “Fengdu: Cité de l'abondance, cité de la malemort.” *Cahiers d'Extrême-Asie* 10: 287–339.

Couvreur, Séraphin. 1950. *Mémoires sur les bienséances et les cérémonies*, tome 1. Paris: Cathasia.

Dai Yuanchang 戴元長. 1962. *Xianxue cidian* 仙學辭典 [Dictionary on the study of immortality]. Taibei: Jianyu yinshua gongchang.

Darga, Martina. 1999. *Das Alchemistische Buch von Innerem Wesen und Lebensenergie: Xingming guizhi*. München: Eugen Diederichs Verlag.

Davis, Tenney L. and Ch'en Kuo-fu. 1942–43. “Shang-yang tzu, Taoïst Writer and Commentator on Alchemy.” *Harvard Journal of Asiatic Studies* 7: 126–129.

Davis, Tenney and Chao Yün-ts'ung. 1939–1940. “Chang Po-tuan of T'ien-t'ai, his *Wu Chên P'ien*, Essay on the Understanding of the Truth. A Contribution to the Study of Chinese Alchemy.” *Proceedings of the American Academy of Arts and Sciences* 73: 97–117.

De Bruyn, Pierre-Henri. 2010. *Le Wudangshan. Histoire des récits fondateurs*. Paris: Indes savantes.

Despeux, Catherine. 1979. *Physiologie et alchimie taoïste. Le Weisheng shenglixue mingzhi*, introduction and translation. Paris: Les Deux Océans.

Despeux, Catherine. 1990. *Immortelles de la Chine ancienne. Taoïsme et alchimie féminine*. Paris: Pardès.

Despeux, Catherine. 1994. *Taoïsme et corps humain. Le Xiuzhen tu*. Paris: Trédaniel.

Despeux, Catherine. 1996. “Le corps, champ spatio-temporel, souche d'identité.” *L'Homme* 137: 87–118.

Despeux, Catherine. 2000. “Talismans and Sacred Diagrams.” In *Daoism Handbook*. Ed. Livia Kohn. Leiden: Brill. 498–540.

Despeux, Catherine. 2006. “ Métaphores et processus d'intégration: la symbolique du corps dans l'alchimie interne de la Chine des Song (Xe–XIIe siècles).” In *Alchimies. Occident-Orient*. Eds. Kappler Claire and Suzanne Thiolier-Méjean. Paris: l'Harmattan. 291–314.

Despeux, Catherine. 2007a. “The Body Revealed. The Contribution of Forensic Medicine to Knowledge and Representations of the Skeleton in China.” In *Graphics and Text in the Production of Technical Knowledge in China. The Warp and the Weft*. Eds. Francesca Bray, Vera Dorofeeva-Lichtmann and Georges Métailié. Leiden: Brill. 637–684.

Despeux, Catherine. 2007b. “Ames et animation du corps. La notion de *shen* dans la médecine chinoise antique.” In *De l'esprit aux esprits: Enquête sur la notion de shen. Of Self and Spirits. Exploring shen in China, Extrême-Orient-Extrême-Occident* 29: 71–94.

Despeux, Catherine. 2015. *Le chemin de l'éveil illustré par le dressage du buffle dans le bouddhisme Chan, le dressage du cheval dans le taoïsme et le dressage de l'éléphant dans le bouddhisme tibétain*. Paris: l'Asiathèque.

Diény, Jean-Pierre. 1987. *Le symbolisme du dragon dans la Chine ancienne*. Paris: Collège de France/ Institut des hautes études chinoises.

Diény, Jean-Pierre. 1989–90. "Le *Fenghuang* et le phénix." *Cahiers d'Extrême-Asie* 5: 1–13.

Doré, Henri. 1915. *Recherches sur les superstitions chinoises*, Vol. IX. Shanghai: Variété sinologiques, Imprimerie de la Mission catholique à l'orphelinat de T'ou-sé-wé.

Esposito, Monica. 1993. "La porte du dragon: L'école du Longmen du Mont Jin'gai et ses pratiques alchimiques d'après le Daozang xubian [Sequel to the Taoist Canon]." Ph. D. diss. Paris VII University.

Esposito, Monica. 2001. "Longmen Taoism in Qing China: Doctrinal Ideal and Local Reality." *Journal of Chinese Religions* 29: 191–231.

Esposito, Monica. 2004. "The Longmen School and its Controversial History during the Qing Dynasty." In *Religion and Chinese Society*. Ed. John Lagerwey. Hong Kong: Chinese University Press and École française d'Extrême-Orient. 621–698.

Feng, Han-chi. 1936. "The Origin of Yü Huang." *Harvard Journal of Asiatic Studies* 1: 242–250.

de Foucaux, Philippe. 1988. *Le Lalitavistara. L'histoire traditionnelle de la vie du Bouddha Çakyamuni*. Paris: Les Deux Océans.

Gauchet, Louis. 1941. "Le *Tou-jen king* des Taoïstes: son texte primitif et sa date probable." *Bulletin de l'Université Aurore*, 3rd series, 2: 511.

Gilson, Étienne. 1988. *La philosophie au Moyen Âge*. Paris: Payot.

Goossaert, Vincent. 1998. "L'alchimie intérieure réhabilitée? Notes critiques." *Revue d'histoire des religions*. Paris: Armand Colin. 493–507.

Goossaert, Vincent. 2007. *The Taoists of Pe-king, 1800–1949: A Social History of Urban Clerics*. Cambridge, MA: Harvard University Press.

Grmek, Mirko, ed. 1995–1997. *Histoire de la pensée médicale en Occident. 1. Antiquité et Moyen Âge. 2. De la Renaissance aux lumières*. Paris: Seuil.

Grmek, Mirko and Barnabeo Raffaele. 1997. "La machine du corps." In *Histoire de la pensée médicale en Occident. 2. De la Renaissance aux lumières*: 7–36.

Grootaers, Willem. 1952. "The Hagiography of The Chinese God Chen-wu." *Folklore Studies*, 11.2: 139–181.

Gyss-Vermande, Caroline. 1984. *La vie et l'oeuvre de Huang Gongwang* (1269–1354). Paris: Collège de France/ Institut des hautes études chinoises.

He Zhiguo and Vivienne Lo. 1996. "The Channels: A Preliminary Examination of a Lacquered Figurine from the Western Han Period." *Early China* 21: 81–123.

Hodous, Lewis. 1929. *Folkways in China*, London: Probsthain.

Hu Daojing 胡道靜. 2011. *Mengqi bitan jiaozheng* 夢溪筆談校證 [Brush talks from the river brook, a critical edition]. Shanghai: Shanghai renmin chubanshe.

Hudson, Clarke. 2008. *Spreading the Dao, Managing Mastership and Performing Salvation: The Life and Alchemical Teachings of Chen Zhixu.* Ph.D. diss. Indiana University.

Ikeda, Suetoshi 池田末利. 1953. "Konpaku kō—sono kigen to hatten" 魂魄考—その起源と發展 [A Study on *hun* and *po*: its origin and development]. *Tōhō shukyo* 東方宗教 1–3: 5–31.

Joly, Robert. 1970. *Hippocrate*, vol. 11. Paris: Les Belles Lettres.

Kalinowski, Marc. 1983. "Les instruments astro-calendériques des Han et la méthode *Liu-ren.*" BEFEO 72: 309–416.

Kalinowski, Marc. 1991. *Cosmologie et divination dans la Chine ancienne. Le Compendium des cinq agents* (Wuxing dayi, *VIth century*). Paris: EFEO.

Kaltenmark, Max. 1953. *Le Lie-sien tchouan. Biographies légendaires des immortels taoïstes de l'antiquité.* Pékin: Centre d'études sinologiques franco-chinois. Réédition 1987. Paris: Collège de France/ Institut des hautes études chinoises.

Kaltenmark, Max. 1960. "Ling-pao: Note sur un terme du taoïsme religieux." In *Mélanges publiés par l'Institut des hautes études chinoises, Collège de France*, 559–588. Paris: PUF/Institut des hautes études chinoises/ Collège de France.

Kaltenmark, Max. 1961–1963. "Au sujet du *Ling-pao tou-jen king.*" *Annuaire de l'École pratique des hautes études chinoises*, V[e] section, 1961–1962: 53–54; 1962–63: 50; 1963–64: 54.

Kaltenmark, Max. 1967. "Au sujet du *Houang-t'ing king.*" *Annuaire de l'École pratique des hautes études chinoises*, V[e] section. 68: 80–81.

Kaltenmark, Max. 1981. "Grottes et labyrinthes en Chine." *Dictionnaire des mythologies*, 480–81. Paris: Flammarion.

Kaltenmark, Max. 1982. "Quelques remarques sur le *T'ai-chang ling-pao woufou siu.*" *Zinbun, Memoirs of the Research Institute for Humanistic Studies* 18: 1–10.

Kohn, Livia and Sakade Yoshinobu, eds. 1989. *Taoïst Meditation and Longevity Techniques*. Ann Arbor, MI: Center for Chinese Studies.

Kohn, Livia, ed. 2000. *Daoism Handbook*. Leiden: Brill.

Komjathy, Louis. 2008. "Mapping the Daoist Body (1): The Text of the *Neijing tu.*" *Journal of Daoist Studies* 1: 67–92.

Komjathy, Louis. 2009. "Mapping the Daoist Body (2): The *Neijing tu* in History." *Journal of Daoist Studies* 2: 64–108.

Koyanagi Shikita 小柳司氣太. 1928. 1934. *Hakuunkan shi* 白雲觀志 [Monograph on the Baiyun Temple]. Tokyo: Tōhō bunka gakuin Tōkyō kenkyū jo.

Kroll, Paul. 1996. "Body Gods and Inner Vision: *The Scripture of the Yellow Court.*" In *Religions of China in Practice*. Ed. Donald S. Lopez. Princeton: Princeton University Press. 149–55.

Lackner, Michael. 1990. "Zur Verplanung des Denkens am Beispiel der T'u." In *Lebenswelt und Weltanschauung in Frühneuzeitlichen China*. Ed. Helwig Schmidt-Glintzer. Stuttgart: Franz Steiner Verlag. 133–156.

Lagerwey, John. 1987. *Taoist Ritual in Chinese Society and History*. New York and London: Macmillan Publishing Company.

Lagerwey, John. 1991. *Le continent des esprits. La Chine dans le miroir du taoïsme.* Bruxelles: La Renaissance du Livre.

Lagerwey, John. 1992. "The Pilgrimage to Wu-tang shan." In *Pilgrims and Sacred Sites in China*. Eds. Susan Naquin and Yü Chün-fang. Berkeley: University of California Press. 293–332.

Legeza, Laszlo. 1976. *Magie du Tao. Le langage secret des diagrammes et de la calligraphie*, french translation, Paris, Sté Nelle des éditions du Chêne, 1976. English edition, London: Thames and Hudson.

Levi, Jean. 2006. Les *Œuvres de Maître Tchouang*. Paris: éditions de l'Encyclopédie des nuisances.

Li Fengmao 李豐楙 and Huang Chaohan 黃兆漢. 1988. *Mingdai daoshi Zhang Sanfeng kao* 明代道士張三豐考 [Research on the Ming Taoist Zhang Sanfeng]. Taipei: Xuesheng shuju.

Li Jingwei 李經緯 *et al.* 1992. *Zhongguo gudai yishi tulu* 中國古代醫史圖錄 [Drawings and paintings on the ancient medical history of China]. Beijing: Renmin weisheng chubanshe.

Li Jingwei 李經緯 *et al.* 2003. "Neijing tu shi" 內經圖釋. http://www.tcm-china.info/index/neijing/njts.htm. Accessed on March 1, 2017.

Li Jingwei 李經緯 *et al.* 2003. *Xinbian Beijing Baiyun guan zhi* 新編北京白雲觀志 [New edition of the monograph of the Baiyun Temple in Beijing]. Beijing: Zongjiao wenhua chubanshe.

Li Yuanguo 李远國. 1991. "Daojiao leifa chutan" 道教雷法初探 [Research on the thunder rites in Taoism]. *Shanghai daozhi* 上海道志 3. Shanghai: Shanghai shi daojiao xiehui chuban. 22–24.

Li Yuanguo 李远國. 2003. *Shenxiao leifa* 神霄雷法 [Thunder rites of the divine empyrean]. Chengdu: Sichuan renmin chubanshe.

Li Yuanguo 李远國. 2009. "Shenxiao jing shuolüe" 神霄經說略 [Summary on the scriptures of the divine empyrean]. In *Daozang shuolüe* 道藏說略. Ed. Zhu Yueli. Beijing: Yanshan chubanshe. 661–685.

Li Zhaosheng 李兆生. 2008. *Xiuzhentu poyi yu zhijie* 修真圖破疑與直解 [Direct explanations and resolutions of the doubts about the *Chart for the Cultivation of Perfection*]. Changchun: Jilin renmin chubanshe.

Li Zhiyong 李志庸. 1988. *Zhongguo qigong shi* 中國氣功史 [History of Chinese *qigong*]. Zhengzhou: Henan kexue jishu chubanshe.

Lin Jiexiang 林洁祥. 1983. *Daojiao wenxian* 道教文獻 [Documents on Taoism]. Taipei: Danqing tushu.

Lin Shuzhong 林树中. 1977. "Jiangsu Danyang Nanqi mu zuanyin bihua tantao" 江蘇丹陽南齊墓磚印壁畫探討 [Research on the mural paintings and engraved stones of the Nan Qi Tomb in Danyang, Jiangsu]. *Wenwu* 文物 issue 1: 64–77.

Liu Lan 瀏覽. *Wenzhou daojiao shilüe* 溫州道教史略 [History of Taoism in Wenzhou]: http://www.zjwztrdg.com/show/3/42.html.

Loewe, Michael. 1979. *Ways to Paradise. The Chinese Quest for Immortality*. London: George Allen and Unwin.

Lu Ch'iang-wu and Davis, H. Tenney. 1939. "Chang Po-tuan of Tien-t'ai. His *Wu Chen Pien*, Essay on the Understanding of Truth." *Proceedings of the American Academy of Arts and Sciences* 73: 5.

Lü Guangrong 吕光榮, ed. 1988. *Zhongguo qigong cidian* 中國氣功辭典 [Dictionary of Chinese *qigong*]. Beijing: Renmin weisheng chubanshe.

Lu K'uan-yu (Charles Luk). 1970. *Taoist Yoga. Alchemy and Immortality*. London: Rider and Company.

Lu K'uan-yu (Charles Luk). 1971. *Ch'an and Zen Teachings*, second series. Berkeley and London: Shambala.

Ma Shutian. 1990. *Huaxia zhushen* 華夏諸神 [Gods of China]. Beijing: Beijing Yanshan chubanshe.

Maspero, Henri. 1971. *Le taoïsme et les religions chinoises*. Paris: Gallimard.

Mathieu, Rémi. 1983. *Étude sur la mythologie et l'ethnologie de la Chine ancienne. Traduction annotée du* Shanhai jing. Paris: Collège de France/Institut des hautes études chinoises.

Mathieu, Rémi. 1989. *Anthologie des mythes et légendes de la Chine ancienne*. Paris: Gallimard.

Miyashita, Saburô 宮下三郎. 1967. "Sogennō iryō" 宋元醫療 [Medical therapies of Song and Yuan]. In *Sōgenjidaino kagaku gijitsu shi* 宋元時代科學技術史 [History of technics and sciences of the Song and Yuan periods]. Ed. Yabuuchi Kiyoshi 藪内清. Kyōto: Kyōto daigaku Jimbun kagaku kenkyūjo. 123–170.

Mollier, Christine. 1997. "La méthode de l'empereur du Nord du mont Fengdu: une tradition exorciste du taoïsme médiéval". *T'oung p'ao* 83: 329–385.

Nakamura, Shōhachi 中村璋八 and Yasui Kōsan 安居香山. 1971 to 1977. *Jūshū isho shūsei* 重修緯書集成 [Collection of the apocryphal texts, newly revised]. Tōkyō: Meitoku shuppansha 明德出版社.

Naquin, Susan and Chün-fang Yü. 1992. *Pilgrims and Sacred Sites in China*. Berkeley: University of California Press.

Needham, Joseph. 1983. *Science and Civilisation in China*, vol. 5: *Spagirical Discovery and Invention: Physiological Alchemy*. Cambridge: Cambridge University Press.

Ōfuchi, Ninji 大淵忍爾. 1974. "On *Ku Ling-pao ching*" 古靈寶經 [On the old scripture of the numinous treasure]. *Acta Asiatica* 27: 35–56.

Okanishi Tameto 岡西為人. 1969. *Sō izen iseki kō* 宋以前醫籍考 [Research on the old medical documents from the Song and before]. 4 vols. Taibei: Nantian shuju.

Overmeyer, Daniel and David Jordan. 1986. *The Flying Phoenix: Aspects of Chinese Sectarianism in Taiwan*. Princeton: Princeton University Press.

Peizhen Changsheng 培真長生. 1988. "Wudang neigong xiulian tushi shijie" 武當內功修煉圖示試解 [Essay of explication of the *Chart on the Inner Cultivation* of Mount Wudang]. *Wudang* 4: 8–10.

Pregadio, Fabrizio. 1991. "The Book of the Nine Elixirs and its Tradition." In *Chūgoku kodai kagakushi ron* 中國古代科學史論 [Studies on the history of ancient Chinese science]. Eds. Yamada Keiji 山田慶兒 and Tanaka Tan 田中淡. 2 vols. Kyōto: Kyōto daigaku jinbun kagaku kenkyūjo. 543–639.

Pregadio, Fabrizio. 1995. "The Representation of Time in the *Zhouyi cantongqi*." *Cahiers d'Extrême-Asie* 8: 155–173.

Pregadio, Fabrizio. ed. 2005. *The Encyclopedia of Taoism*. 2 vols. London: Curzon Press.

Pregadio, Fabrizio. 2009. *Awakening to Reality: the Regulated Verses of the* Wuzhen pian, *a Taoist Classic of Internal Alchemy*. The Golden Elixir Press.

Pregadio, Fabrizio. 2014. *The Way of the Golden Elixir. An Introduction to Internal Alchemy*. Golden Elixir Press.

Reiter, Florian. 1988. *Grundelemente und Tendenzen des Religiösen Taoïsmus*. Stuttgart: Franz Steiner Verlag.

Reiter, Florian. 1990. "Some Remarks on the Chinese Word *Tu* 'Chart, Plan, Design.'" *Oriens* 32: 308–327.

Ren Jiyu 任繼愈, ed. 1990. *Zhongguo daojiao shi* 中國道教史 [History of Chinese Taoism]. Shanghai: Shanghai renmin chubanshe.

Robert, Jean-Noël. 1997. *Le Sutra du lotus*. Paris: Fayard.

Robinet, Isabelle. 1979. *La méditation taoïste*, Paris: Dervy Livres.

Robinet, Isabelle. 1984. *La révélation du Shangqing dans l'histoire du taoïsme*, 2 vol. Paris: École Française d'Extrême-Orient.

Robinet, Isabelle. 1990. "The Place and Meaning of the notion of Taiji in Taoist Sources prior the Ming Dynasty." *History of Religions* 29.4: 373–411.

Robinet, Isabelle. 1991. "Sur le sens des termes *waidan* et *neidan*." *Taoist Resources* 3.1: 3–40.

Rousselle, Erwin. 1933. "Ne Ging Tu: Die Tafel des inneren Gewebes. Ein taoistisches Meditationsbild mit Beschriftung." *Sinica* 8: 207–216.

Rudolph, Richard and Wen Yu. 1951. *Han Tomb Art of West China: A Collection of First and Second Century Reliefs*. Berkeley: University of California Press.

Sakade Yoshinobu 坂出祥伸. 1991. "Neikeizu to sono enkaku" 內經圖とその沿革 [The *Neijing tu* and its evolution]. In *Chūgoku kodai kagaku shiron, zokuhen* 中國古代科學史論, 續篇. Eds. Yamada Keiji 山田慶兒 and Tanaka Tan 田中淡. 45–85. Kyoto: Jinbun kagaku kenkyūjo.

Schafer, Edward. 1967. *The Vermilion Bird*. Berkeley: University of California Press.

Schipper, Kristofer. 1965. *L'Empereur Wou des Han dans la légende taoïste. Han Wou-ti nei-tchouan*. Paris: École française d'Extrême-Orient.

Schipper, Kristofer. 1975. *La concordance du Houang-t'ing king*. Paris: École française d'Extrême-Orient.

Schipper, Kristofer. 1982. *Le corps taoïste*. Paris: Fayard.

Schipper, Kristofer. 1987. "Master Chao I-chen 趙宜真 (?–1382) and the Ch'ing-wei School of Taoism." In *Dōkyō to shūkyō bunka* 道教と宗教文化 [Taoism and religious culture]. By Kan'ei Akizuki 秋月觀暎. Tokyo: Hirakawa Shuppansha. 715–734.

Schipper, Kristofer. 2008. *La religion de la Chine. La tradition vivante*. Paris: Fayard.

Schipper, Kristofer and Franciscus Verellen. 2004. *The Taoist Canon: A Historical Companion to the Daozang*, 3 vols. Chicago: University of Chicago Press.

Seidel, Anna. 1969. *La divinisation de Lao-tseu dans le taoïsme des Han*. Paris: École française d'Extrême-Orient.

Seidel, Anna. 1970. "A Taoist Immortal of the Ming Dynasty: Chang San-feng." In *Self and Society in Ming Thought*. Ed. Theodore de Bary. New York: Columbia University Press. 483–531.

Seidel, Anna. 1983. "Imperial Treasures and Taoist Sacraments. Taoist Roots in the Apocrypha." In *Tantric and Taoist Studies in Honour of R.A. Stein*, vol. 2. Ed. Michel Strickmann. Bruxelles: Institut Belge des Hautes Études Chinoises. 291–371.

Seidel, Anna. 1989. "Chronicle of Taoïst Studies in the West 1950–1990." *Cahiers d'Extrême-Asie* 5: 223–347.

Shi Weixue 石維學. 1988. "Wudang xiuzhen tu poyi" 武當修真圖破譯 [Translation of the *Chart for the Cultivation of Perfection* of Mount Wudang]. *Wudang* 12.2: 2–3; issue 3: 6–7.

Sivin, Nathan. 1977. "Chinese Alchemy and the Manipulation of Time." *Science and Technology in East Asia*. New York: Science History Publications.

Stein, Rolf. 1987. *Le monde en petit*. Paris: Flammarion.

Stein, Rolf. 1988. "Grottes-matrices et lieux saints de la déesse en Asie orientale." *BEFEO* 151: 2–83.

Strickmann, Michel. 1975. "The Thunder Rites of the Sung. Notes on the Shen-hsiao Sect and the Southern School of Taoism." *Toho Shukyo* 东東宗教 46: 15–28.

Strickmann, Michel. 1978. "The Longest Taoist Scripture." *History of Religions* 17: 331–354.

Strickmann, Michel. 1983. *Tantric and Taoist Studies in Honour of R. A. Stein*, vol. 2. Bruxelles: Institut Belge des Hautes Études Chinoises.

Unschuld, Paul. 1986. *Nan-ching. The Classic on Difficult Issues*. Berkeley: University of California Press.

Thompson, Laurence. 1989. "On the Prehistory of Hell in China." *Journal of Chinese Religions* 17: 27–41.

Van der Loon, Piet. 1979. "A Taoist Collection of the Fourteenth Century." In *Studia Sino-mongolica. Festschrift für Herbert Franke*. Ed. Wolfgang Bauer. Wiesbaden: Franz Steiner Verlag. 401–405.

Van der Loon, Piet. 1984. *Taoist Books in the Sung Libraries*. London: Ithaca Press.

Wang Ming 王明. 1980. *Baopuzi neipian jiaoshi* 抱朴子內篇校釋 [Translation and annotation of the works of the master who embraces simplicity]. Beijing: Zhonghua shuju.

Wang Ming 王明. 1984. "*Huangting jing* kao" 黃庭經考 [A study of the *Huangting jing*]. In *Daojia he daojiao sixiang yanjiu* 道家和道教思想研究 [Studies on Taoist thought]. Beijing: Zhongguo shehui kexue chubanshe. 324–371.

Wang Ming 王明. 1984. *Daojia he daojiao sixiang yanjiu* 道家和道教思想研究. Beijing: Zhongguo shehui kexue chubanshe.

Xiao Dengfu 蕭登福. 1989. *Han Wei liuchao fodao liangjiaozhi tiantang diyu shuo* 漢魏六朝佛道兩教之天堂地獄說 [Buddhist and Taoist views on hells and paradises in the Han, Wei and Six Dynasties]. Taibei: Xuesheng shuju.

Xiao Xinzhu 蕭新鑄. 1985. "Wudang lianxing xiuzhen quantu qianshuo" 武當煉性修真全圖淺說 [Summary and explanation of the *Complete Chart for the Cultivation of Perfection and the Sublimation of the Innate Nature of Mount Wudang*]. *Wudang* 35.

Xu Dishan 許地山. 1961. *Fuji mixin de yanjiu* 扶乩迷信的研究 [A study of the superstition of spirit writing]. Taipei: Shangwu yinshu guan.

Yamada Toshiaki. 1989. "Longevity Techniques and the Compilation on the *Lingbaowufu xu*." In *Taoist Meditation and Longevity Techniques*. Eds. Livia Kohn and Sakade Yoshinobu. Ann Arbor, MI: Center for Chinese Studies, 99–124.

Yang Yanming 楊彥明. 2004. *Wutan hua Yang Bing yu Wuxi xu* 武探花楊炳與習武序 (Introduction to the "Military Exercices" by Yang Bing). Beijing: Zhongguo wenshi chubanshe.

Yin Zhihua 尹志華. 2014. *Qingdai Quanzhen dao lishi xintan* 清代全真道歷史新探 [New research on the history of the Quanzhen school in the Qing dynasty]. Hong Kong: Xianggang zhongwen daxue chubanshe.

Zheng Chenghai 鄭成海, ed. 1971. *Laozi Heshang gong zhu jiaoli* 老子河上公註校理 [Laozi, annotated by Heshang gong, a critical edition]. Taibei: Zhonghua shuju.

Zheng Hong 鄭洪, "Daojiao 'Xiuzhen tu' banben xitong ji liuchuan qingkuang" 道教《修真图》版本系统及流传情况 [Different editions of the *Chart for the Cultivation of Perfection* and the circumstances of its diffusion], *Zongjiaoxue yanjiu* 宗教學研究 (Researchs on Religions), 2017, 2:58–63.

*Zhongguo daojiao* 中國道教 [Chinese Taoism], review edited by the Baiyun Temple, first number in 1992.

Zhu Yueli 朱越利, ed. 2009. *Daozang shuolüe* 道藏說略 [Short presentation of the Taoist Canon]. 2 vols. Beijing: Yanshan chubanshe.

# Index

www.ingramcontent.com/pod-product-compliance
Lightning Source LLC
LaVergne TN
LVHW010544300926
849162LV00002B/229